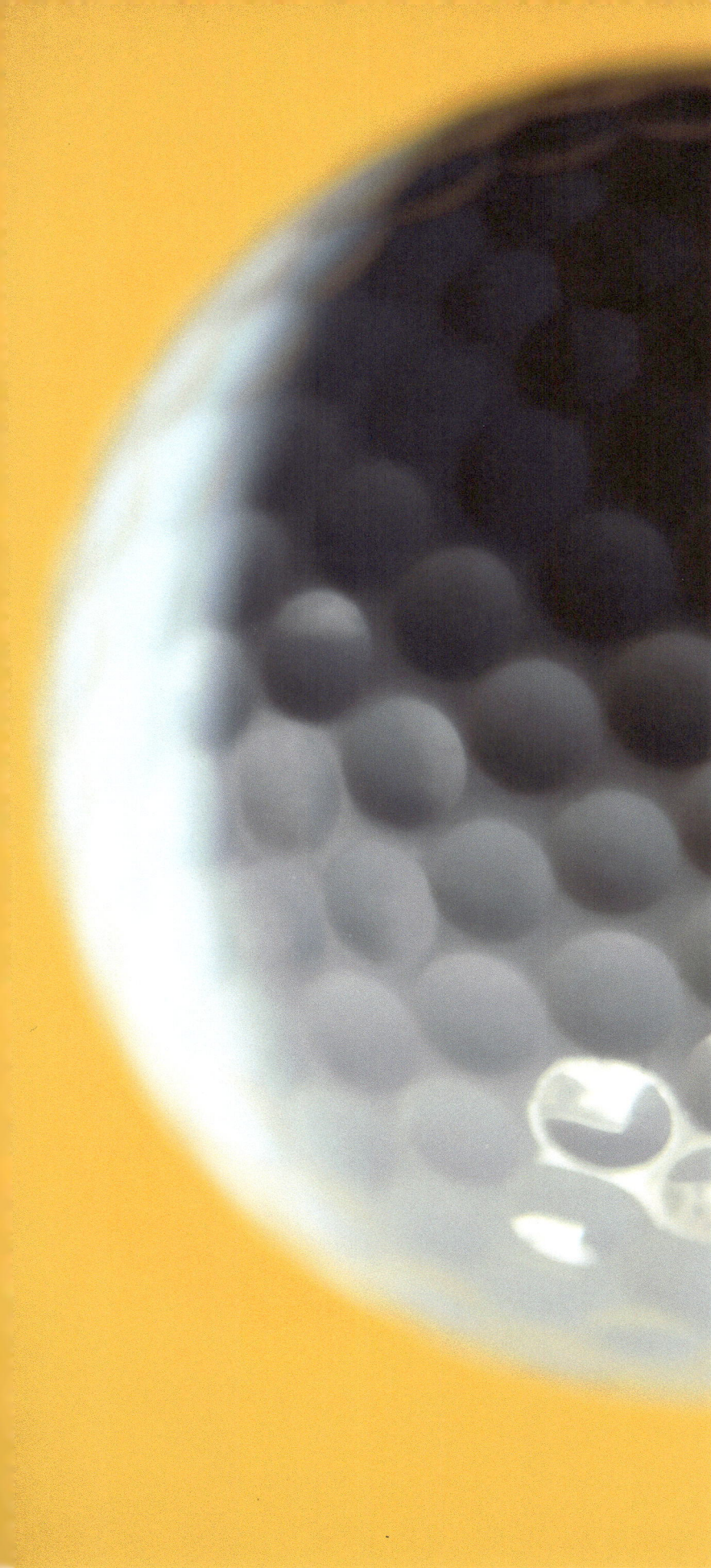

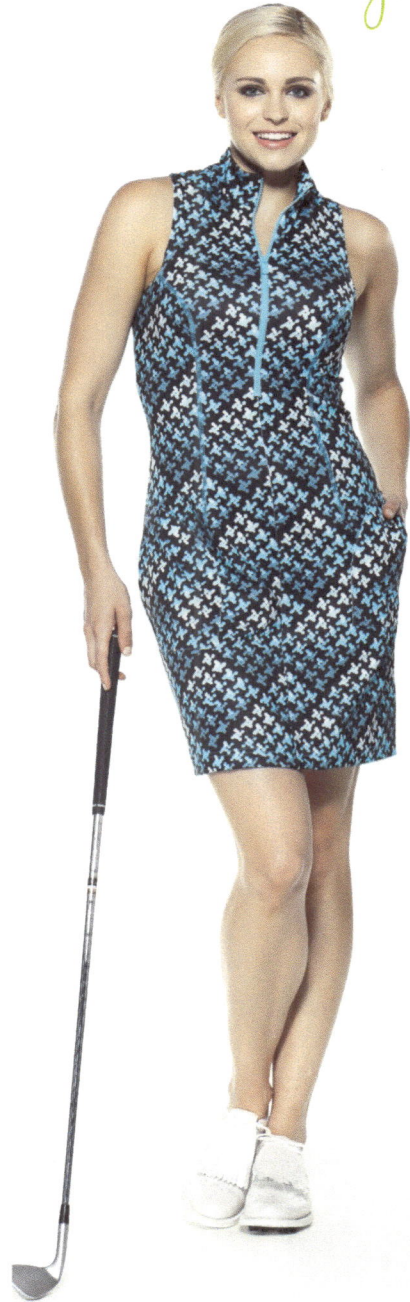

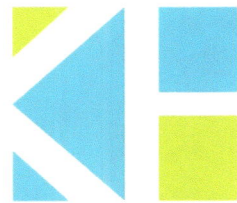

AGENDA Collector's Issue
Fitness Couture 2016

Contents

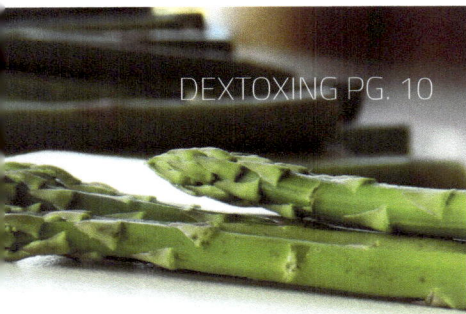

DEXTOXING PG. 10

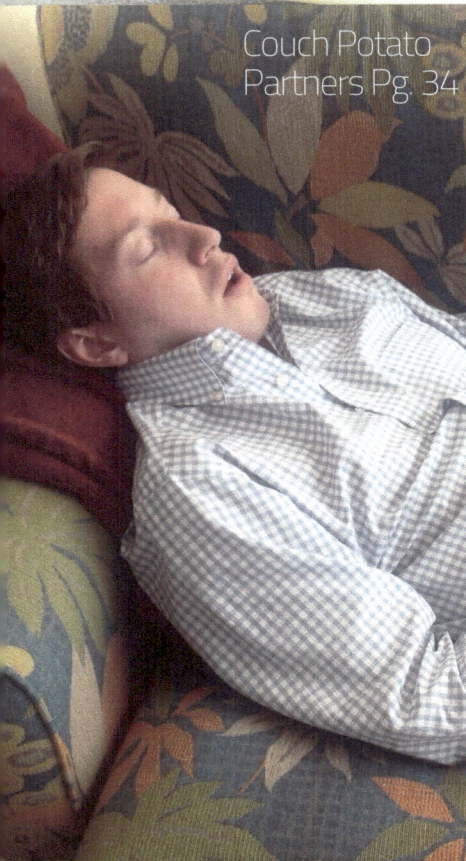

Couch Potato
Partners Pg. 34

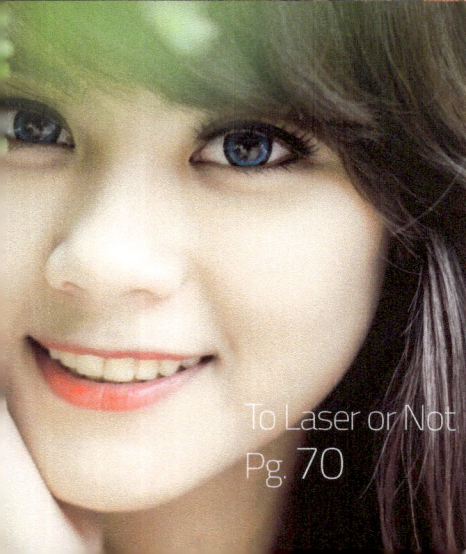

To Laser or Not
Pg. 70

AGENDA Collector's Issue
Fitness Couture 2016

Contents

Spa Massage Etiquette Pg. 94

Home Made into Gym Pg. 150

Editorial

KAYLENE PEOPLES
Publisher/Editor-in-Chief

LETTER FROM A TIME-CHALLENGED EDITOR-IN-CHIEF
HERE'S TO TIGHT ABS!

Dear Readers,

A few years ago I went to a boot camp three times a week at 6:30 a.m.. It was not too far from where I lived, about a 15-minute drive. I had a goal to lose 30 pounds, and I was very motivated! I lost those 30 pounds, fit into a size 4, and looked as good naked as I did with my clothes on. I am a firm believer in boot camps; they work. Now I am in the same place I was before I joined that summer boot camp all those years ago. I am unhappily overweight. I have replaced my size 4s, 6s, and 8s with size 12s—I refuse to go past a 12, even though I am bulging out of those 12s! How could I let that happen to me again, you ask? I had an accident a couple of years ago and fell down stairs, landing on hard slate. I was laid up for almost a year and lost all my lean muscle. The weight didn't start accumulating until summer of last year. That was when I had the outrageous idea to put out a print magazine. So not only was I without my lean muscle, but I was what is called "skinny fat," and I started gaining weight from sheer lack of movement. It took almost six months to publish the magazine, and I have been carrying an extra 30-40 pounds of *Agenda* in Print "baby fat" ever since.

Now here are the real issues: 1) I lost my motivation to work out because I started going to the gym and ended up over-exerting myself, causing re-injury—this happened twice, creating a major setback; 2) I was exhausted from non-stop long days which turned into non-stop long nights staring at a computer screen, and getting eye strain; 3) I was squeezing into too small clothing, making me look even bigger than I was, thus resulting in a bad body image. And from there everything started falling apart. I hated looking at myself in full-length mirrors; shopping for clothes became my biggest nightmare. I used to be an athlete and couldn't bring myself even to watch a tennis match on television, let alone get back on the tennis court myself. Not only did my body change, so did I.

Now I have recently joined a gym. I told myself having a gym membership would get me motivated; but it has been four days since I joined, and I still haven't paid my 24-Hour Fitness (only a seven-minute drive) a visit. My excuse is that I need to finish *Agenda* **Magazine Collector's Issue (Fitness Couture)** first, and I'm opting to do that before finally focusing on my weight, health, well-being, happiness, and everything else that should be a priority. As I write this letter, I realize the excuses not to exercise are endless. There are always reasons we don't, won't, or can't do something important. For some of us the reasons are sheer laziness, lack of motivation; or we are over-worked, exhausted and have no time. In putting together this issue, I have discovered there is no excuse that is good enough to prevent us from taking better care of ourselves. I invite all of you, whether fit or not, to read the informative content flowing on each page and take control of your own health and well-being. I admit it took me 2 ½ years and endless excuses, but now I have all the resources available to work out and eat healthy right here . . . and now so do you! So here's to you and your health from Fitness Couture . . . I see tight abs in all our futures!

Sincerely,

Kaylene Peoples

Kaylene Peoples- Editor-in-Chief

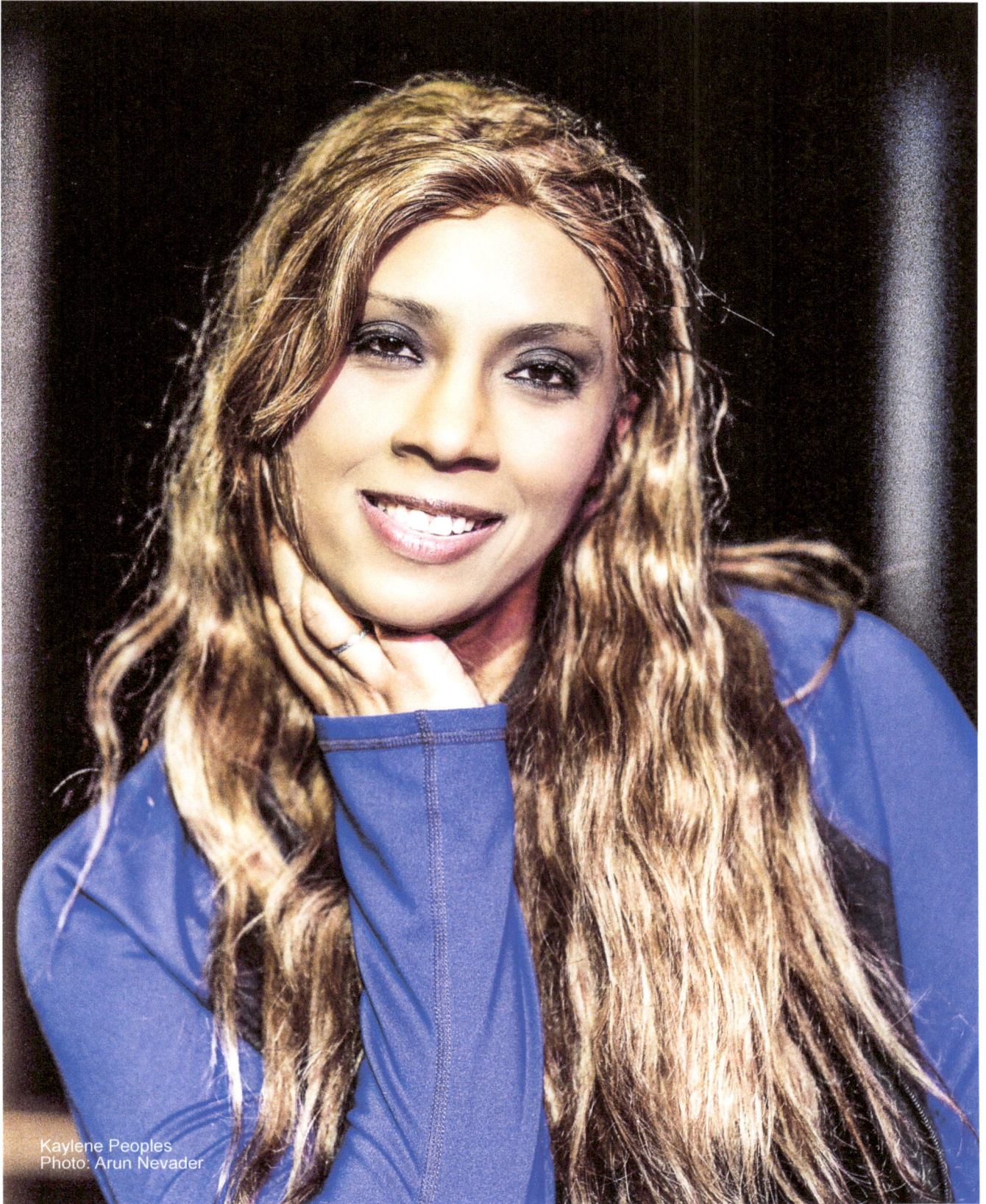

Kaylene Peoples
Photo: Arun Nevader

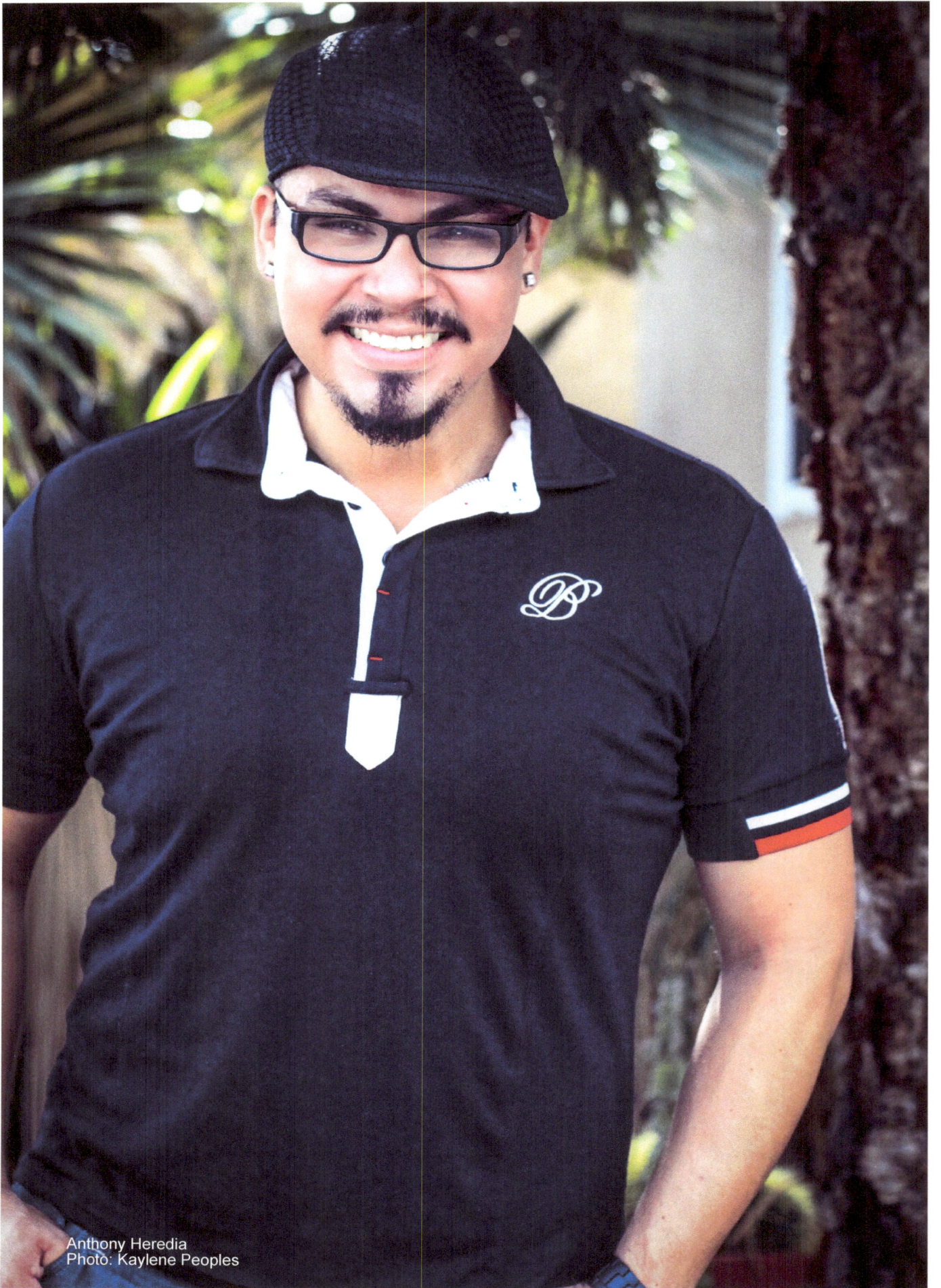

Anthony Heredia
Photo: Kaylene Peoples

Insights

ANTHONY HEREDIA
Health/Fitness Editor

LETTER FROM YOUR FITNESS EDITOR
LET'S GET YOU MOTIVATED!

Hello Fitness Family,

Welcome to the very first wellness- and fitness-focused edition of *Agenda* magazine, appropriately dubbed **Fitness Couture**. Our mission? To help you reach and conquer your personal wellness. It takes more than a mountain of DVDs, magazines, and health books to find your way to fitness utopia. Fitness Couture is a health community of expert fellow wellness enthusiasts who are leveraged to offer you wisdom and support in the areas of fitness, health, and nutrition. I personally believe there is no better teacher than life experience itself, and my fourteen years in the health industry have granted me a number of failures, followed quickly by even greater improvements and successes from those failures. I lost over 80 pounds to save my life. How did I do it? By making positive, dramatic changes to my world on every level. The process was far from perfect, but I have proudly kept the weight off for 10 years; and I learned through trial and error just like everyone else. Fitness Couture will guide you to becoming and maintaining the very best you. We will help you have great health in spite of any previous failures.

Mental, physical, and spiritual health can be complicated topics, and the more you learn, the more you realize there's a lot to learn! The monumental goal of obtaining your physical ideal is enough to intimidate even the most seasoned health enthusiasts. If you make mistakes, be kind to yourself . . . you are not a health/fitness pro (even we "pros" don't know enough about everything when it comes to a perfect performance). The long-term goal here is balance, not perfection. Accept the fact that you will slip. So when you do, be ready to dust yourself off and learn from the fall, coming back twice as strong and wiser now from the experience! With this mentality you are guaranteed to go the distance. Mentally prep (not just for some program that has a beginning and end) and adjust your thoughts toward a permanent new positive way of life. There is no such thing as a "master" plan. And a panacea for the best diet, fitness routine, or health product does not exist. But in the coming pages, you will learn what's best for you and yours. Remember, when you find a great formula you love, it inevitably will evolve over time. Our job is to bring to you powerful content and our expert opinions on various wellness and fitness topics. Together we can be a team and motivate each other to start this fitness journey and get in better shape today!

Sincerely,

Anthony Heredia

Anthony Heredia - Health/Fitness Editor

On the Cover

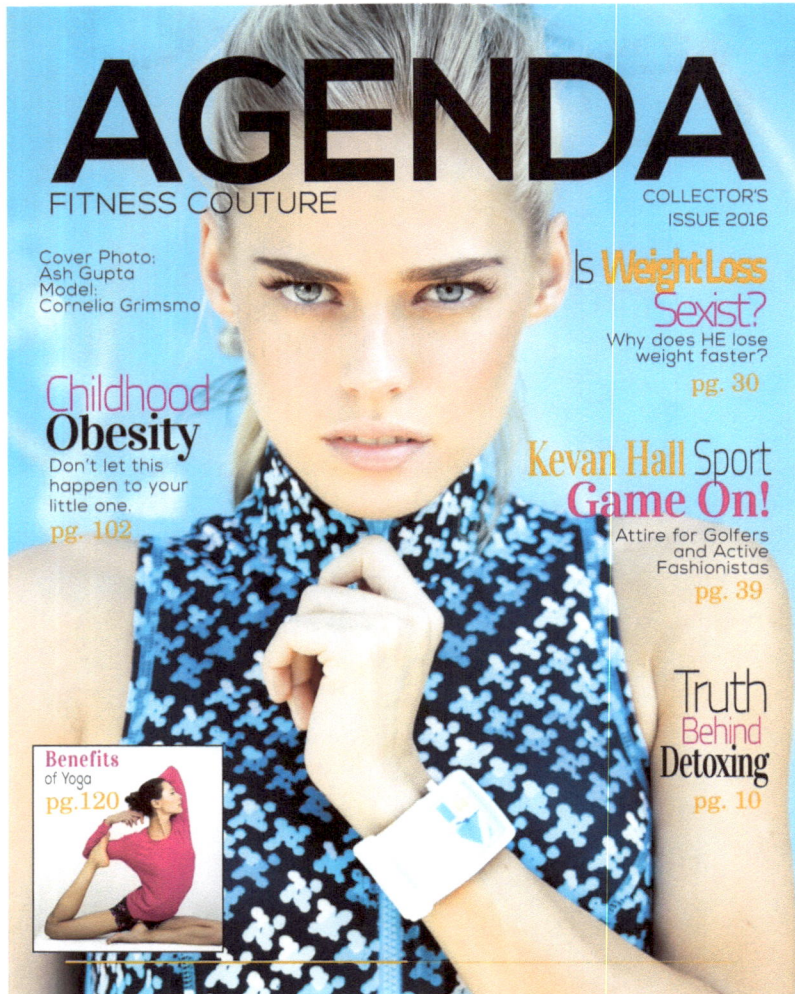

Photographed by Ash Gupta for 838 Media Group, model **Cornelia Grimsmo** wears designer Kevan Hall's newest line "Kevan Hall Sport." The line features golf attire that doubles as fashionable activewear. In the accompanying editorial the models (Cornelia Grimsmo and Summer de Almeida) wear hats and gloves, which are all a part of the Kevan Hall Sport line. The cover was chosen for this *Agenda Magazine Collector's Issue 2016* titled **Fitness Couture** because of the line's sporty, yet fashionable appeal.

For this shoot, the 838 Media Group team also includes additional photographer Tuhan Bedi with hair and makeup by Inara Lopetaite Akin, and model Summer de Almeida. Check out the full editorial on page 42 and read the interview with Kevan Hall on page 39.

ADDITIONAL IMAGES INSIDE THIS ISSUE

PG. 23-27 (MODEL JEREMY CROWE, NTA MODELS - LA) PHOTO BY GLENN GORDON

PG. 30 (MODEL DREW LIPSON, NTA MODELS - LA) PHOTO BY GLENN GORDON

PG. 40-41 (MODELS SUMMER DE ALMEIDA, CORNELIA GRIMSMO) PHOTOS BY ASH GUPTA

PG. 50 (MODEL) PHOTO BY ARUN NEVADER

PG. 51 (GIRL WORKING OUT) PHOTO BY MADZINDIA

PG. 55 (GIRL JOGGING) PHOTO BY DEVINO TRICOCHE

PG. 66-67 (BOTTOM IMAGES OF MODELS) PHOTOS BY ARUN NEVADER

PG. 70 (RUNWAY MODEL) PHOTO BY ARUN NEVADER

PG. 76 (GIRL LEAPING AT BEACH) PHOTO BY GLENN GORDON, MODEL GEORGENE SMITH

PG. 79 (MODEL) PHOTO BY ARUN NEVADER

PG. 107 (BOY AT POOL "HUNTER JUNE THOMPSON") PHOTO BY MICHAL AMI THOMPSON

PG. 114 (1. GUY SURFING) PHOTO BY DEVINO TRICOCHE; (2. GIRL GYMNAST) PHOTO BY ARUN NEVADER; (3. WOMEN KAYAKING) PHOTO BY DEVINO TRICOCHE

PG. 132 (DOG CROSSING STREET) PHOTO BY DEVINO TRICOCHE

(STOCK IMAGES: MORGUEFILE.COM, IMAGEBASE.NET, STOCKVAULT.NET)

A Little About Us

KAYLENE PEOPLES

Kaylene Peoples , the Founder/Publisher/Editor-in-Chief of *Agenda* magazine online and now in print (since Fall 2014), has spearheaded and cultivated a rare, niche audience since *Agenda's* launch back in 2004. *Agenda* has garnered an audience of fashion/lifestyle savvy readers whose thirst for information has kept the magaizne thriving for over 11 years.

ANTHONY HEREDIA

The main contributor of health/fitness content, Anthony Heredia is saddled with plenty of nutrition and fitness education, and a full application of those skills in the real world. Anthony Heredia has trained countless celebrities and even some of us "regular" folks. His love and passion for the world's well-being and health is reflected on the pages of *Agenda*..

SHAHADA KARIM

Beauty editor Shahada Karim has contributed incredible content with "tried" and "true" reviews. Yes, she tests each product herself. Nothing gets past her, or her promise to write the most honest review on each beauty product in *Agenda*. As the creator of her own beauty line, Shahada practices what she preaches and has an infectious passion for skin care and beauty.

ASH GUPTA

Ash Gupta's stunning editorials have helped to define the look of the magazine. His team (838 Media Group) raises a bar that is out of reach for many photographers. Ash not only mentors young photographers, but due to his global reach as a photographer, he is one of India's most revered citizens. He was recently honored by his country for his worldwide, artistic contributions.

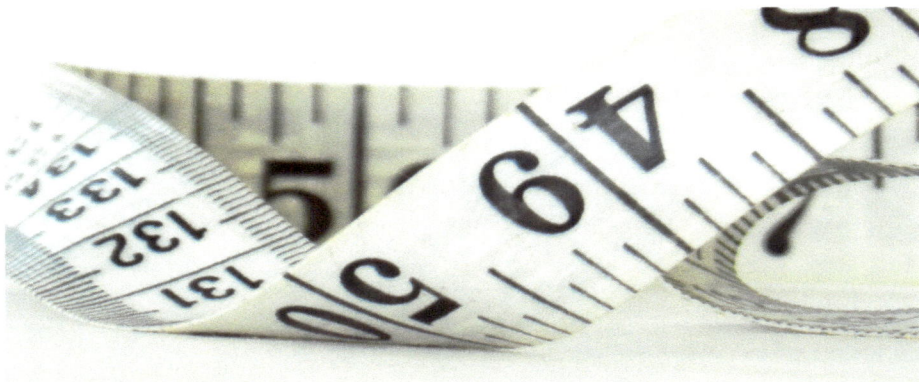

AGENDA COLLECTOR'S ISSUE Fitness Couture 2016

Agenda Magazine
P.O. Box 65053
Los Angeles, CA 90065

contact@agendamag.com
www.agendamag.com

CONTRIBUTORS

Kaylene Peoples
Editor-in-Chief, Journalist,
Creative Director, Layout

Lee Peoples
Executive Editor, Copy Editor

Anthony Heredia
Health/Fitness Editor, Journalist

Shahada Karim
Beauty Editor, Journalist

Ash Gupta
Photographer

Glenn Gordon
Photographer

Arun Nevader
Photographer

Devino Tricoche
Photographer

Publicity
First Take PR
www.firsttakepr.com
contact@firsttakepr.com

Truth Behind Detoxing
Cleansing HOW-TOs

BY ANTHONY HEREDIA

FIRST THINGS FIRST, DETOXING IS A BUNCH OF BULL, PARDON MY FRENCH. THERE IS ACTUALLY NO SUCH THING AS "DETOXING," WHICH IS ACTUALLY CONSIDERED NONSENSE IN MEDICAL TERMS.

According to Dr. Frank Sacks of the Harvard School of Public Health, the need for your body to rid itself of toxins has "no basis in human biology." Our bodies have their own cleaning systems that detoxify regardless of how we eat. It's time to replace the word "detoxing" with the word "cleansing." Most health professionals agree that it is just better to do a cleanse and eat healthier. Doing so hits the reset button and guides us to improved health and fitness.

Cleansing removes harmful environmental and dietary substances from our diets so that our body's natural systems and detoxification process can function properly and thrive. We are exposed to countless environmental pollutants (smog, emissions, pesticides) as well as nutritional toxins (artificial preservatives, animal hormones, trans fats, large amounts of sugar, excess sodium). Over time these impurities threaten to overwhelm our organs, making them less functioning. It's spring cleaning time. So clean out your kitchen and you will clean house in your body!

Keep in mind that there is no "one" set way to cleanse or to improve eating habits. But this article offers a safe and easy approach; it is not a cureall. You should eat food that is low in processing and is as fresh as possible. The very purpose of a cleanse is to give your body a break, to give your body a chance to heal itself, and to play catch up from the past. Those years of unhealthy eating will eventualy add up to your compromised health one day. You should give yourself approximately two weeks to see if there are any food groups that have a negative effect on your body to kick start your new lifestyle of eating better.

It is astounding the number of expensive detox diets that are available, all promising special herbal blends. Each guarantees a panacea from the inside out. "These diets can give people a false sense of security, a feeling that they've been protective of their health," Dawn Jackson-Blatner, a dietitian at the Northwestern Memorial Hospital Wellness Institute and American Dietetic Association spokeswoman, told WebMD.

CONSULT WITH A DOCTOR BEFORE YOU CLEANSE

". . . I believe in taking the most natural and minimalistic approaches to your body (please, always consult with your physician, though), and a detox (cleanse) is no exception," states Dawn Jackson-Blatner.

The proper cleanse is not a diet but simply making a healthy shift in what you eat and what you expose yourself to for the long run. You take the time to filter out as many artificial substances as possible and usher in a host of natural foods to give your body the time and resources it needs to repair itself. All you will need is fresh natural foods (organic preferably), common low-cost natural supplements, lots of water, patience, determination, commitment, and finally, good advice (provided here, of course).

Cleansing Bad Foods Out and Reducing Inches in Your Midsection

When your body is exposed to potential allergens (environmental & nutritional), it becomes inflamed. It swells from the inside and slows down many processes. This can lead to the appearance of a larger stomach, but this is actually inflammation that your body is battling. When there is heavy inflammation, you are much more likely to gain body fat as well as create a vicious cycle of weight gain.

Regulate True Appetite (Eliminate Fake Hunger & Cravings)

An abundance of artificial preservatives, excess sugar, nutrient imbalances, and toxic foods trigger false chemical signals, making you crave foods you really don't need.

Regulate & Boost Sex Drive

A healthy sex drive is a result of healthy hormone secretion and proper blood flow combining in an internal orchestra that brings your lust to life. Should a problem arise on either the hormonal or circulatory level, your taste for lovemaking might decrease significantly. There are many reasons why your sex drive decreases, but many of those reasons can be significantly helped with self-care.

Regulate True Appetite (Eliminate Fake Hunger & Cravings)

An abundance of artificial preservatives, excess sugar, nutrient imbalance, and toxic food triggers false chemical signals, making you crave foods you really don't need.

Regulate Mental Clarity

Mental clarity is a result of proper neural signals firing cohesively as a result of good blood chemistry. Thinking clearly requires body homeostasis (full body balance) through good oxygen uptake, nutrient balance, and proper circulation, all of which can easily be thrown off by a toxic, malnourished system.

Lessen or Eliminate Bad Breath and Body Odor

You are what you eat. Bad breath comes from bad stomach chemistry and rotting food in your mouth. Bad body odor stems from toxins leaving through your sweat glands. The worse your eating habits, the more potent the offending odor. Both problems can be helped significantly through better diet.

Lessen or Eliminate Allergies, Eczema, Acne, or Psoriasis

Nowadays many allergies and skin conditions are being recognized more as the result of food irritants. This can also be addressed by a medical allergy patch exam. You might be allergic to something you're eating and not know it.

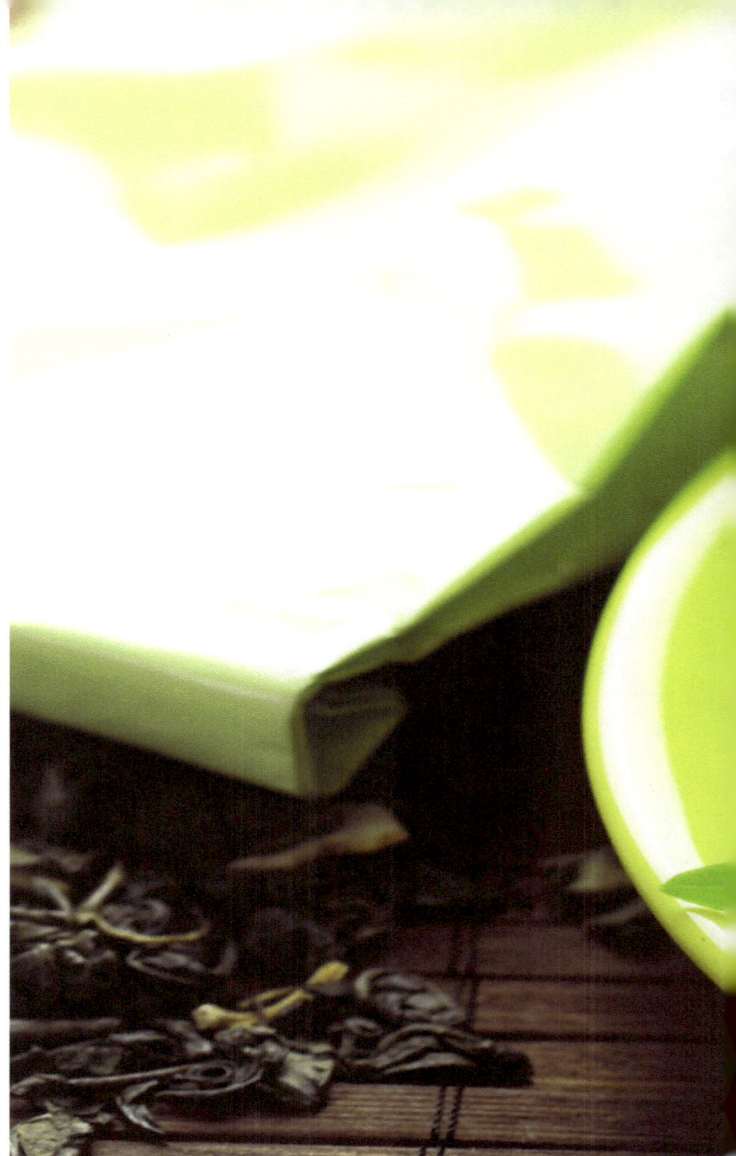

Regulate & Boost Metabolism (Weight Loss)

You basically are able to burn (use) more calories with a cleaner engine (metabolism), thus aiding in your weight loss efforts. It's a bit more complicated than that, but I am sure you get the idea.

Regulate & Boost Energy Levels and Moods

Mood imbalance and lethargy are caused for various reasons, but I am referring here to neural chemical imbalances due to electrolyte, fluid, and nutrient imbalances. Not giving your body what it needs can drastically affect energy levels and cause mood swings. You should always consult your physician for serious scenarios.

Regulate Bowel Movements

Increase fiber. Having regular bowel movements is crucial to your health because if you aren't regular, the toxins in your colon are given time to be reabsorbed into your healthy system.

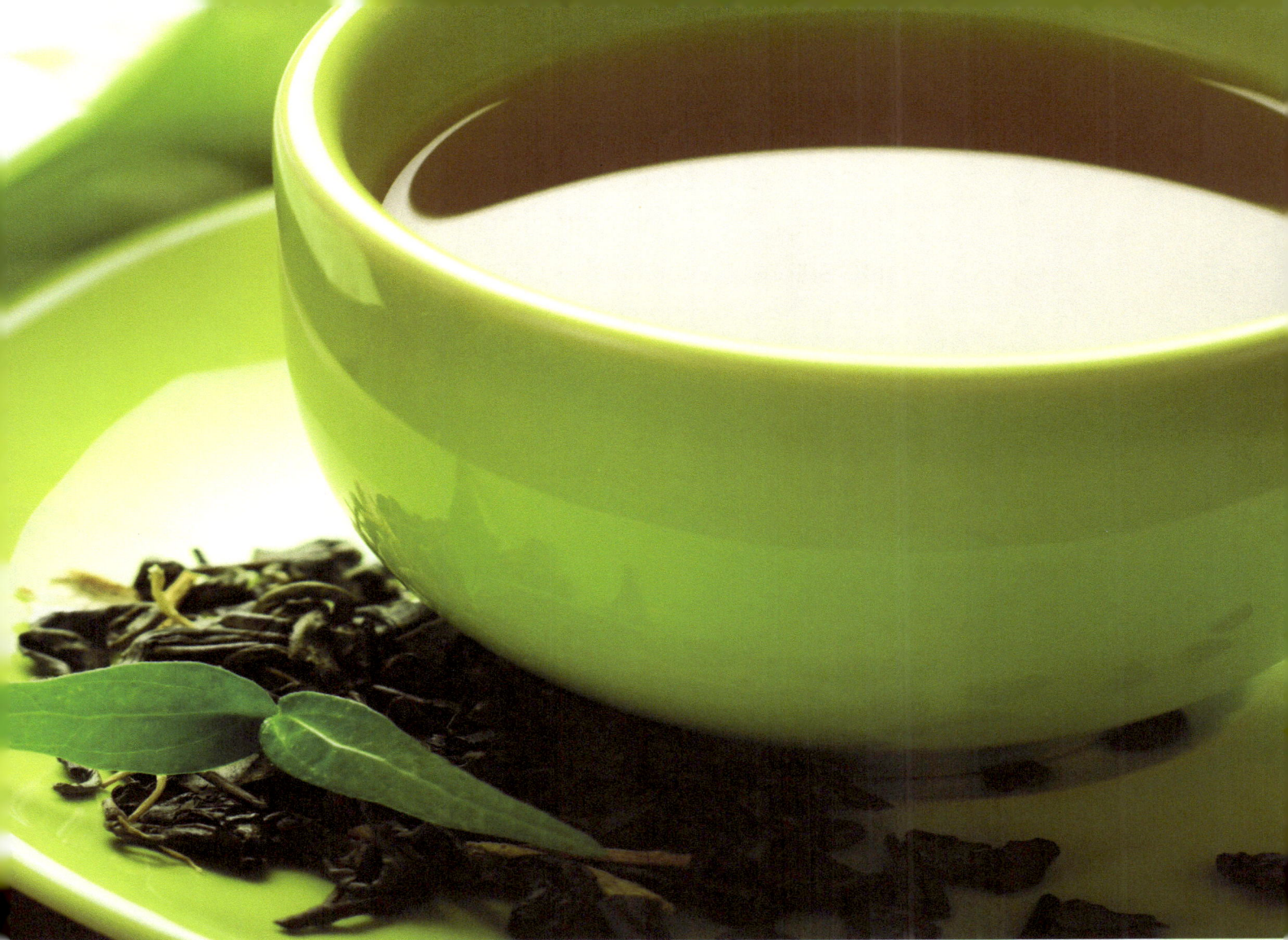

False chemical signals make you crave foods you don't really want.

Improve Skin Health
Restore proper moisture and oils to skin, allowing healthy collagen to keep your skin smooth and youthful.

Slow Aging
Fight deterioration of collagen (main cause of aging) and combating free radicals (the destroyers of healthy cells).

Regulate or Eliminate Bloating, Puffiness, Gas, and/or Indigestion
Regulate good to bad bacteria and enzyme ratios in your body that keep you in balance.

Regulate & Boost Immune System

The idea of a proper
cleanse is to create an ideal
foundation for a lifelong
positive health shift that will in
turn rev your metabolism.

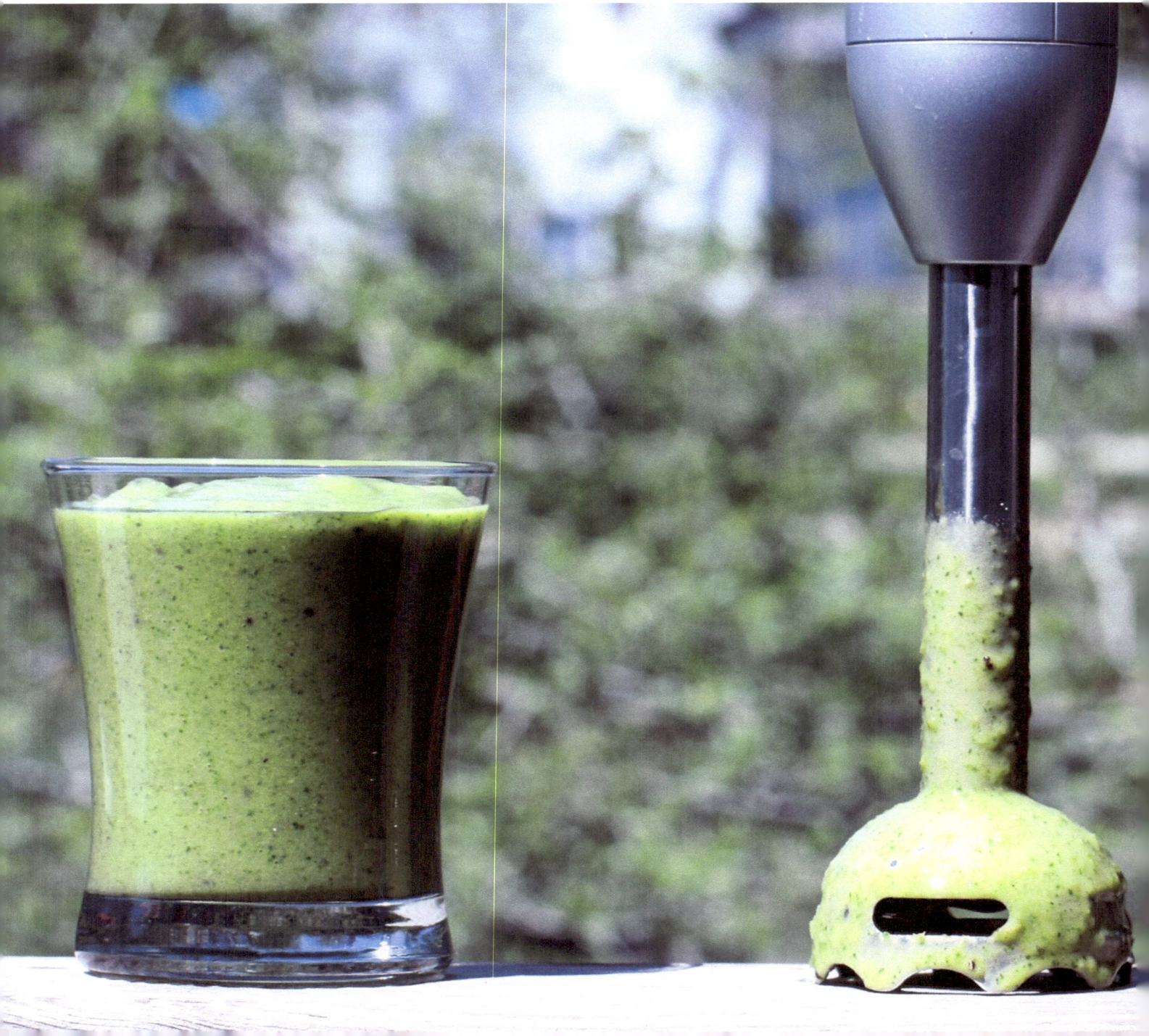

IS DETOXING SAFE?

By my definition of cleansing, yes, but always consult your physician before making dramatic changes to your diet. My definition of cleansing includes pulling away from artificial, over-processed foods, minimizing exposure to environmental toxins, and increasing self-care to give your body the chance it needs to optimize. It is not magic, and you mostly lose water weight and possibly backed up fecal matter (stool) in your colon, both of which drop big weight fast; but still this is vital. You do lose some body fat, but the idea of a proper cleanse is to create an ideal foundation for a lifelong positive health shift that will in turn rev your metabolism.

HOW DO I GET STARTED?

Allergies:

If you are relatively new to taking care of yourself and not very familiar with your body, I would first recommend that you ask your doctor for an allergy patch exam. There are a significant number of people today with food and/or environmental allergens who are none the wiser. You might not be aware of an allergy because some symptoms are as small as headaches, gas, irritation, or lethargy. Allergies become relevant because one symptom you might not be aware of is internal inflammation (which you obviously cannot see). Inflammation can severely affect nutrient absorption and a host of other systems. Make a trip to your doctor and let your doctor know you are interested in finding out whether you have any allergies and if you should worry about intestinal inflammation. (Doctors have a special test.)

WHAT SHOULD I AVOID? (TEMPORARILY)

Sugar

This includes products containing sugar and hidden forms of sugar, such as sucrose, dextrose, corn syrup, brown sugar, and turbinado sugar. Artificial sweeteners are usually not recommended. Stevia and erythritol are allowed natural sweeteners.

Dairy Products

(Milk, butter, cream cheese, sour cream, and other dairy products)

Wheat

(Wheat and products containing wheat, such as pasta and bread)

Gluten

All gluten-containing grains: wheat (including spelt, triticale, and kamut), rye, and barley

Coffee

One cup a day is ok if needed to reduce the occurrence of caffeine withdrawal headaches; but if you can, go without.

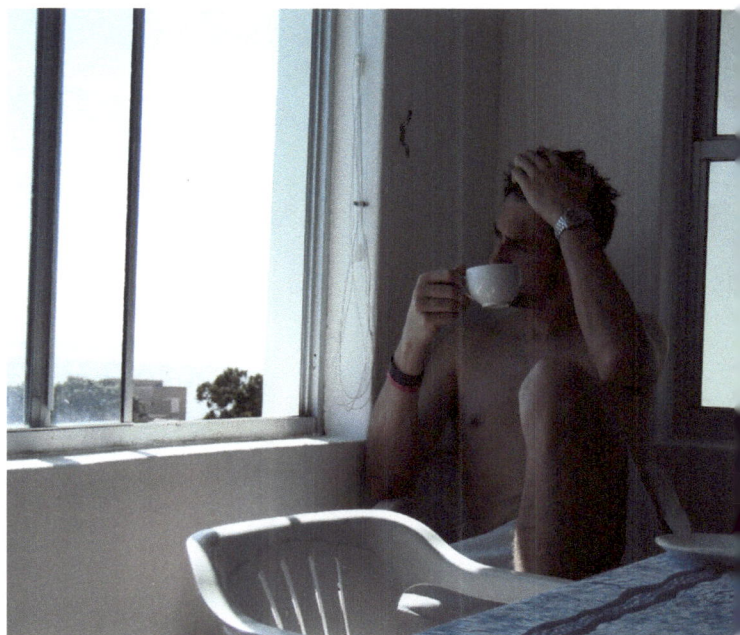

Stress

I can hear you snickering and laughing from here. Stress reduction is important. Stress reduction is scientifically proven to be critical to proper health, longevity, weight management, and a host of other subjects. Try as hard as you can to minimize your stress for this two-week approach with massages, pampering, delegating your work to others temporarily, or just avoiding stressful scenarios temporarily. I know it's easier said than done, but there is logic behind my madness. If after these two weeks your health and mood are significantly enhanced, then it is in your best interest to take the time to create a battle plan to combat stress for the long run, for the sake of your health.

OTHER FOODS TO AVOID

- Yeast
- Alcohol
- Food additives and preservatives
- Chocolate
- High-fat foods

SO WHAT SHOULD I HAVE?

Fruit
(Fresh or frozen fruit)

Vegetables
All fresh, please. Particularly good veggies include broccoli, cauliflower, Brussels sprouts, onions, garlic, artichokes; beets, red and green vegetables.

Rice
All forms of rice, brown rice preferred.

Other Grains
Quinoa, amaranth, millet, and buckwheat can be used instead of rice. These can be found at a health food store or in some grocery stores.

Beans
Split yellow and green peas and lentils are easiest to digest and require the least soaking time. Other good options include kidney beans, pinto beans, mung beans, garbanzo beans (chickpeas) and adzuki beans.

Nuts and Seeds
Good choices include flaxseed, pumpkin seeds, sesame seeds, sunflower seeds, almonds, cashews, and walnuts (usable as snacks or on a salad). Natural nut butters are ok. Peanuts and peanut butter are usually not recommended.

Oil
Extra-virgin olive oil is preferred.

Condiments
Vegetable salt, sea salt, vinegar, soy sauce or tamari, all herbs or spices

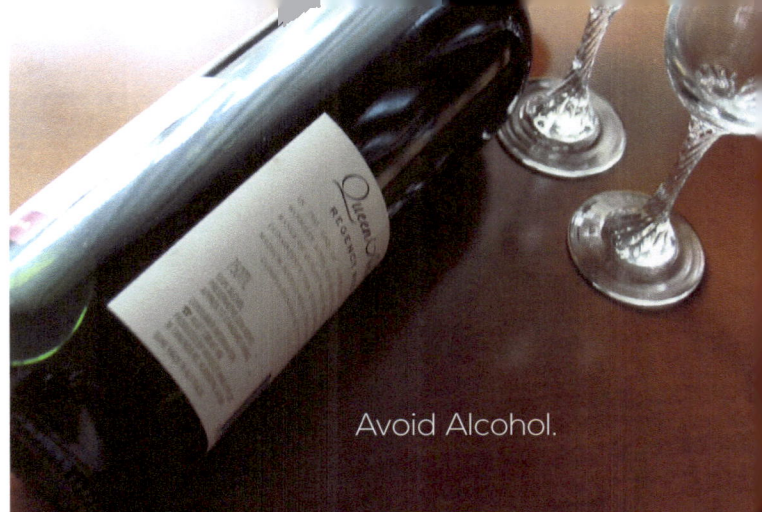

Avoid Alcohol.

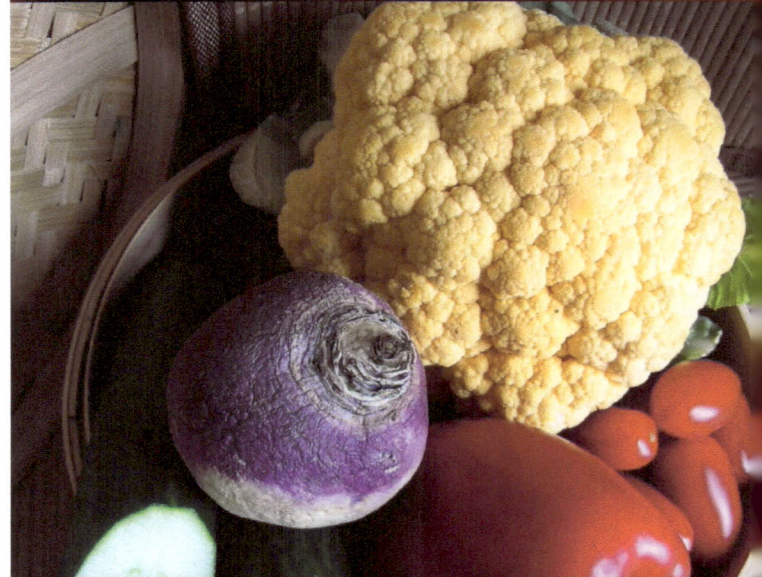

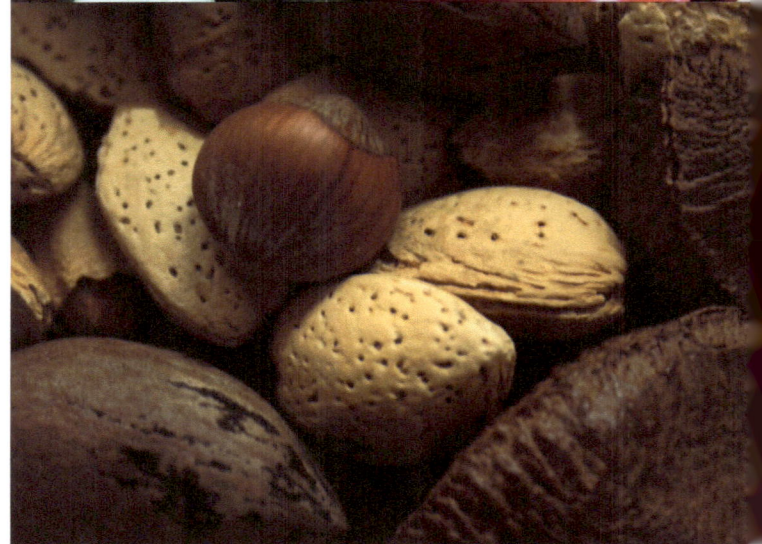

Tea
Herbal teas, green tea

Beverages
Water, lemon water, pure unsweetened fruit and vegetable juices, rice milk

SO NOW HOW DO I DETOX?

It will take two weeks eating five to six equal meals throughout the day. First meal should be within 30 minutes of waking up. I don't recommend starvation, so eat the amount of calories your body requires. Should you want to put some emphasis on weight loss, find out how many calories you should eat and subtract 500 a day (head to our weight loss article for more info). This calorie deficit will give you an approximate 1-2 lb of fat loss a week, given you don't skip meals and are a little active at least. Please note that those of you increasing that 500 calorie deficit should not cut your calories so much that you are starving because it will launch your body into weight storage mode. Stick to a 500 calorie deficit for now. To calculate how many calories, simply multiply your body weight times ten; and that will give you a solid general idea of the calories you use in a day. If you are very sedentary, subtract 300 calories from that number to be more accurate.

Now that you have your allotted calories, split them up evenly over those 5-6 even meals. As for what you should eat, refer to the included list (What Should I Have?) and avoid the "Avoids" list. Have fun and make your own meals, or buy food if you are not a cook; but stick as close as you can to these two lists for two weeks. The idea is to minimize possible negative influences in your health and filter them out in this cleansing time. Stay committed and it will pay off big. After these two weeks, begin to reintroduce all the items from the "Avoid" list one at a time; try to separate the time between each. Notice how your body responds to each of them, and should you not like what happens (i.e., gas, bloating, headache, lethargy, restlessness, mood shift), then eliminate it completely. This is a great simple way to optimize your health and life. There are definitely some items on the "Avoid" list that I highly recommend that you never bring back, though: high fructose corn syrup, white flour, heavy artificial preservatives, and large amounts of sugar. The closer you stay to natural forms of food the easier it is to keep weight down and health up. The body suffers when you mistreat it.

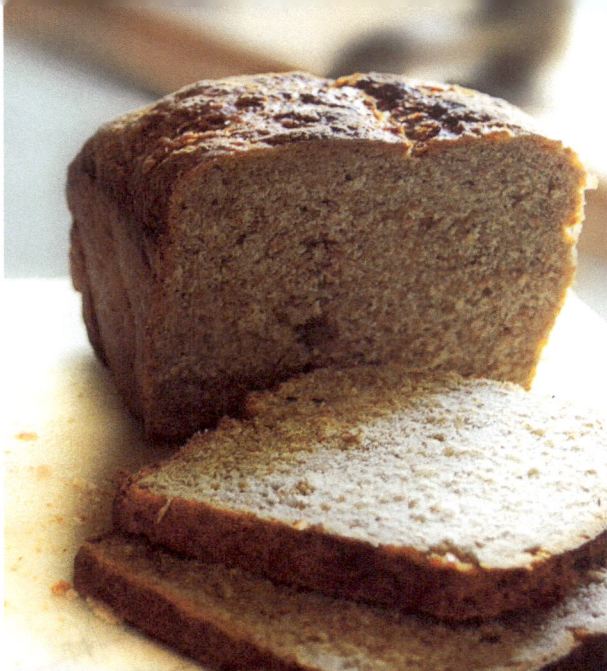

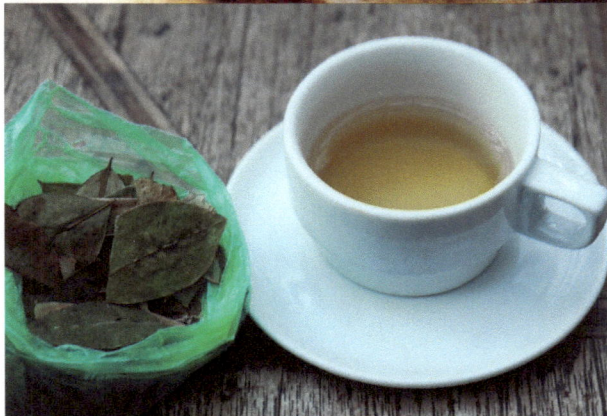

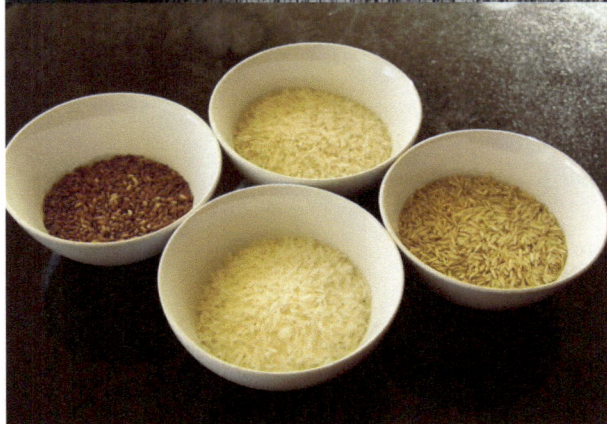

CLEANSE MUST DOs

Fiber – If you are cleaning bad stuff out, it needs to completely leave your system; and only fiber is truly going to take care of the bulk of that work.

Drink a minimum of eight glasses of water per day, warm or room temperature preferred.

(Recommended) A good probiotic to aid in digestion.

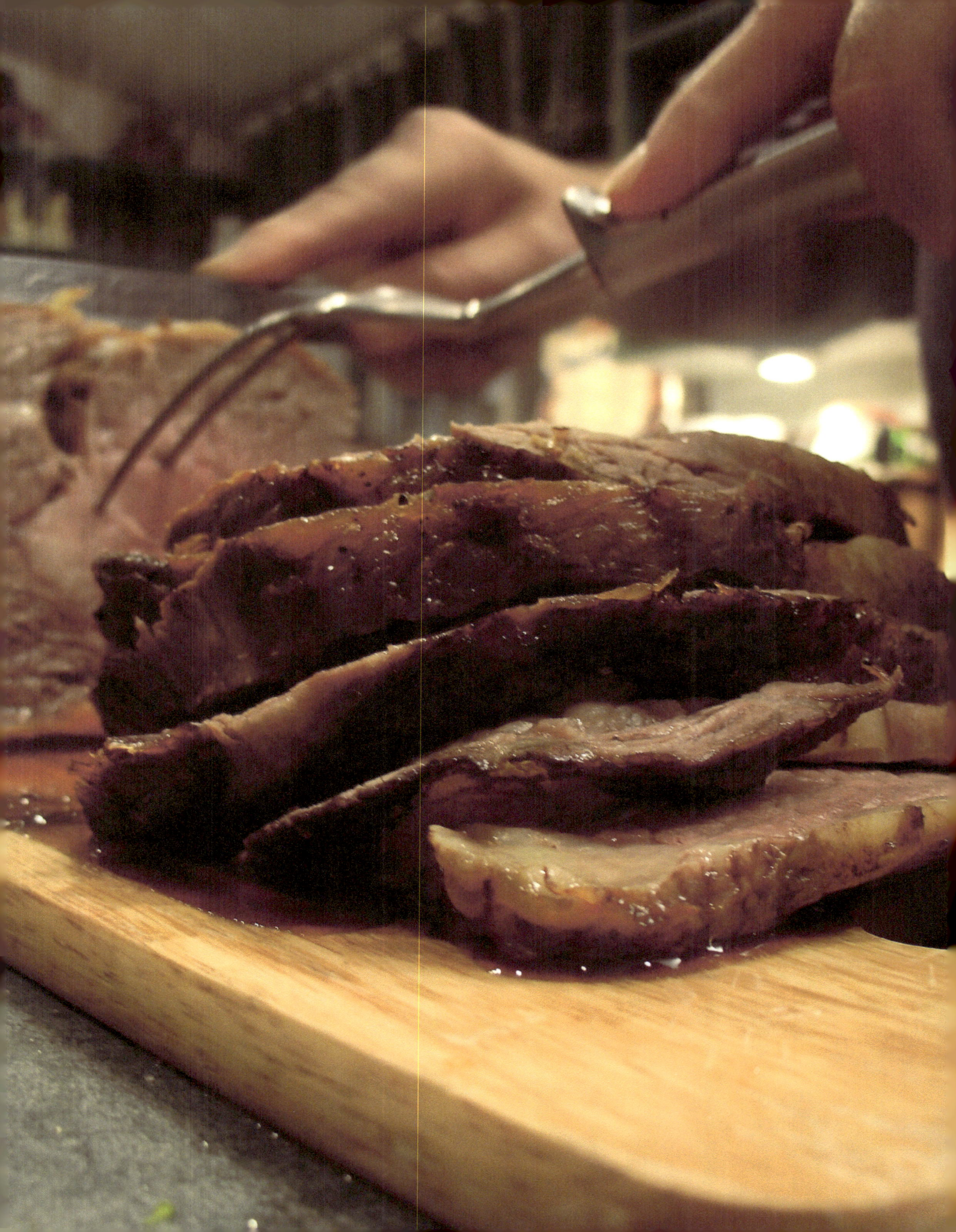

BY ANTHONY HEREDIA

THE POWERS OF PROTEIN

WHAT, WHY, AND HOW?

We all need it for just about everything our bodies do; and if you enjoy proper protein in your diet, you just might discover some new wonderful levels of beauty and health. There are at least 10,000 different proteins that make up our bodies, these ranging from the muscles that move you and down to your nails and hair. Difficulty in muscle gains and brittle nails or hair can often be a cause of low protein levels. It's a vital component of just who we are; and if we lack proper levels of this building block, our bodies have no choice but to build weaker structures or eat some of our healthy muscle to get what it needs. To give you a better understanding of the role of protein in your body and its importance, we will give you some basics to this vital nutrient.

So What Is Protein?

There are three major (macro) nutrients our body requires to keep in balance: fats (lipids), carbohydrates, and protein. All forms of meat are dominantly protein, but you can find variant amounts of protein in just about anything that grows, like vegetables, for example, as protein is the base for the growth of life. Protein's primary function in our bodies is to serve as a building tool. Protein itself is created of subunits called amino acids, the true building blocks. Think of amino acids as puzzle pieces. There are 20 different puzzle pieces in total, and a different combination of puzzle pieces creates a different picture with its own unique purpose. There are nine essential amino acids our body cannot create and must obtain from our diet and 11 that it can acquire all on its own. All 20 puzzle pieces are vital for normal growth and daily function, as well as critical for peak health and fitness. If any of the critical pieces are missing from your diet, your body will need to break down another part of your body, like your hard-earned muscle, to finish its job.

So Why Do I Need Protein?

1) Structure

Each combination of amino acids serves a different purpose in your body, ranging from building your muscles, growing your hair, and repairing you, to helping create hormones and keeping your skin youthful. Protein gives your body structure and the tools to build. It literally keeps your teeth in your gums, keeps your organs together, and shapes come-hither curves that beg for fitted clothes or summer sun. Collagen (the secret to young beautiful skin) actually makes up for 25% of the protein in your body's construction, making protein very significant.

2) Regulation

It also serves to regulate your body's hormones, enzymes, immune system, and fluid balance. Inadequate protein in your diet can cause frequent illness, low energy, poor digestion, dehydration, slow recovery times, reduced sex drive, mental fog, and a host of other problems. These problems are a result of your body simply needing to do a job and not having the building blocks it needs to complete its task. When your body needs any of the 9 essential amino acids due to insufficient diet, it will break down healthy, active muscle or organ tissue to retrieve what it needs. Your body will trade some of your nice arm muscle in order to keep you breathing. Tissue breakdown (catabolism) results from imbalanced nutrition, compared to physical demands, significant calorie reduction, or starvation. Your body will begin to recycle itself to survive. Worst yet is the fact that muscle deterioration dramatically slows down metabolism because muscle tissue is a powerful calorie-burning engine. The less muscle you have the slower your metabolism, meaning you can eat less and gain weight easier. This is very typical in most dieting American women who cut calories too low, sacrificing muscle. Low muscle women who are

on a dieting cycle merely look at food and gain weight because their bodies are less equipped to process the food, leading to greater storage. Yes, these women are losing weight, but muscle weight. In exchange for losing 5 pounds of muscle, they will now need to eat 250 calories a day fewer to stay the same weight. One pound of muscle burns 50 calories a day extra, so a lean, toned, protein-filled body is allowed to eat a lot more to stay a lot more beautiful. Remember that although muscle weighs three times more than fat, it is also three times smaller, creating a fine, tight appearance. Go, protein!

3) Energy

Finally, protein serves as a potential source of energy. Your body loves to use carbohydrates and fat as a primary source of energy, while protein is left for last. Your body stores about 500-1500 calories of carbohydrates throughout your body in the form of glycogen for immediate fuel access, and it stores fat in all the places you love to hate; but your body does not store protein. Your body prefers to use carbohydrates as a primary source of energy for intensive physical demands and higher functions (brain and nerves), as it is a fast and efficient source of fuel. Fat (lipids) is also an excellent source of energy, but it is primarily used for less intensive physical demands and non-glucose dependent cells (like muscle cells). You use fat for energy as you sit at your desk doing your work. Fat burns longer but much slower, obviously, or we would all look like Greek statues. Last on the chain of command is protein which is not a great source of energy as it takes the longest to convert into a usable form of fuel for our bodies, and still it is inferior as fuel, compared to carbs and fat. Your body works three times harder to convert protein into usable fuel in comparison to carbohydrates, one of the reasons for high protein diets becoming so infamous for fat loss.

Protein for Weight Loss?

So how do low carbohydrate/high protein diets work? Well, they basically convert your carb-burning body into a fat-burning body through what most could call stressful manipulation. The science lies in your liver, which converts carbs you ingest into glucose for immediate energy or stores them in your liver as glycogen. The liver will release glucose (immediate fuel) into your blood system for cellular energy and stored lipids (fat) into your system for simpler non-glucose dependent cells (like muscle cells), conserving glucose for needier cells. Your liver can store an estimated 12-hour supply of fuel; but once it runs out, it begins to convert amino acids (protein) into glucose (immediate fuel). The more complex cells (brain & nerve) need more than this protein fuel, so your body begins to convert the released fat energy in your blood into what is known as ketone bodies (upgraded fat energy). Your brain and nerve cells are now forced to partially accept this less effective fat energy (ketones), and the body is now forced to use only fat and protein for energy (ketosis), resulting in dramatic body fat depletion. So basically you convert a carb-burning Ferrari into a hybrid sedan running on fat and protein, which aren't nearly as effective as carbs.

So, What's the Catch?

The catch is that this inferior process forces your liver to do an incredible amount of stressful work, leading to possible permanent liver damage in extended trials. This inferior energy source also causes mental fog, significantly slower reaction times, dramatic fatigue, and a host of other problems as your body is basically being stressed out. Worst of all is once you return to normal eating from a prolonged period of this dieting method, your body will hyper load and retain fat in self-preservation, just in case you attempt this again. You rarely permanently win by manipulating or tricking the human body for extended periods of time. It's a bit smarter than you might think. Remember that these are all merely tricks, gimmicks, and techniques to manipulate your body. No extended trick will ever give you the life and body you dream of. Always ask yourself if you can make whatever you are doing a permanent healthy way of life. Fight your body, and it will fight back and win. The human body has evolved over thousands of years as a sophisticated survival tool, so your best bet is to work with its original settings and instructions. Higher protein methods are fine for small durations as a technique to give fat loss a quick kick, but by no means is it a way of life. Protein is a powerful necessary building and structural tool in your journey towards reaching your health and fitness goals, but for best results I suggest it be used in balance as evolution intended.

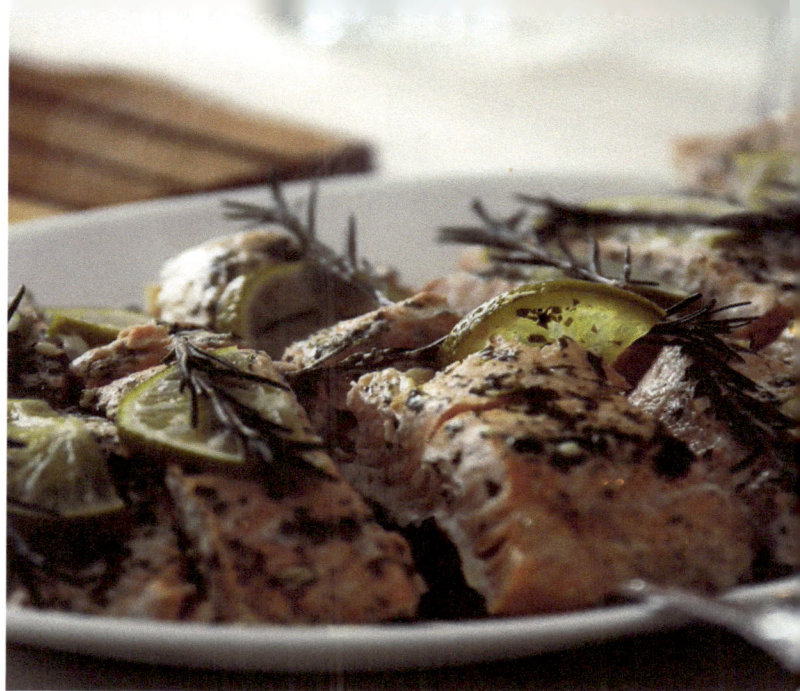

So How Much Protein Do I Need?

A good nutrient balance for the average body by today's standards is 20-30% protein, 15-25% fat (the good kind) and 55-65% carbohydrates. According to the Institute of Medicine, adults need a minimum of 0.8 grams of protein per kilogram of body weight, basically 8 grams for every 20 lbs. Individual needs of each category will always vary according to your current health, fitness regimen/goals, and daily activity; so consult your local health/nutrition professional for some precision, or grab a good nutrition book to take control yourself.

Sleep
Deprivation

BY ANTHONY HEREDIA

THE PRODUCTIVITY AND AESTHETICS ENEMY
YOU ARE GRUMPY, SLOWER, AGE FASTER, AND GAIN WEIGHT; SO SLEEP!

There is a critical correlation between your sleep and the effects on your overall health when you don't get enough of it, including weight gain. Isn't sleep overrated in these high-paced days? No, it is not. Let us explain why. Successful weight loss consists of fitness, balanced nutrition, along with giving the body what it needs to recover and thrive. The body needs down time to make the positive changes you ask of it; no recovery time means trouble for you. Sleep deprivation has been proven to significantly accelerate the aging process, increase fat storage, along with a plethora of other adverse effects that are very avoidable.

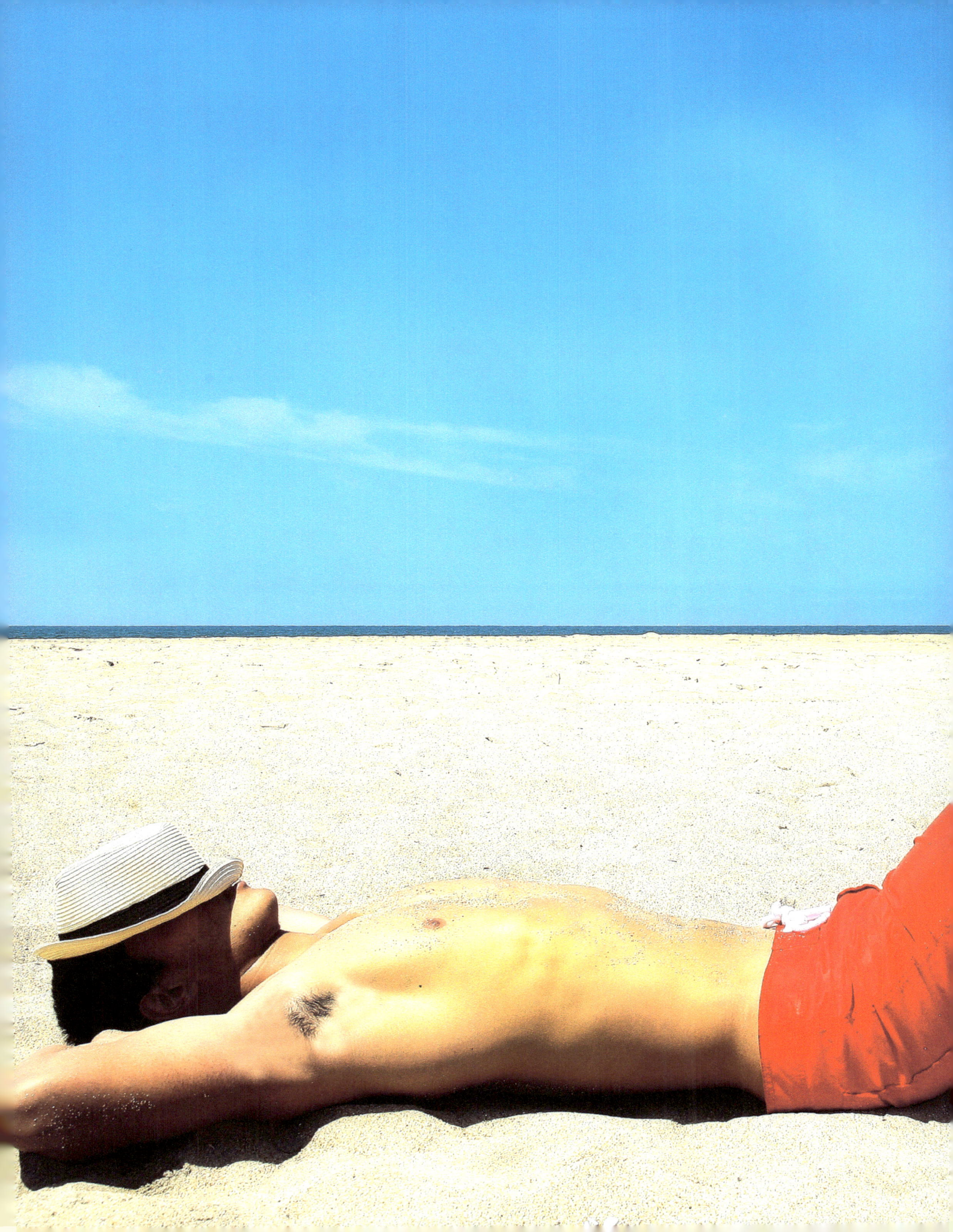

Adverse Effects of Sleep Deprivation

Self-Sabotage

o **Mood Swings**

o **Chronic Fatigue**: Repairs occur in the REM or Delta phase of sleep, the deepest level of sleep where you dream. If you can't reach a deep enough level of sleep, your body cannot properly refresh you, leaving you to still feel exhausted after a night of sleep.

o **Accelerated Aging**: During the deep stages of REM sleep, the body repairs and regenerates tissues, builds bone and muscle, and strengthens the immune system. As you get older, you sleep more lightly and get less deep sleep. The less sleep you incorporate the less time your body has to keep you young, thus prematurely aging you.

o **Clouded Mind, Foggy Thoughts**

o **Hindered Work Performance**

o **Affected Mental Health**: Sleep deprivation has mental as well as physical complications. While those with depression are more likely to suffer from insomnia, insomniacs or those suffering from other sleep disorders are also more likely to develop depression, impaired memory and thought processes.

o **Decreased Immune Response**: As part of the immune system, cytokines play a key role in fighting disease and infection. As the body's levels of cytokines drop, you become more susceptible to illness and infection.

o **Increased Alcohol Sensitivity**: Sleep deprivation also magnifies alcohol's effects on the body, so a fatigued person who drinks will become much more impaired than someone who is well-rested.

o **Increased Pain Perception**

o **Increased Cortisol Levels**: Cortisol levels are increased in your body during stressful times, promoting fat storage as a form of self preservation.

o **Unbalanced Hunger**: An imbalance in the hormones Ghrelin increasing (Hunger Hormone) and Leptin decreasing (Satiety Hormone), causing the body to crave carbohydrates and sugar.

o **Significantly Slower Reaction Time**: After 24 hours of no sleep, you are as impaired as if you had enough alcohol to be legally drunk in most states.

o **Restricted Nutrient Absorption**: Sleep deprivation interferes with the body's ability to metabolize carbohydrates and causes high blood levels of glucose, which leads to higher insulin levels and greater body fat storage.

o **Reduced Levels of Growth Hormone**: GH is a protein that helps regulate the body's proportions of fat and muscle. You will be more likely to store fat and use lean muscle tissue for energy.

o **Insulin Resistance (Possible)**: Since hormone levels are not allotted proper time to regulate themselves, an imbalance can contribute to increased risk of diabetes as the body is less receptive to insulin.

o **Increased Blood Pressure (Possible)**: When the body is not allotted the proper time to recuperate, it is forced to work harder under these stressful circumstances. The hours you don't sleep add up in debt that your system adapts to by pushing harder.

o **Increased Risk of Heart Disease**: Due to body systems working overtime with a non-recuperated body and reduced immune system, heart disease is more likely.

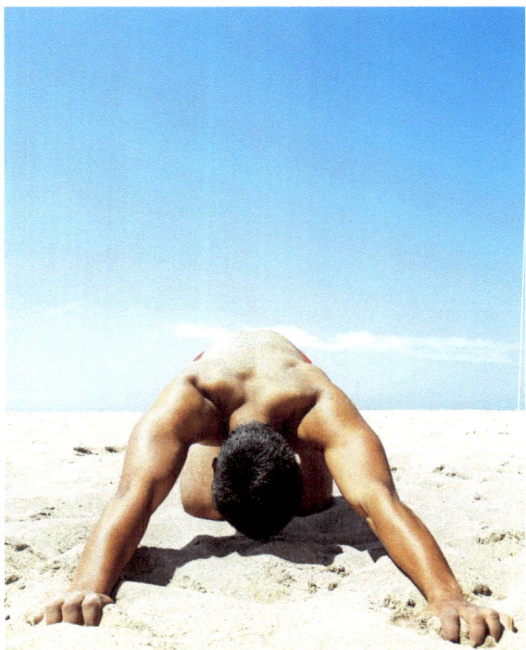

SLEEP DEPRIVATION IS AS BAD AS BEING INTOXICATED

Working yourself to the edge of your limits on no sleep is no better than working intoxicated. After staying awake for 24 hours straight, a person will be as impaired as if he/she had had enough alcohol to be legally drunk in most states.

In one Australian study, researchers created a blood alcohol equivalent test with 40 volunteers for different levels of impairment from sleeplessness. Group one stayed awake for 28 hours while group two drank alcohol every half hour until reaching a blood alcohol concentration of 0.10 percent, the drunken-driving standard in most American states. Every half hour the subjects took a computerized test of hand-eye coordination. "Results showed that after 24 hours of sleeplessness, participants were about as impaired as they were at the 0.10 percent level of blood alcohol. After 17 hours, they were about as impaired as they were with an alcohol level of 0.05 percent, which many Western countries define as legally drunk, the researchers said."
– National Sleep Foundation

HELP ME! WHAT IS GOING ON INSIDE ME?

Deep sleep is repair time. Your body needs to catch up from the day's toils. Should you deprive it, it has no choice but to defend itself, resulting in a destructive attack on your health and appearance. This is not personal; it is survival. Yes, I know that in today's fast-paced busy world sleep can be a very inefficient and inconvenient part of your schedule, but consider the price you are paying. "Sleeping is so overrated" seems to be the modern mantra. Sleep deprivation interferes with the body's ability to metabolize carbohydrates and causes high blood levels of glucose (sugar), which leads to higher insulin levels and greater body fat storage. The hormonal imbalance between leptin and ghrelin is actually the largest internal battle, transforming you into a carbohydrate/sugar craving, fat storing machine. You also begin to produce reduced amounts of growth hormone, which is what helps regulate the body's proportions of fat to muscle. This is reducing the muscle that helps you burn that evil fat in the first place.

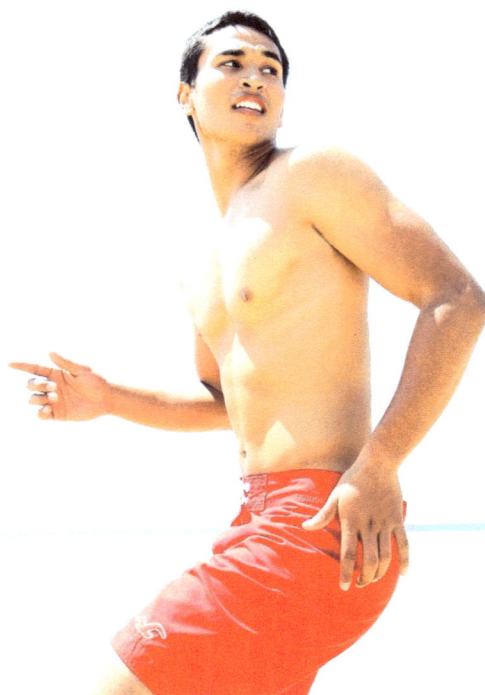

WHAT IS ALL THIS HORMONE IMBALANCE TALK ABOUT?

Leptin and ghrelin are our focus. They work in a kind of "yin and yang" system to balance the feelings of hunger and fullness. Ghrelin is produced in the gastrointestinal tract and stimulates appetite, while its counterpart leptin is produced in fat cells and sends the signal to our brains that we are full and have no need to store fat. Leptin and this full feeling are triggered exclusively by good fats (Omega-3s, fish, nuts, oils, etc.) and fiber. This all ties together as we introduce low amounts of sleep. Sleep deprivation drives leptin levels down, resulting in its taking longer to feel satisfied while eating, driving you to overeat. Lack of sleep also causes ghrelin levels to rise as a self defense mechanism, increasing your appetite for high-fat foods to hit that satiety sweet spot. I am sure I do not need to clarify how stressful it can be not to be able to get much needed sleep. Stress itself increases your cortisol levels, a stress hormone that also puts our bodies in self defense mode by turning the fat storage dial up a few notches in bad times. I hope by now I have convinced you that sleep is not a luxury; it's a necessity, ladies and gentlemen.

WEIGHT GAIN FROM NO SLEEP?

Stanford University held a study in which 1000 volunteers were surveyed on their sleeping habits and then had their ghrelin (hunger hormone) and leptin (satiety hormone) levels measured. "After eight hours of no sleep all volunteers showed increased levels of ghrelin (weight gain hormone) and decresed levels of leptin (weight control hormone). Results conclusively proved that those who slept the fewest hours per night also weighed the most, holding larger amounts of body fat," the study found. The body is simply adapting to a stressful environment, it is doing what it knows best. This is one reason you are more likely to eat more when you are not feeling at your best. "One thing I have seen is that once a person is not as tired, tired, they don't need to rely on sweet foods and high carbohydrate at your best. "One thing I have seen is that once a person is not as tired, they don't need to rely on sweet foods and high carbohydrate snacks to keep them awake — and that automatically translates into eating fewer calories," says Dr. Michael Breus of

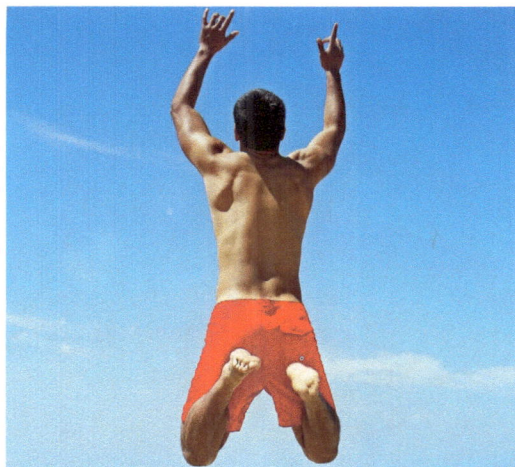

the Atlantic School of Sleep Medicine.

Sleep! More specifically, you need deep recuperative sleep, also known as Delta sleep or NREM sleep. This is the stage in sleep where you dream. This is also the time all repairs take place. Deep sleep is your goal to reverse this process. "Infants can spend up to 50% of their sleep in the REM stage of sleep, whereas adults spend only about 20% in REM," states the National Sleep Foundation. Please take the time at night to make an event of sleep. Turn off all ambient light and rude distractions in the room (including those with whom you share your bed) so that your body can reach this delta stage of sleep. If you need white noise (TV or sound) in the room to fall asleep, you will be fine as long as you set a timer for your appliances. You will need to consistently achieve a full night's sleep for at least one solid week for your body to begin to regulate itself once more. When your body receives consistent rest, it will do the work for you. Combine good rest, proper nutrition, and some regular fun exercise, and I guarantee you a summer body to die for. Look forward to a future article on tips and tricks to getting in a full night's sleep without sleeping the whole night.

HOW MUCH SLEEP DO I NEED?

According to the National Institute of Health, infants usually require about 16-18 hours of sleep per day, while teenagers need about 9 hours per day on average. Most adults need about 7-8 hours of sleep per day. According to Dr Colette Bouchez of WebMD, "A presentation at the 2006 American Thoracic Society International Conference showed that women who slept 5 hours per night were 32% more likely to experience major weight gain (an increase of 33 pounds or more) and 15% more likely to become obese over the course of the 16-year study, compared to those who slept 7 hours a night." Reaching your 6-8 hours of sleep a night I know is easier said than done; but as you can see, it is critical to your health, beauty, and in this case, your waistline.

More Solutions

Whether your sleep issues exist due to your work life, family life, medical reasons, or simply lifestyle in general, you must tend to this in order to keep yourself healthy. Treatment options depend on your particular circumstances, but here are some suggestions to help you begin your rejuvenation. The key is to create new habits and improved consistent sleep patterns. Normalize your amounts of sleep. Infants usually require about 16-18 hours of sleep per day, while teenagers need about 9 hours per day on average. Optimal sleep for health improvements are between seven and nine hours of sleep a night.

WAYS TO IMPROVE SLEEP INCLUDE

Exercising regularly earlier in the day to help regulate energy levels

Consuming low levels of liquids before bed

Finding a non-habit forming sleep aid, for example, melatonin

Relaxing with a hot bath before bed

Avoiding alcohol, nicotine, or caffeine before bed

Avoiding treating heartburn at night

Creating an ideal sleep environment by removing media distractions and making the bedroom as dark as possible to fall asleep faster and remain asleep.

In conclusion, sleep!

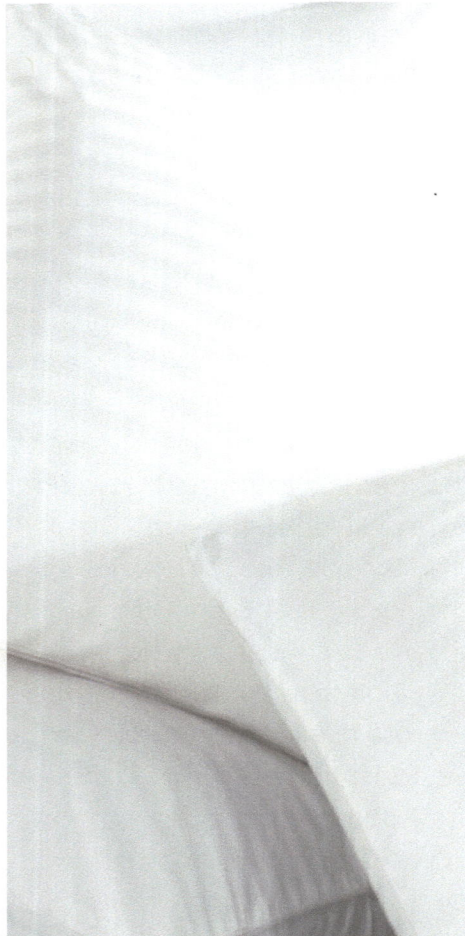

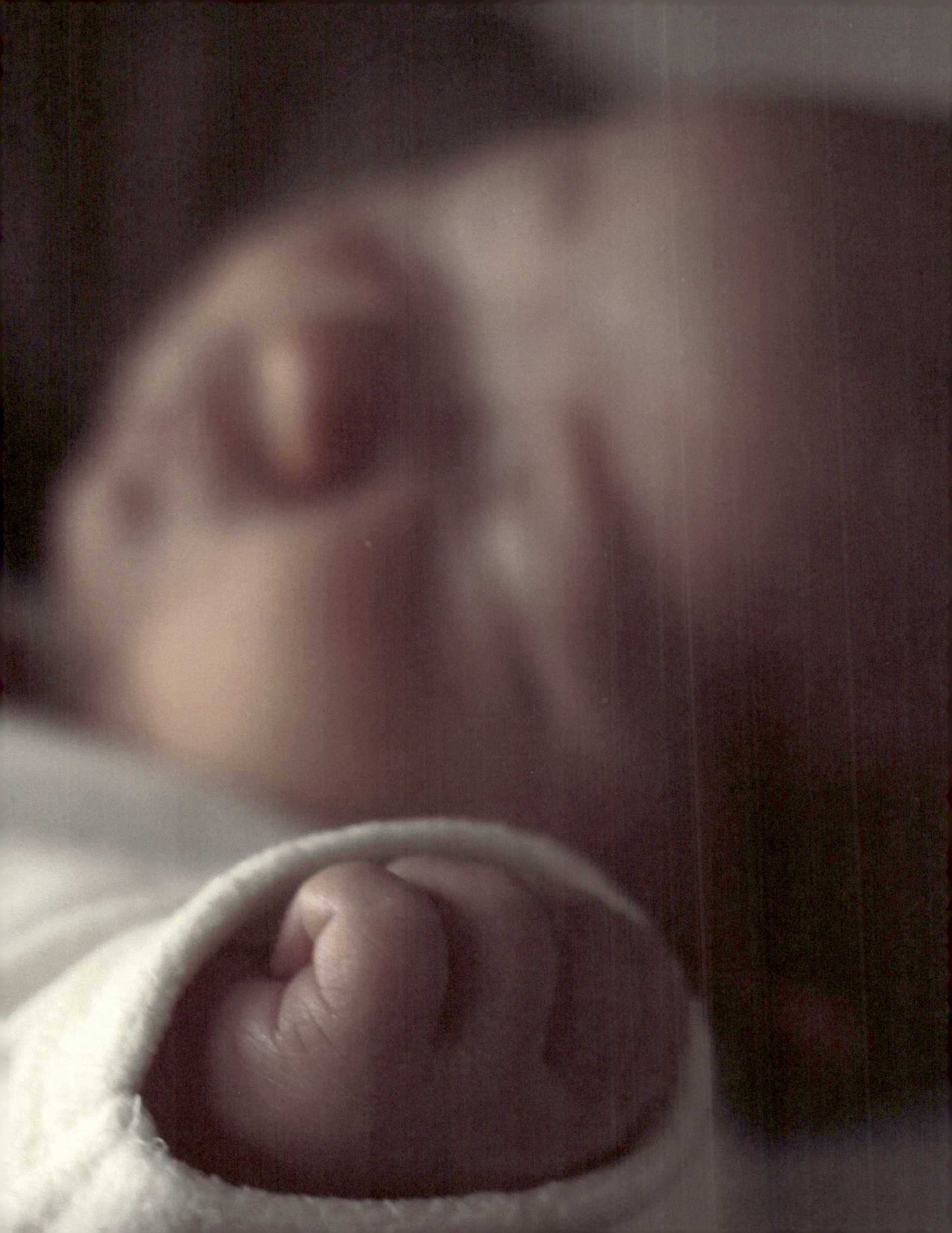

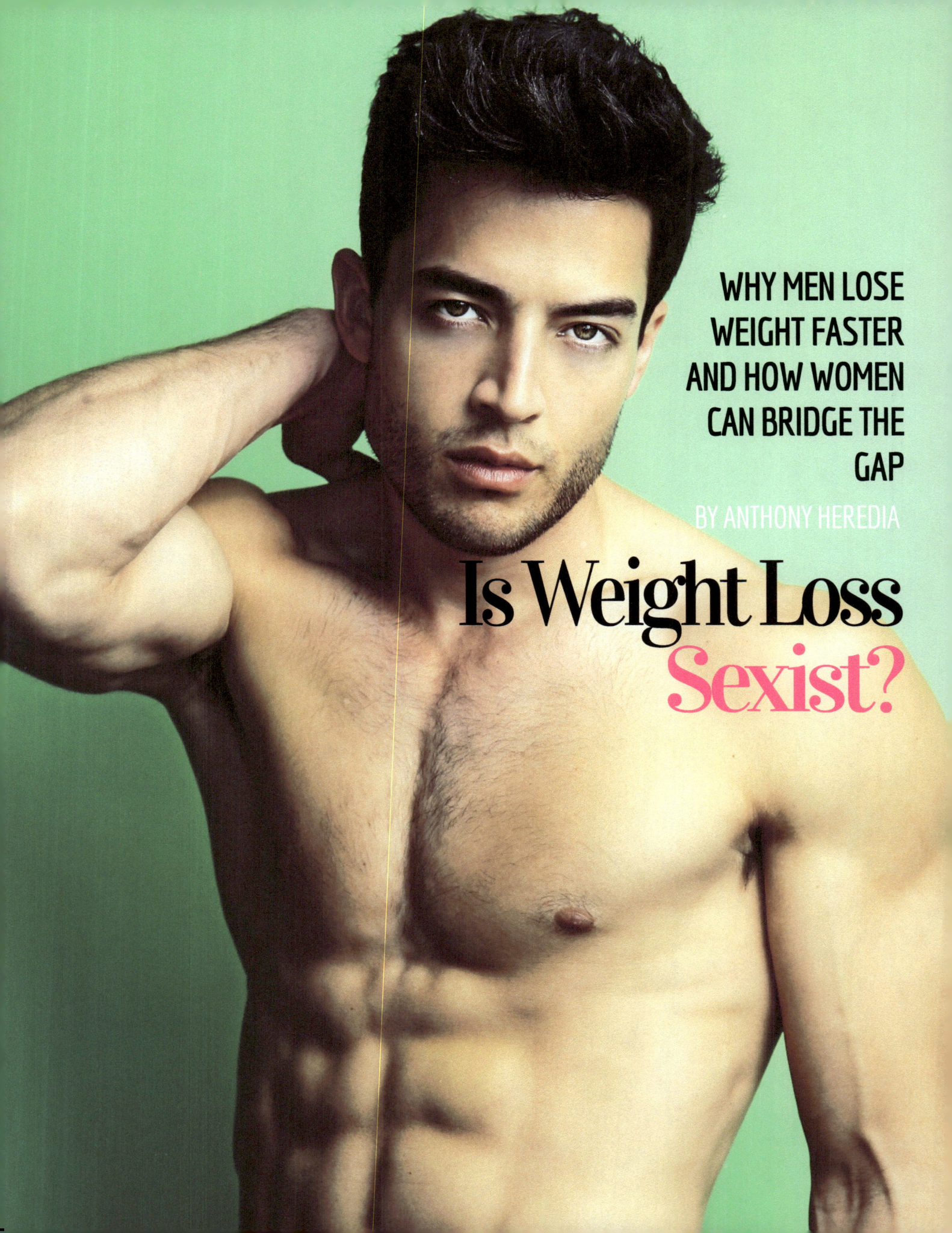

WHY MEN LOSE
WEIGHT FASTER
AND HOW WOMEN
CAN BRIDGE THE
GAP

BY ANTHONY HEREDIA

Is Weight Loss Sexist?

We address the age-old question of why we men hold this unfair advantage in the battle of the bulge, and further yet, how to help women close the gap. The truth is that men do have major fitness advantages over women, and that women are built with some hurdles, thanks to good old Mother Nature and genetic design. Fret not, though. If there's a will there's a way! The first male advantage involves body composition, enabling men to burn calories at an accelerated rate in comparison to women. Specifically, I am referring to the fact that men have greater amounts of muscle mass, making them extremely efficient fat burning machines. Every extra pound of lean muscle devours an extra 50 calories a day by simply existing. Might not sound like much, but should you add an extra 5 lbs of lean muscle mass to your body (which visually is one toned leg), you would burn an extra 500 calories a day doing what you already do. In one week's time you will have burned 3500 calories, 1 lb of fat, simply due to your having one well-toned leg. (I recommend you tone both legs together, though.) This either means you can eat an extra sandwich with two pieces of fruit, staying exactly the same size, or change no eating habits and naturally lose nearly 1 lb a week. Not bad, right?

Men were genetically designed by nature to hold and build more muscle mass, testosterone being the key player in all of this. Women, on the other hand, are predisposed to store and retain fat due to higher levels of estrogen, a hormone that works to keep the fat on a woman's body so it's easier for her to become pregnant. That means women have to work harder to lose weight at the same rate as men. Realistically, women do take longer to add on the same muscle a man undergoing the same approach would; yet she will reap the same benefits once packing that not so gorgeous muscle. Do take note to remember that the male body originated as an expendable yet efficient hunting, gathering, defending machine. Ladies, you were beautifully designed to survive and bring in new and wonderful life into our world. Aesthetics were unfortunately not part of the original grand scheme of things. Take up any complaints with the big architect on that one.

A second grand advantage revolves around men naturally designed for more active lives, combined with faster response to exercise. Women have a lower tolerance for exercise due to smaller lung capacity, leading women to feel as though they are working harder than men even if the women are working at the same level. This makes exercise feel extra difficult in heat and high humidity. Under strenuous, unbalanced conditions, a woman's body will enter starvation mode easier than a male's, slowing the metabolism to hang onto more fat in the hopes of self-preservation. Research has found that on average the metabolism of a man is 5 to 10 percent higher than that of a woman of the same weight and height. The American Journal of Physiology found that women burn an average of 16 percent fewer daily calories than men. Researchers found that a woman's resting metabolic rate was 6 percent lower than that of a man, along with 37 percent fewer calories burned during physical activity. A woman's edge in weight management stems from her uncanny intuition. Women tend to be more attentive to what's going on with their bodies and are better able to make the connection between food and emotions, a male weakness.

Men have more muscle mass, making them extremely efficient fat burning machines. Every extra pound of lean muscle devours an extra 50 calories a day by simply existing.

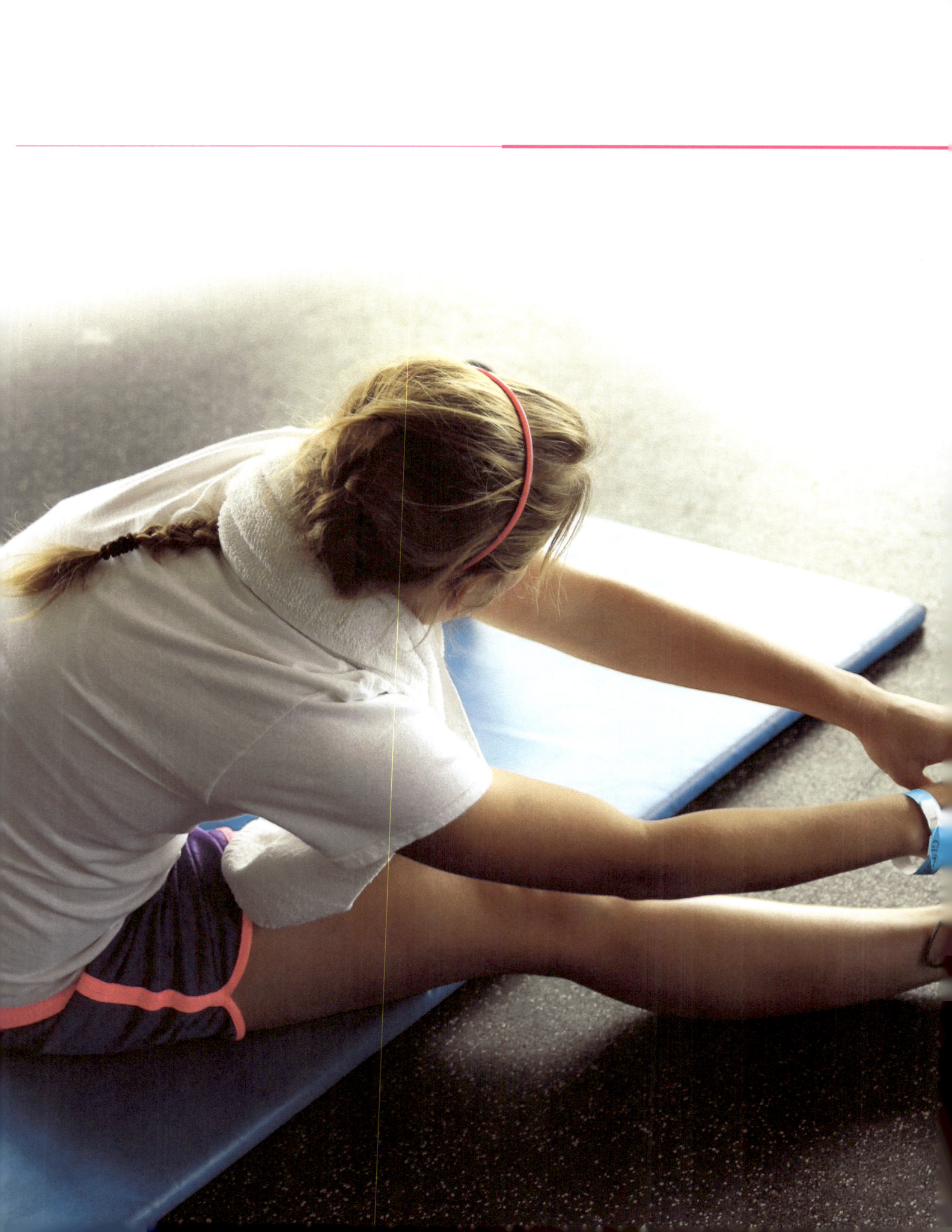

BOTTOM LINE: NOW HOW TO LEVEL THE PLAYING FIELD

The key lies in building fat-incinerating muscle. Build that fat-burning body-sculpting muscle mass so that you can eat more guilt-free and reach the highest tiers of your physical goals. A woman with added lean muscle can burn much higher levels of calories and more effortlessly maintain upper tiers of health. Women are generally afraid that building muscle means getting bulky as their partner strives for, but it's not true. First off, 1 lb of muscle is 3 times smaller than 1 lb of fat. It is denser, so you might weigh the same, but you get so much smaller and firmer. Also, to build bulky muscle you need to eat far more than you burn so that the body has building blocks to make the bulk; so even if you were to leave your workout in agony daily, you wouldn't grow without eating more than you take in. One pound of fat is 3500 calories, while 1 lb of muscle is 2500 calories; so to add even one pound of muscle a week, you would need to eat 800-1000 calories above your basic need and push hard enough that your body builds new tissue. Basically, ladies should not be afraid of bulking up, as I promise it's very hard for us guys alone to add 1 lb, eating everything in sight and pushing as hard as we can. Ladies, to get stronger and not bulky, simply push hard to the point of feeling that light soreness; and eat six balanced meals a day, getting in the base calories you need (more on exact calories in "Health 101-How to Lose Weight" article). Calories should be just a few hundred above what your body needs on workout days especially so that your body has the bricks to build the house (muscle). I recommend finding a good challenging class in your gym, an experienced credentialed trainer, or a fun yet butt-kicking DVD program to start with if you aren't sure where to begin. Strength training can be tricky and one of those things you don't want to learn by trial and error, as you can get very hurt. Be safe, but go hard. You won't regret it.

Extend Your Cardio.

Studies show that 60 minutes per day minimum for 5 days a week is what's needed to reap the max benefits for slimming down and building stronger lungs for endurance and increased metabolism. Once you are happy with the body that is unfolding, you can pull back to maintenance workout time, which is 3 times a week at your 60 minutes. If you have trouble with that, increase your time incrementally, or dividing up the time in the same day is fine, as well. As you trade more muscle for fat, you will burn more and more doing the same as muscle powers up your calorie-fueled engine.

Set Realistic Goals.

A realistic rate of loss is 10 percent of your body weight over a few months or 1/2 to 2 pounds a week. Pushing your body to lose too much too fast with unhealthy tricks is the reason people yo-yo. As previously mentioned, 1 lb of fat is 3500 hundred calories, so losing 2 lbs would be 6000 calories or the equivalent of nearly 18 typical ham sandwiches as perspective. That is a lot to lose in just a week, so be kind to yourself and treat your body right.

Make healthy living a routine.

Women are much more disciplined and patient than most men, so make sure to capitalize on this fact. Keep a food diary to keep yourself accountable; make healthy choices a habit as brushing your teeth so that you no longer think about it. It becomes second nature. Even if you only have 15 minutes to work out, make sure you do it more so to maintain the habit and routine, which is so easy to lose. Choose water over empty calories, and educate yourself on all your new changes. Don't just listen to us health nuts. We read the books, but if your interest should spark, ask why and find your answer. By educating yourself, you become that much more committed to yourself. Not a bad investment, I say.

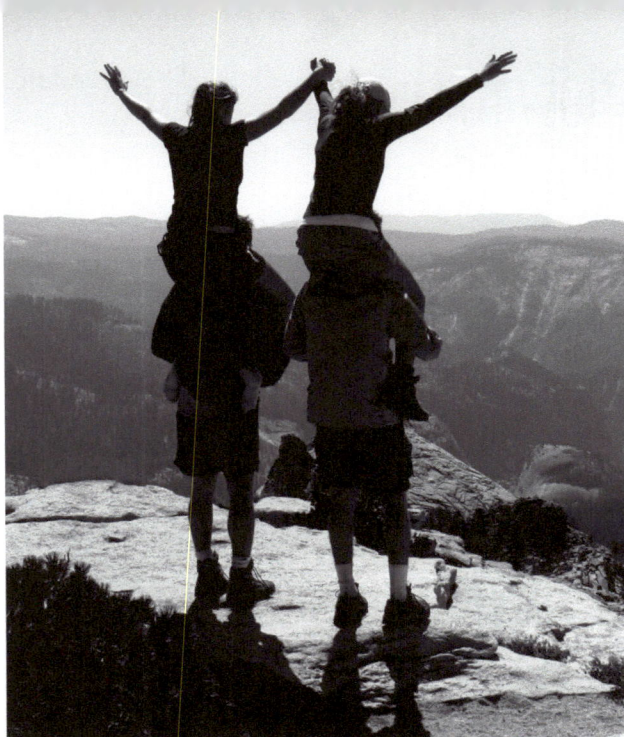

GET YOUR INACTIVE PARTNER OFF THE COUCH NOW!

BY ANTHONY HEREDIA

The average American reaching age 77 will have viewed over 150,000 hours of TV in his/her lifetime. (Are you kidding me!?) That equates to spending roughly 17 years of one's precious life in front of a glowing box. According to the surgeon general, more than 60 percent of American adults don't exercise regularly, and 25 percent aren't active at all. The Center for Disease Control says that 34 percent of Americans are overweight, and more than 28 percent were severely obese in 2010. Inertia has become a national emergency. We all know even without statistics that being sedentary is bad for countless reasons, but it is so much worse when you are in a relationship with someone who doesn't seem to share your passion for taking care of yourself.

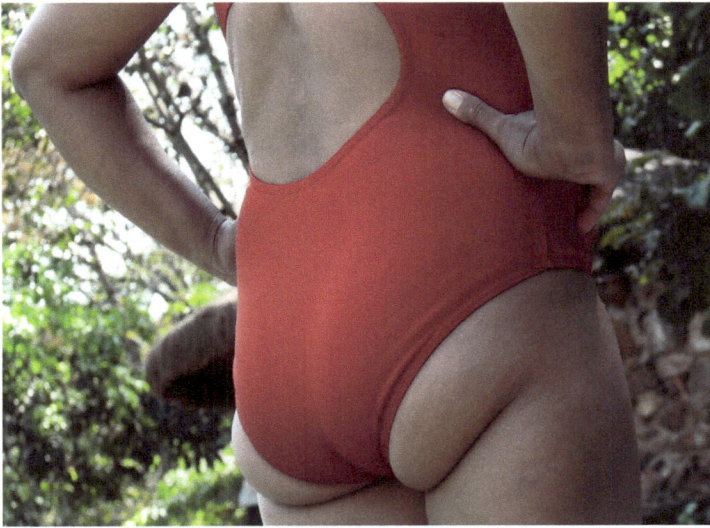

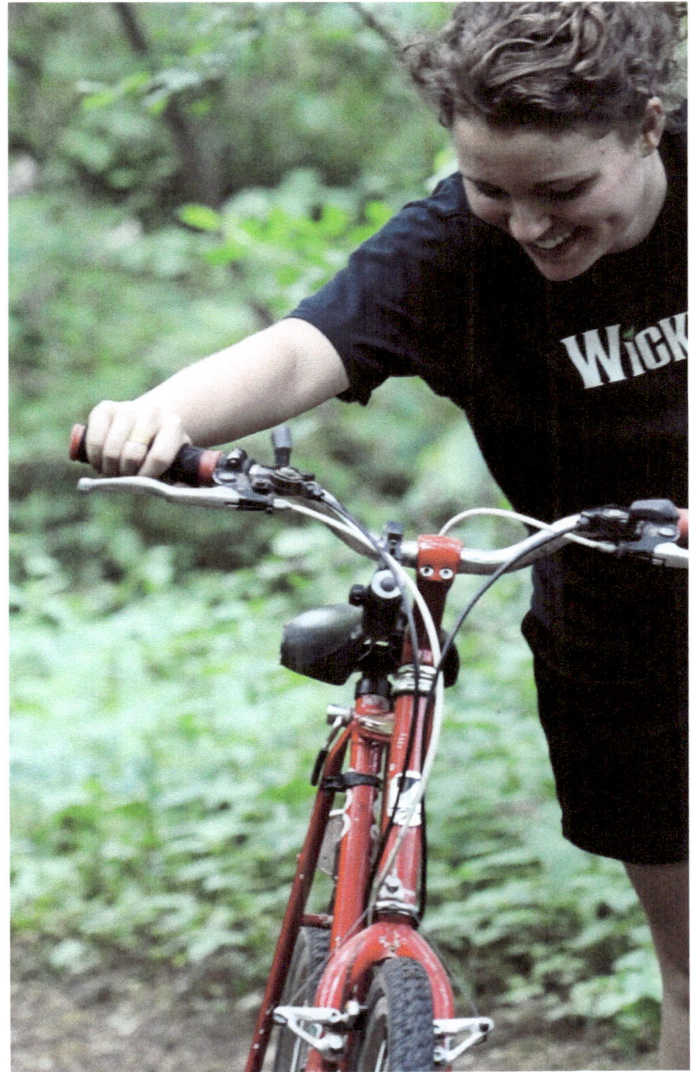

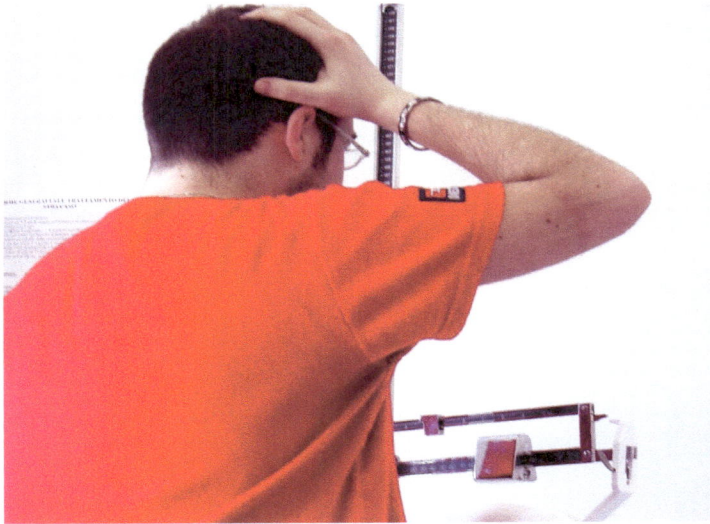

So how do you get your loved one off the couch in a way that won't result in the cops showing up at your door? Let's just avoid that scenario, shall we? Exercise is omnipotent. It enhances every single aspect of your life. Being fit improves self esteem and energy levels, promotes better sleep patterns, clearer thinking, promotes getting promoted at work (yes, you read that right); relieves depression, and improves your complexion. Living fit slows aging, regulates sex drive, stamina, and even hormone levels. It increases work productivity, enhances the immune system, and so much more. And these are just a few examples why someone should get fit, but for now we are going to highlight the fact that couples who live a fit life together

stick to their programs longer, remain together longer, and are happier. Once you're motivated to help your partner, head over to my Health 101 article for a battle plan to get him/her moving.

Exercise can be an outlet. I consider my workout time "me" time. I don't carry my cell phone or tell anyone I'm out running, so I can disappear while exercising. But there are always those times when I would love some company. It's about balance. You might love exercise as "you" time, which is fine; but that doesn't mean you can't share a workout or two; let's get your potato of a spouse motivated. Here are just 6 benefits to exercising with your partner that you might not have thought of.

GETTING FIT

Balance – With many couples, one partner tends to favor cardio (typically women), while the other tends to favor strength training (typically men). By working out together, you can balance your workout program to include more of both while educating each other. Let your partner teach you about the areas of fitness you're unsure of, and be open to new fitness experiences.

Quality Time – Couples spend most of their time apart due to careers and regular responsibilities. Instead of working out alone every time, why not plan a little workout time that fits both of your schedules. The couple that sweats together stays together after all. You'll reach your fitness goals without sacrificing that one-on-one time every partnership needs.

Respect and Pride – These topics are immense deal breakers. Getting in shape for someone who doesn't appreciate the work has ended many a relationship. By working out together at least once a week, you both can respect each other more by seeing what it takes each other to be healthy. Taking care of your body and your health also shows your other half that you care about him/her by wanting to be around for years to come.

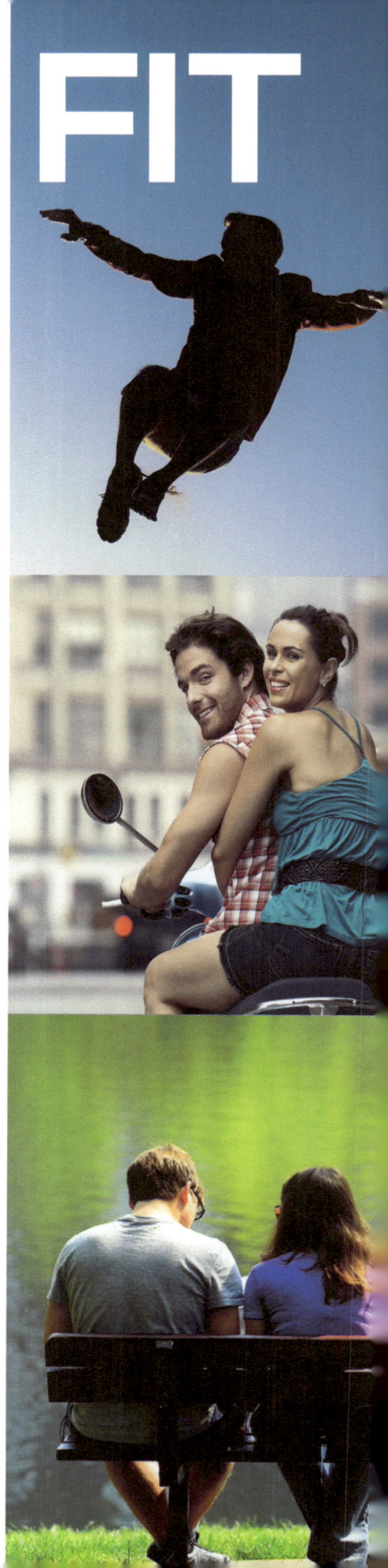

BENEFITS

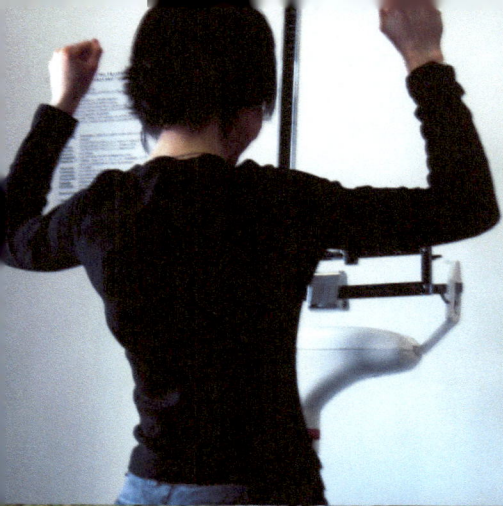

Inspiration and Support – Getting encouragement and praise from your partner is one of the best motivators. When he/she sees you sweating bullets, it creates admiration. The absolute best compliment anyone can give someone is, "You make me want to be a better person." You become inspiration. It helps both of you to remain consistent, take care of one another, and inspires you to continue your workout program.

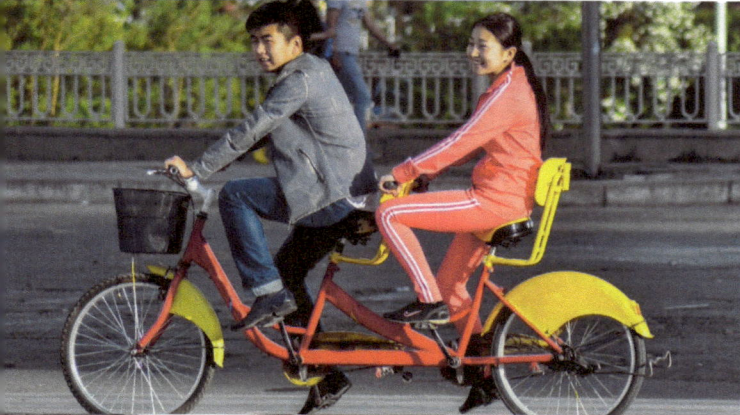

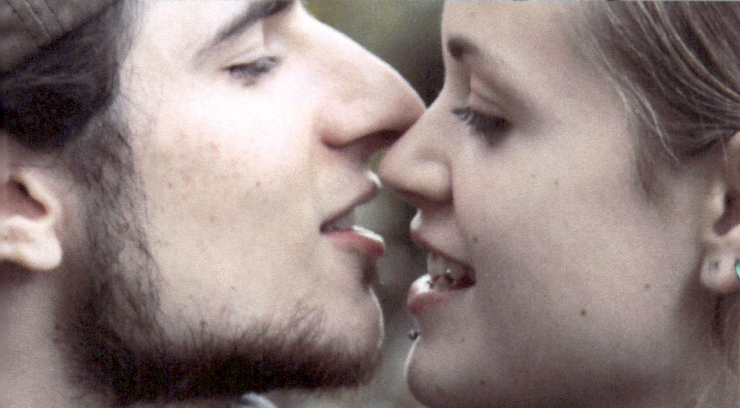

Teamwork and Safety – Working out together gives you a chance to work on your communication skills and teamwork. With someone else watching your form and being there to spot you when you need it, you'll exercise more safely than if you were alone. This creates fantastic bonding and trust.

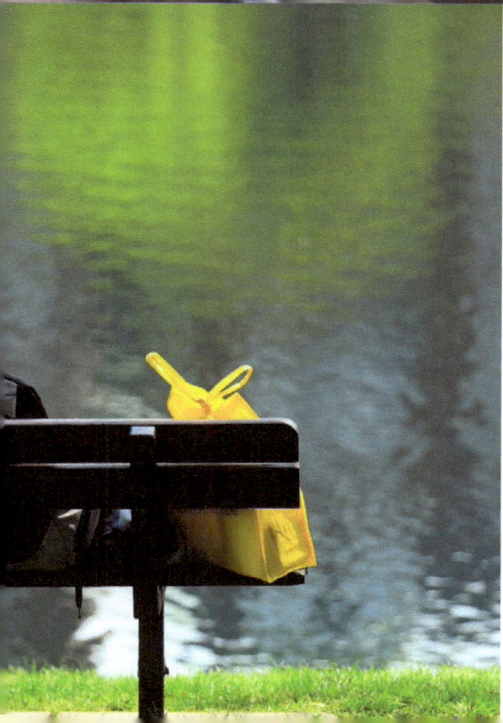

Sexual Desire – Exercise produces chemicals in the brain that evoke feelings of happiness, reduce stress, and also increase arousal and libido. Several studies show that men and women who exercise regularly report better (and more frequent) sex with their partners. Watching your partner grunt, sweat, and combat a hard workout regimen can be a powerful aphrodisiac, but don't take my word for it.

With these workout ideas for couples, you and your partner can spend quality time together while you stay on track to reaching your goals. Let me know how this all turns out. Don't forget to check out the other articles for details on fitness and calories for a better battle plan. Until we meet again, I bid thee all adieu.

AGENDA

FITNESS COUTURE

COLLECTOR'S
ISSUE 2016

Cover Photo:
Ash Gupta
Model:
Cornelia Grimsmo

Is **Weight Loss** Sexist?
Why does HE lose weight faster?
pg. 30

Childhood **Obesity**
Don't let this happen to your little one.
pg. 102

Kevan Hall Sport
Game On!
Attire for Golfers and Active Fashionistas
pg. 39

Benefits of Yoga
pg.120

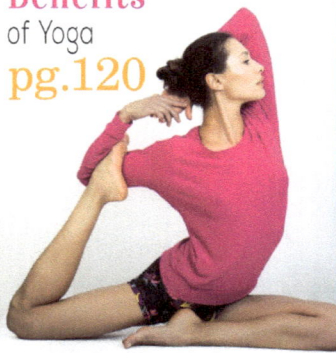

Truth Behind **Detoxing**
pg. 10

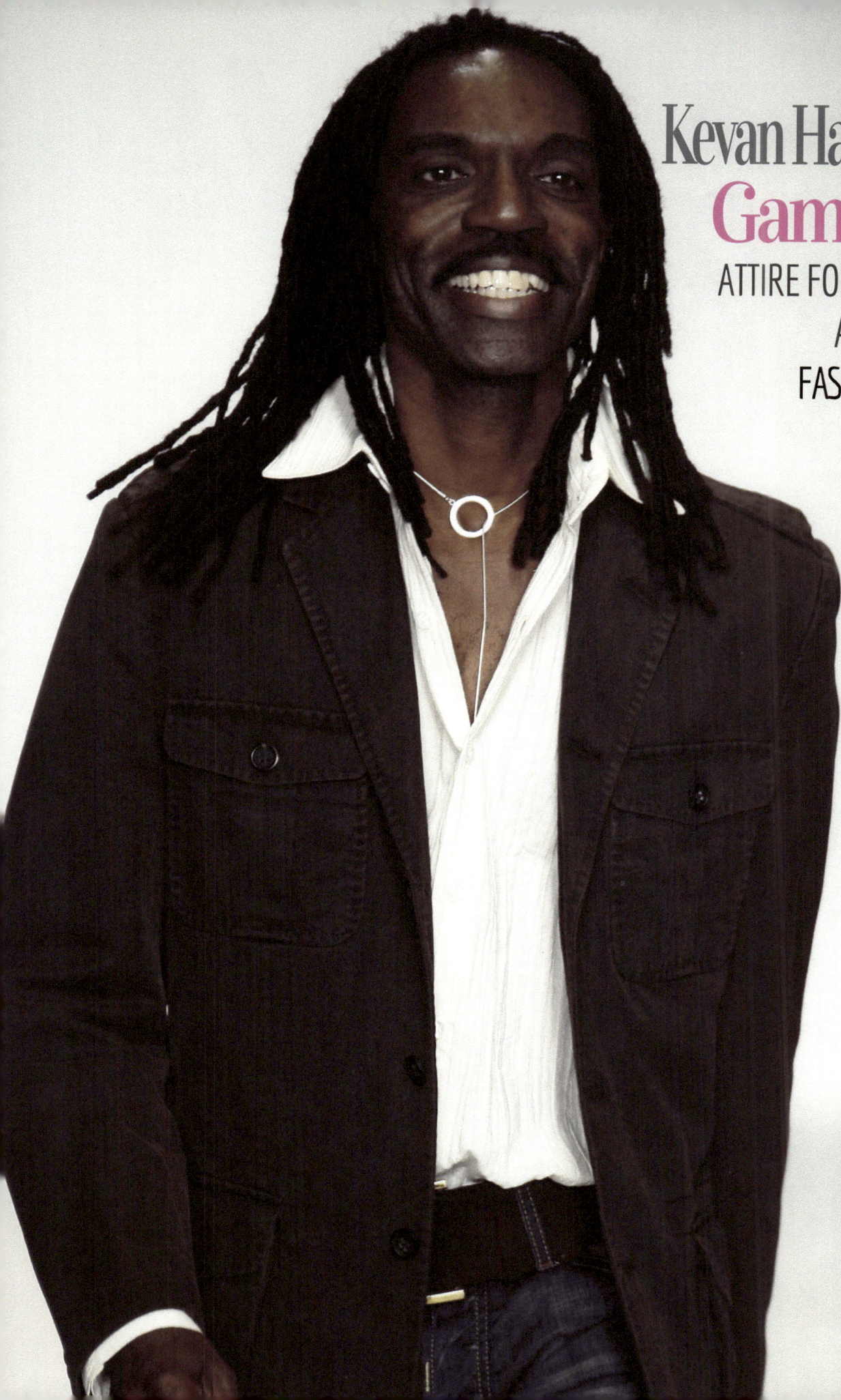

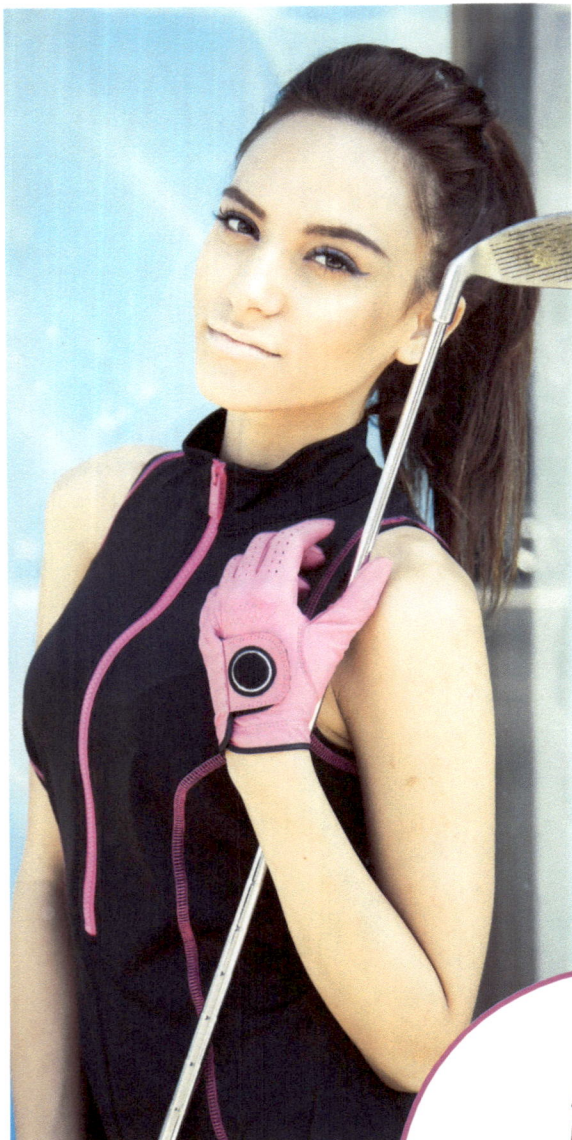

We use athletic fabrics that have all the necessary qualities like UV protection, moisture wicking, stretch . . .

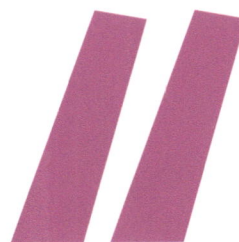

Designer Kevan Hall is known for his couture collection of exquisite gowns and formal wear. His designs have graced the pages of many fashion magazines, and have been worn by the Hollywood A-listers. I have known Kevan Hall for 11 years now and watched his designs on the runways, and I have always loved his work. So how exciting it was for me to learn that the couture fashion designer is now making clothes for the active fashionista—a fabulous golf line. This line is also conveniently wearable for the woman who wants to be comfortable, and look cute. She can toss those signature Kevan hall golf shoes and throw on some cute wedges. Introducing Kevan Hall Sport, our cover, and featured fashion interview.

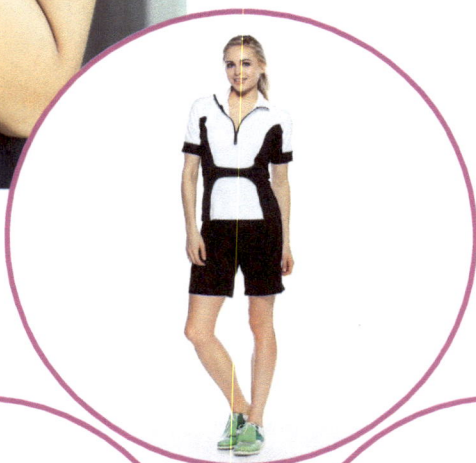

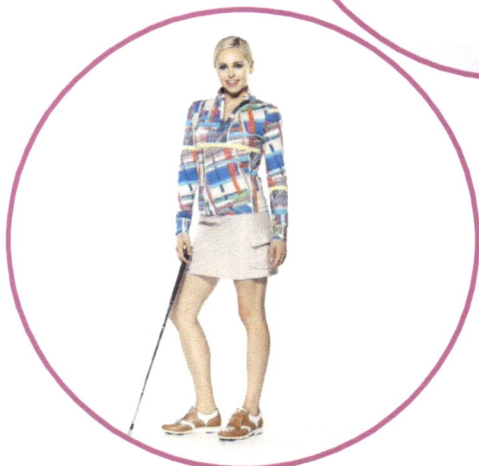

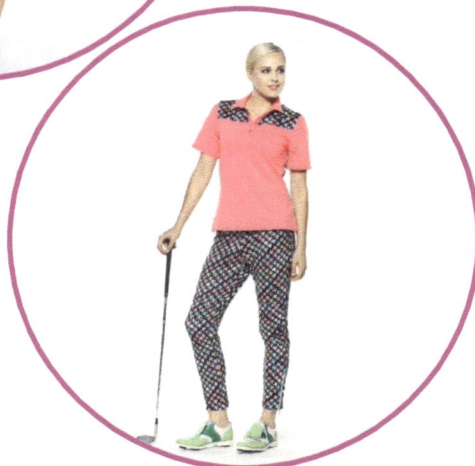

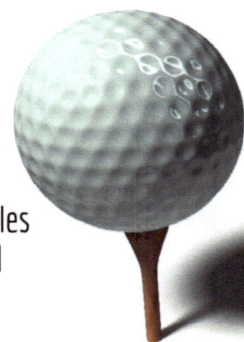

Questions by Kaylene Peoples
Responses by Kevan Hall

What a beautiful, colorful collection of golf-wear, as well as just "active wear." Why and how did you come up with this line?

Many of my best clients approached me to create a golf collection for women who want to look fashionable on the golf course. I decided to design a lifestyle collection for the golf course that could be easily worn to the fairway and then to lunch or other activities planned for the day looking fabulous!

What fabrics are you using?

Athletic fabrics that have all the necessary qualities like UV protection, moisture wicking, stretch, and that feel comfortable yet luxurious.

What was the creative inspiration for your designs?

My partner Beth is my inspiration. She has incredible style and taste in helping to create this line. She also is an avid golfer.

Any challenges developing an active wear line for women?

Golf is a different market for my brand, so the challenge is to reach out to new clientele and educate them about Kevan Hall Sport.

I understand you have an affiliation with the PGA? Tell me a little about that, and what events do you have coming up?

We just returned from the PGA show, and Kevan Hall Sport was a hit! Buyers lined up to see this new, exciting collection of women's golf wear that included our stylish dresses. They also loved our exclusive prints and vibrant colors. We're thrilled to be able to offer women a new fresh look on and off the golf course.

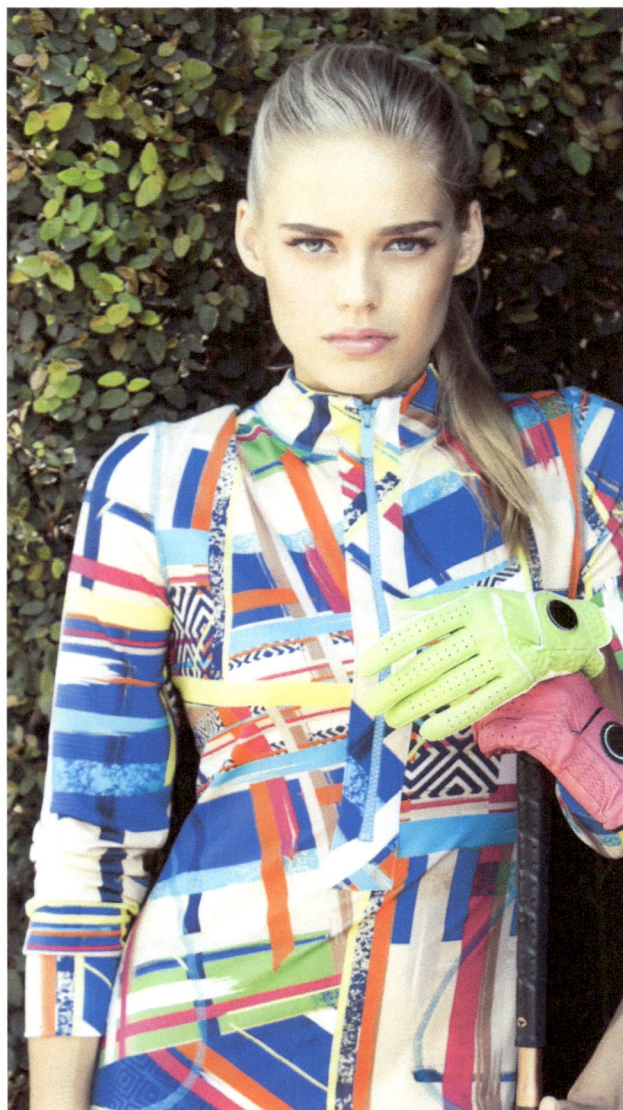

What are your price points? Tell me about any accessories that go along with Kevan Hall Sport.

Prices range from $90 - $190 retail, mostly sized XS, S, M, L, XL, with the exception of some of our bottoms, which are sized 2 - 14. We have accessories planned to debut this year, which include golf shoes, bags, and scarves.

Do you play golf, or any other sports?

I'm a golf enthusiast! I do love the outdoors and enjoy hiking.

Visit www.kevanhallsport.com to learn more.

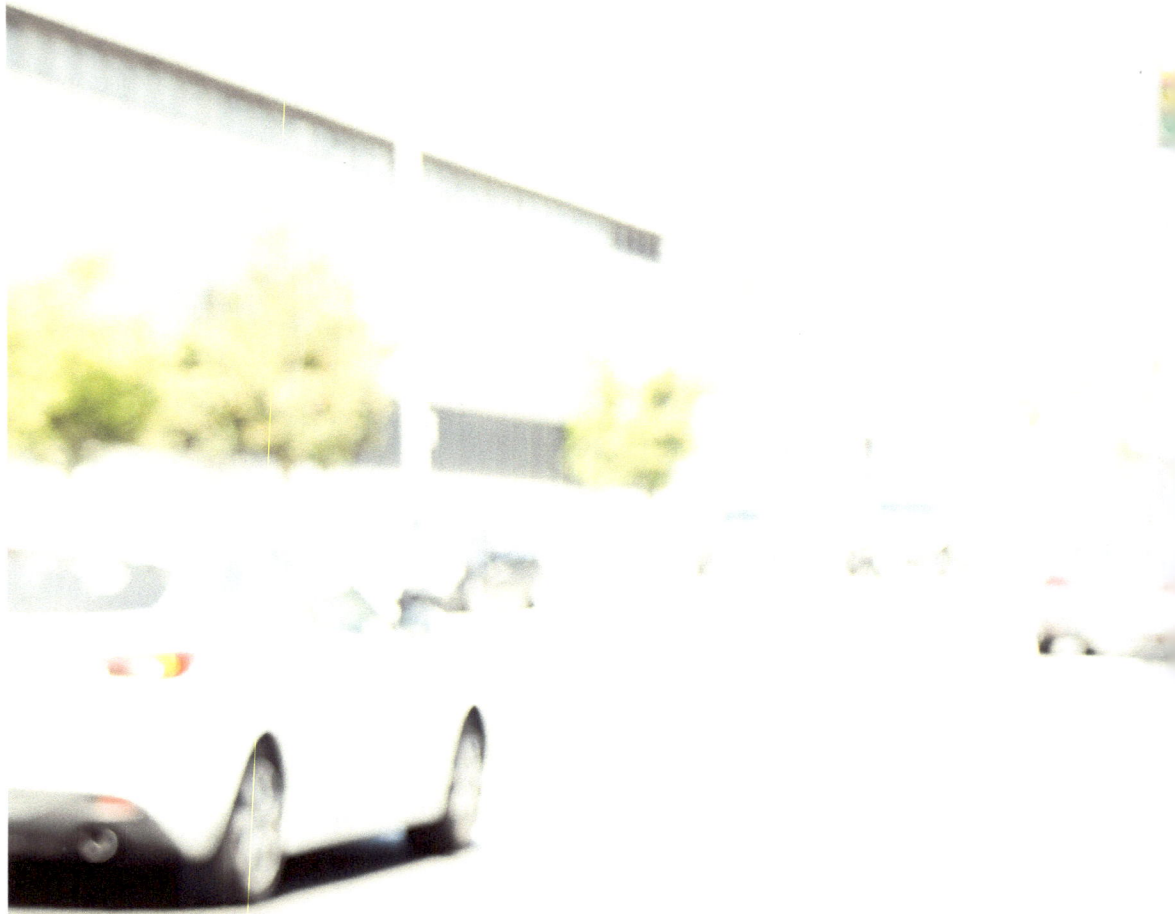

Kevan Hall
Sport

Photographed by Ash Gupta with Tuhan Bedi for 838 Media Group
Hair and Makeup by Inara Lopetaite Akin
Models: (L-R) Summer de Almeida, Cornelia Grimsmo
Clothes and Accessories by Kevan Hall
Written by Kaylene Peoples

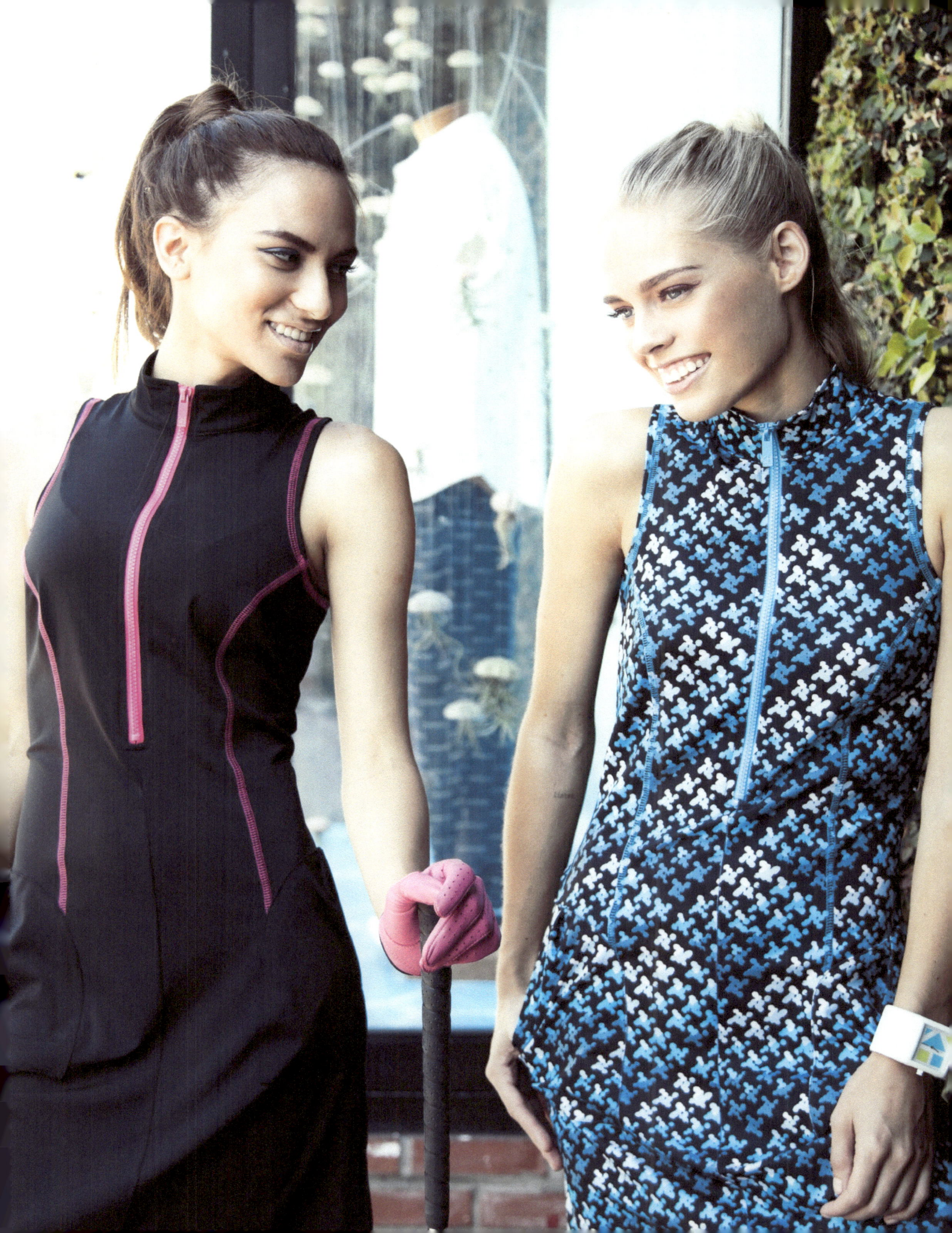

Walking and Golf

Walking is a great exercise when preparing to play golf. Remember, with 9 holes or 18 holes you will be giving your legs quite a workout. Give yourself the advantage and walk.

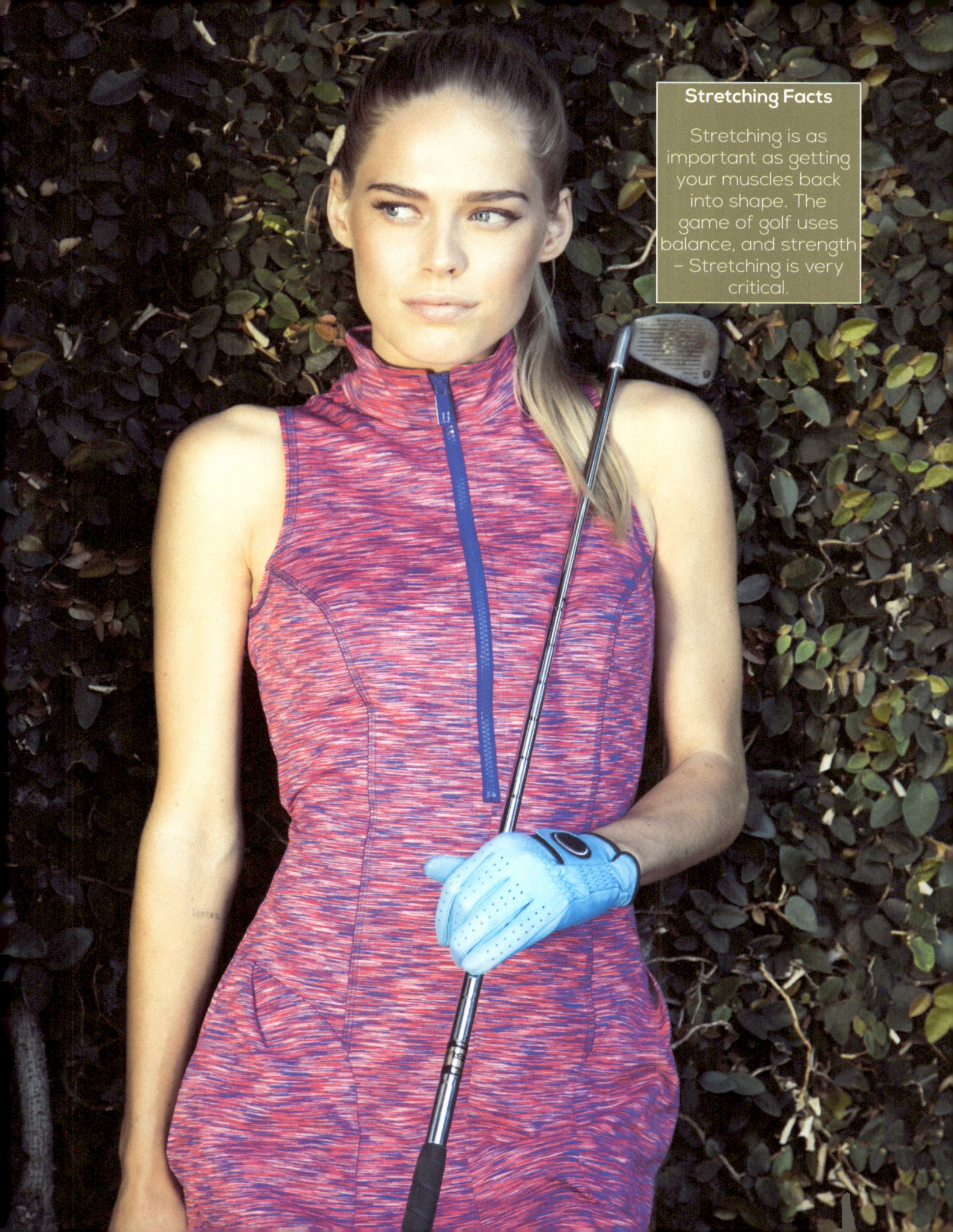

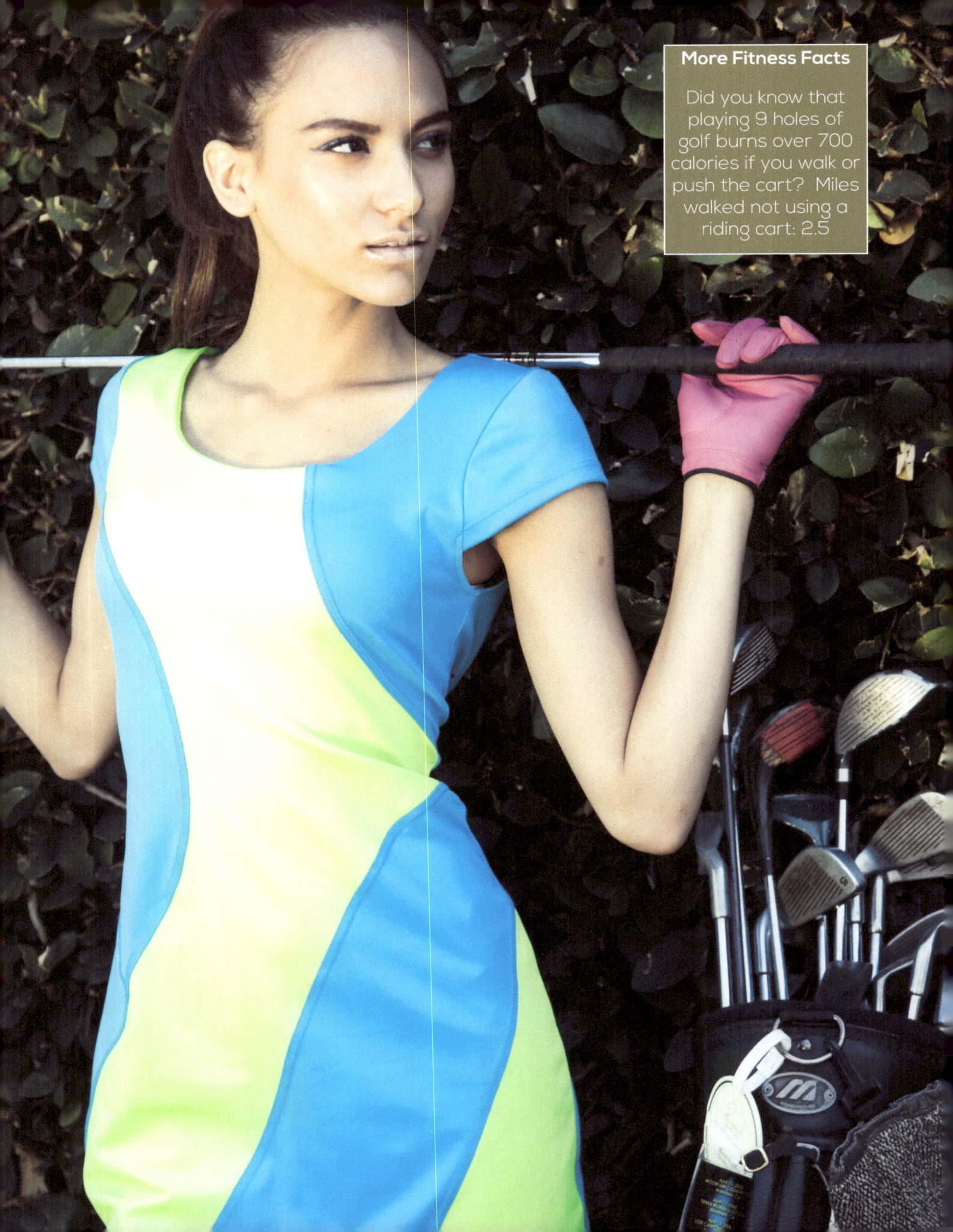

Sports That Teach Focus

Sports that teach you self-control and focus will be of great value to you on the golf course. Joining sports such as tennis, yoga, and martial arts are great complements to help you improve your golf game and lower your handicap.

(Model: Summer de Almeida)

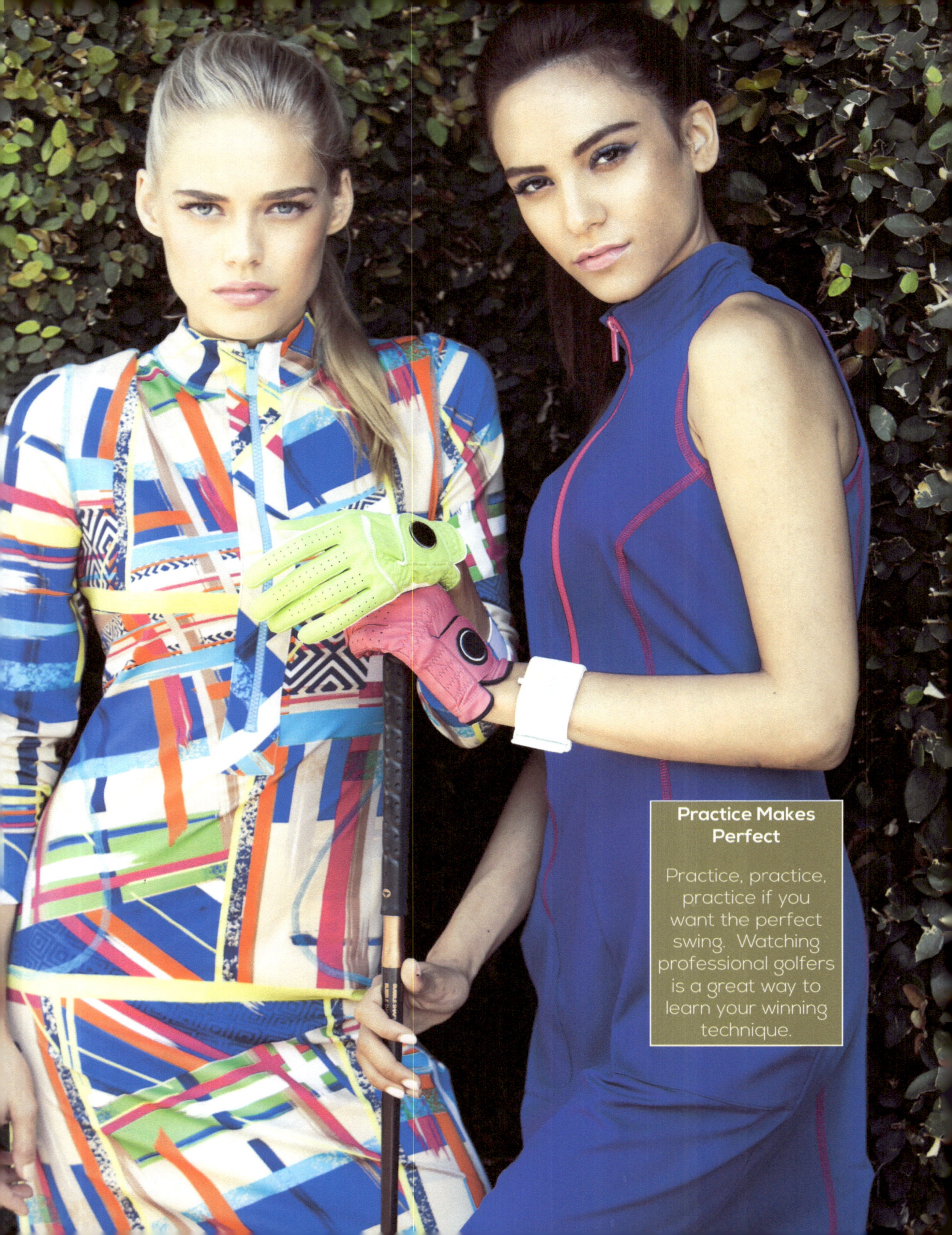

Practice Makes Perfect

Practice, practice, practice if you want the perfect swing. Watching professional golfers is a great way to learn your winning technique.

AGENDA

FITNESS COUTURE

COLLECTOR'S ISSUE 2016

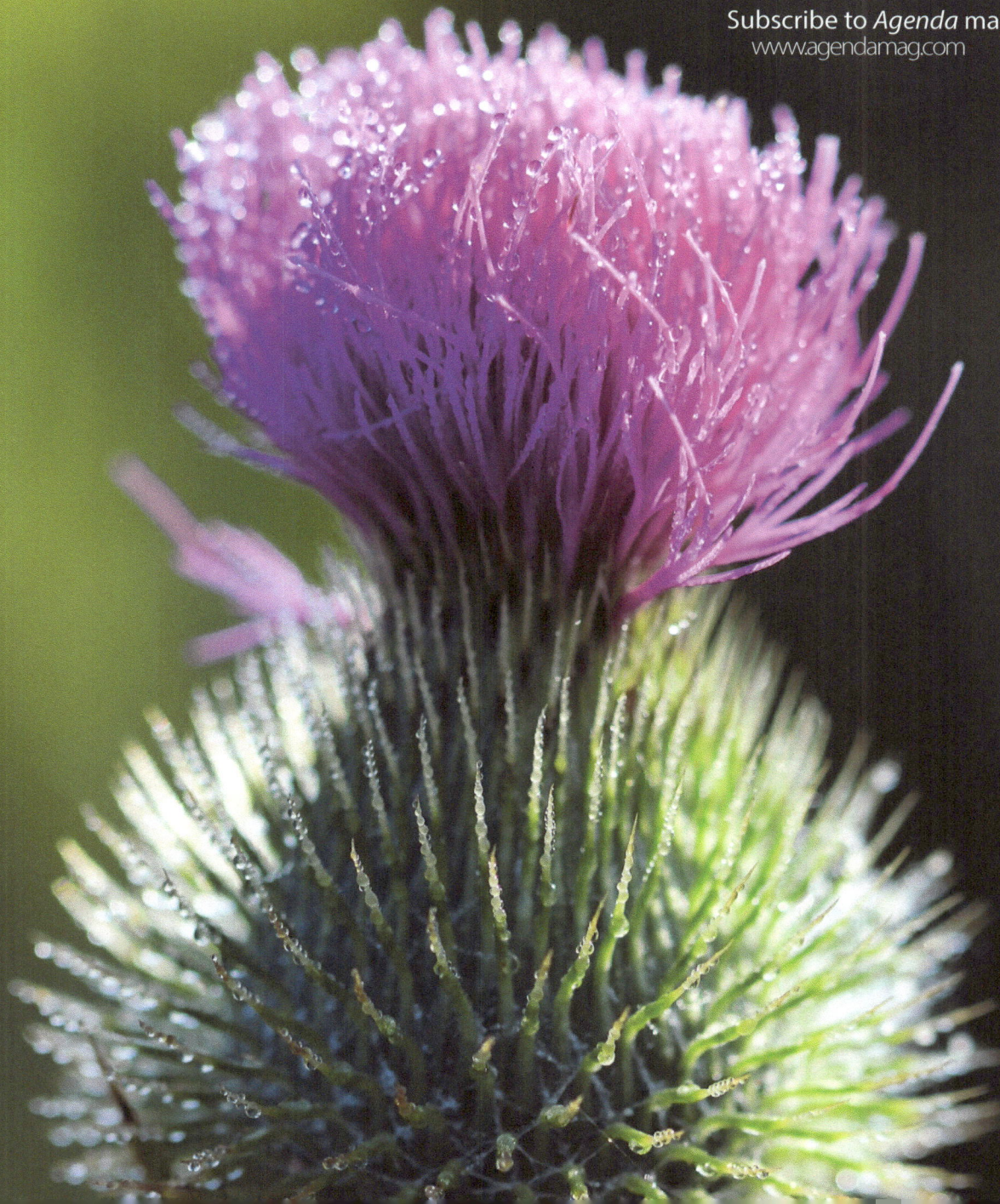

Welcome to what will become an elegant cooperative relationship between you and your figure, soon to be your even healthier slender figure. I would love to focus on empowering you on all levels of health awareness; so, first, let us give you a simple overview to starting the weight drop in this month and continuing thereafter for ultimate life goals. We will keep it light and simple in this article; but for those nutrition buffs who love to get down to the more technical details and numbers, head over to my "Health 101" article for an in-depth look at everything mentioned here. Now back to that pesky weight we want to cast off into some remote, dark bottomless cavern. The easiest way to get your bodies to lose those bothersome pounds is to make your body feel **safe**. Force change on the body, and it will comply; but it will always want to go back to what it knows. Negotiate and your hard work will stay! Now isn't that a radical concept, keeping your hard-earned results! What will they think of next?

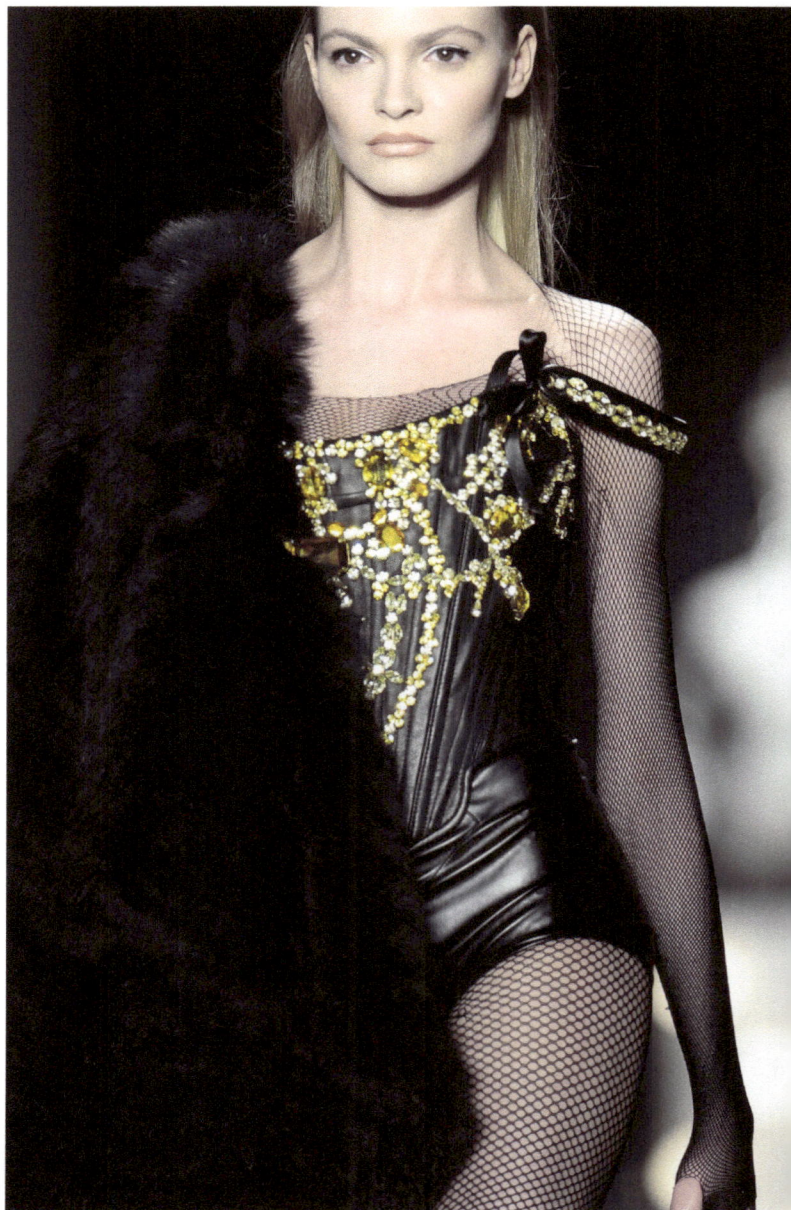

Drop a
Clothing Size

DROP A CLOTHING SIZE IN A MONTH
DO IT RIGHT AND IT STAYS!

BY ANTHONY HEREDIA

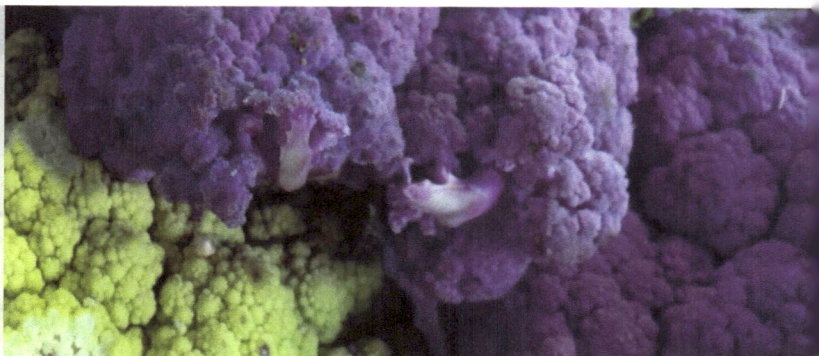

So what do you mean by safe? Why doesn't my body feel safe?

Your body holds onto body fat for what it believes to be good reasons and not just to give you a hard time, as you might think. Remember, your body doesn't care what you look like. It doesn't care what car you drive, what job you have, what designer name you're wearing; who you know, what style is in fashion, what color hair you have, or even whom you married. Your body has better things to worry about, like, hmmm, survival. You know, that whole pesky keeping you breathing thing? So you have to work with your body to get it to do what you want. Your body doesn't like change, such as weight loss, if it is forced. It hates unnecessary change because your body sees it as stress, its sole purpose is to become as efficient as possible by reaching homeostasis (consistent balance). This is why, when you find a quick way to drop some weight, it comes back with a vengeance; because your body is basically rebelling. It didn't know you were trying to look good for a wedding. It believed times were rough, so

hold tight until bountiful times come back when it can catch up and then prep for the next "hard times." The question then is, so how do I get my bratty body to do what I want without putting it in self-defense mode? You give it what it needs. Yup, that's it! The big secret is out now. Cars need gas, oil, coolant, steering fluid, etc.; and your body is a bit more complicated, so it needs a few things, too.

> Your body doesn't like change, such as weight loss, if it is forced . . . because your body sees change as stress.

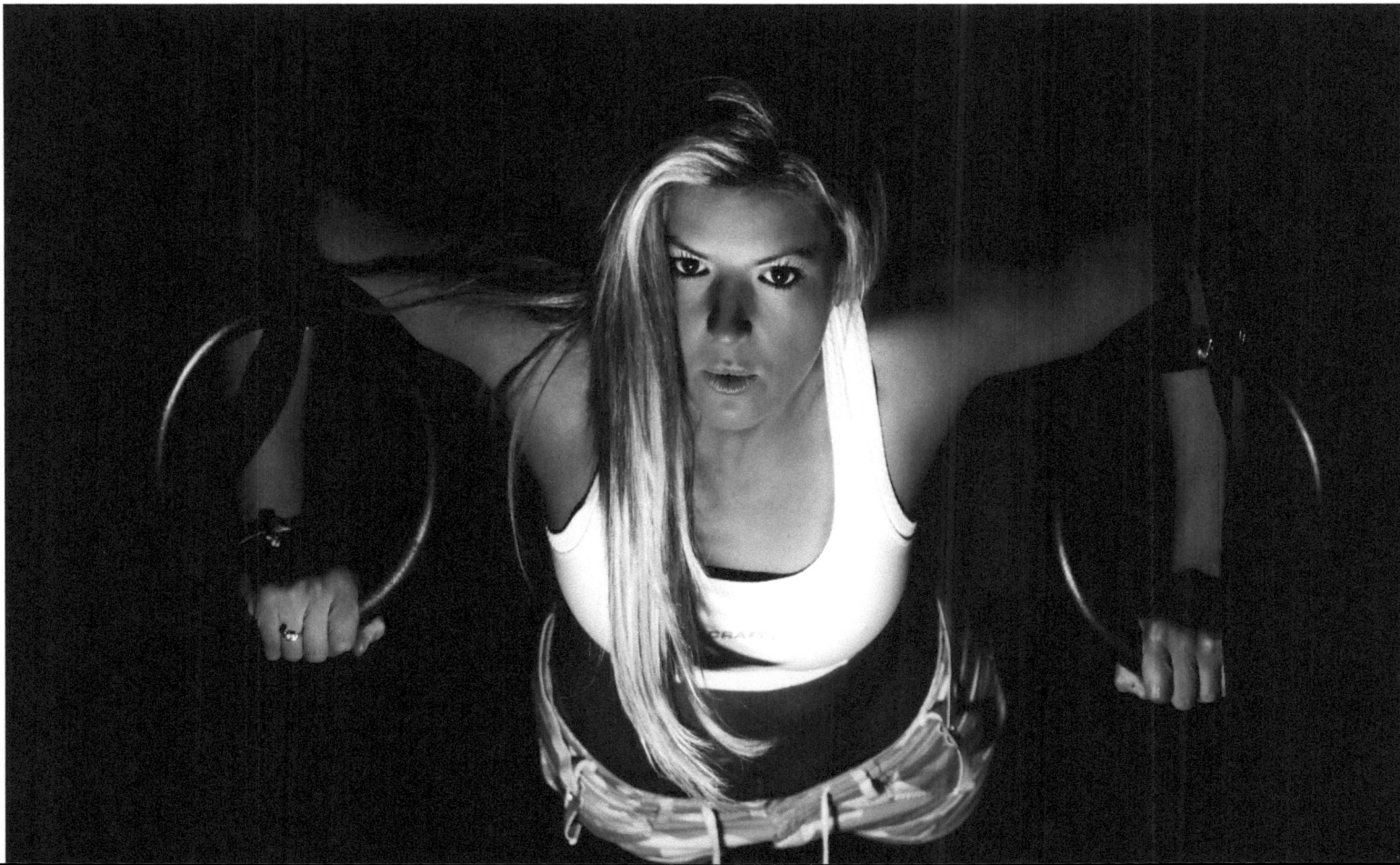

So get to it, you say. How do I make it feel safe to get what I want!?

The answer is simple. Eat! I know you have heard it before, but it's true, and here is how. The in-depth answer to why will be in our Health 101 article. First thing you should do is start by eating every 2-3 hours. Start with breakfast within 30-60 minutes of getting up in the morning to kick start your metabolism. What this will do is train your body not to hold onto the weight because there is a constant supply of food. Thus, it has no reason to hold onto excess. You basically tell your body through balanced consistency that times are good, so you give it permission to lean out. If you eat a little something every 2-3 hours, then there is a steady stream of nourishment coming into your body, and it has no strong reason to hold onto its storage, your body fat.

We gain fat for countless reasons, but the main ones are taking in more than we use up and starving the body, combined with nutritional inconstancy, creating a defensive response. You can find out how much you should eat at www.caloriecontrol.org/calcalcs.html. Eating every 2-3 hours is easy, so no excuses. It's as easy as: cereal with milk and a 2-3 egg white omelet for breakfast; fruit and 7 almonds as a next snack; a sandwich or hearty salad with meat midday; fresh baby carrots and celery sticks, cherry tomatoes, or tons of others, as a next snack; a nice 3-part dinner with half the plate being a favorite veggie, one part 3-4 oz. of lean meat, a cup of rice, beans, pasta, or any other starch of your choice; and finally, some cottage cheese with a little fruit as a night snack. And you've got a full, on-track day. More ideas for menus to come!

First, start eating 5-6 smaller daily healthier meals every 2-3 hours as foundation, which makes a drastic impact on weight loss or even just feeling good (specifics on calories in Health 101 article). Step two is to start drinking water. A study done by the Journal of Clinical Endocrinology and Metabolism discovered how just 17 oz. of water increases metabolic rate by 30% in healthy adults. On the other hand, even mild dehydration proved to reduce metabolism by up to 3%. Step three is exercise, which can actually be enjoyable, I promise. The trick to keeping at your fitness regimen is realizing the fact that the best kind of exercise is the kind that keeps you coming back for more! You don't have to be stuck in a gym staring at the wall and being gawked at to get a good workout, unless you love that (then more power to you).

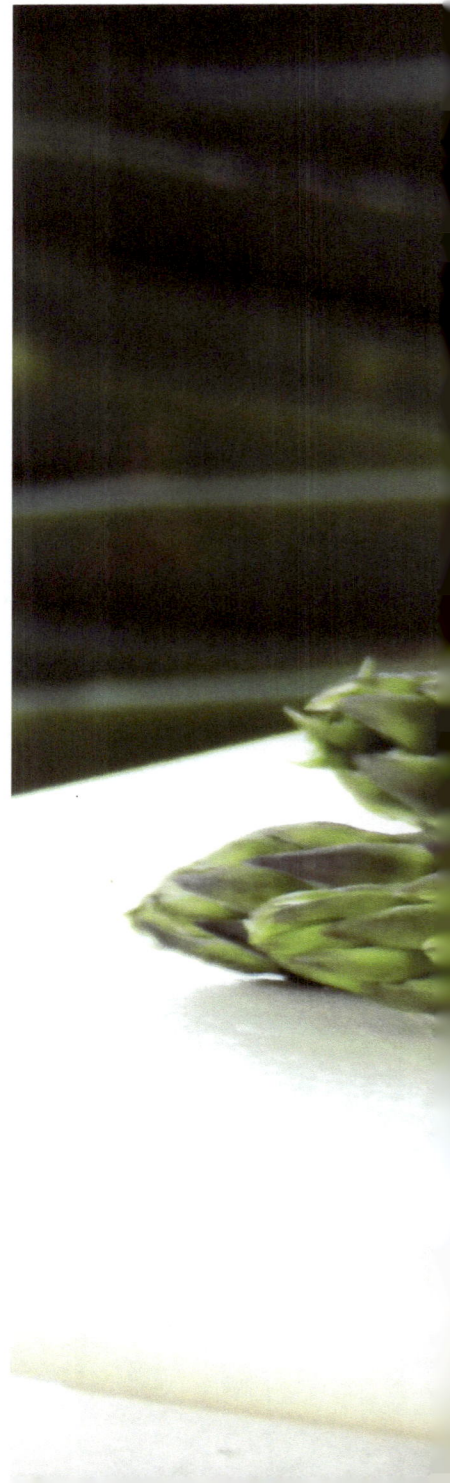

We gain weight for countless reasons, but the main one is taking in more than we use up.

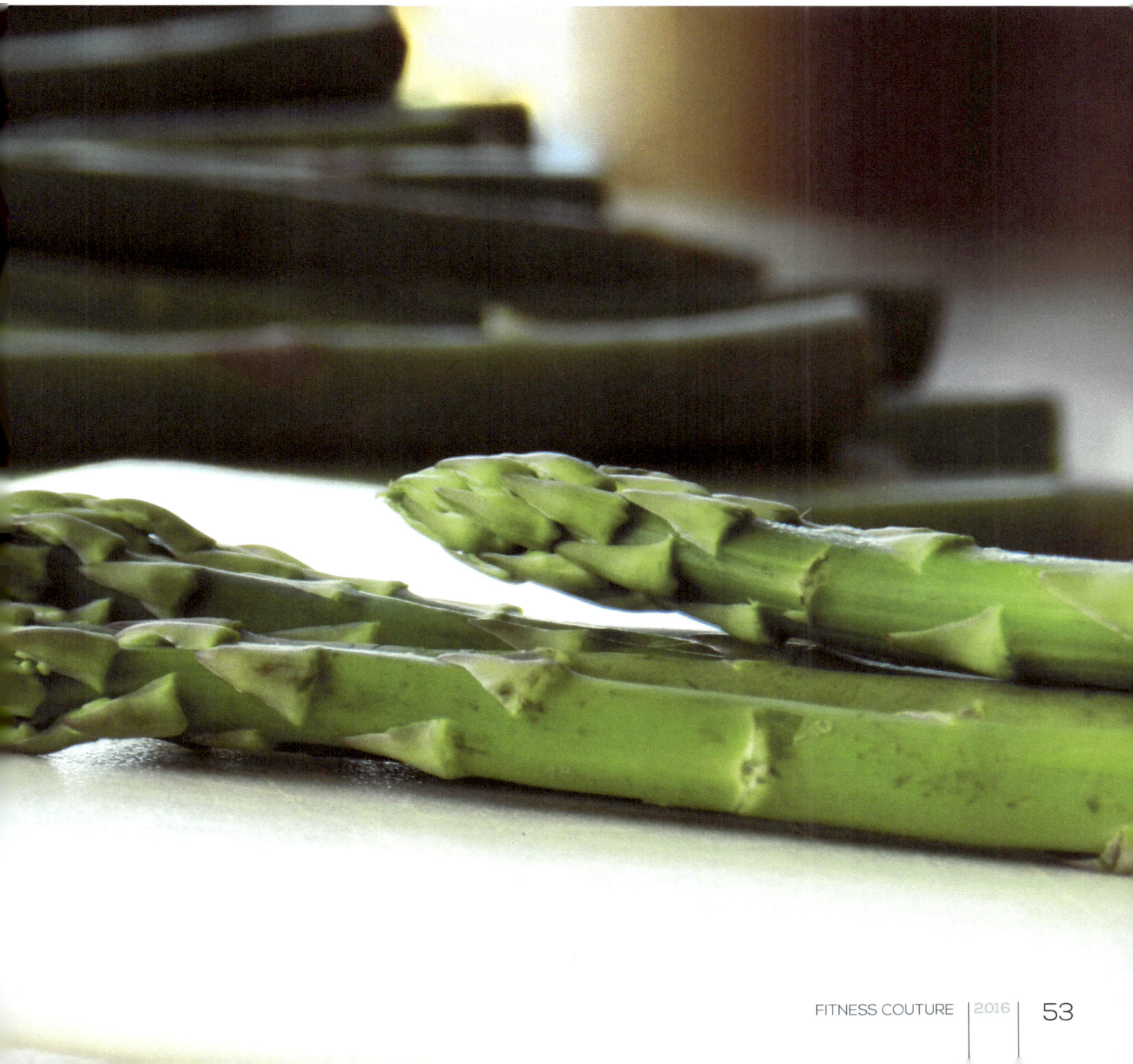

Your body needs the building and recovery time, or your engine will not be at its full potential.

Exercise in anything that gets you moving; think outside the box and expand your horizons. You can swim, bike, jog; take a hike, take a boot camp; power walk with a friend; fly (well maybe not); roller blade, take up a martial arts, play with your kids, play a sport; or my favorite, dance the night away with a feverish step and a fire in your eye. Dance at home for goodness sake! The idea is move! If you have kids, use them as weights. No, seriously though, they are weight that you can lift and (safely) toss to play with and work out! Drag your best friend to take dancing lessons, which burn immense calories. There is no right or wrong way to start, as the hardest part to exercise is getting started and creating the habit. Even an Olympian after not working for a length of time is going to drag himself/herself back into it. But once one starts and finds his/her rhythm, it becomes dramatically easier. Aim to do something that involves resistance at least twice a week and hit the workout of your choice at least 3-5 times for the best results starting off. Final step is to sleep. Dr. Michael Breus, clinical director of sleep division for Arrowhead Health in Glendale, Arizona, and author of *Beauty Sleep: Look Younger, Lose Weight*, explains that it's not so much that you will gain weight from not sleeping, but the metabolism will significantly slow down for the day's operations after a night lacking proper sleep.

Aim for your 6-8 hours, and if you simply can't sleep, then make sure to have a catch up day and don't feel bad for sleeping in. Your body collects sleep debt; it adds up, and your body keeps count like an angry bookie. Pay your debt off to get your fat burning engine at its max. Remember that your body is a fine Ferrari motor. It needs nutrients, water, fitness, and rest to be at its best, or how can you expect it to look and feel the way you dream of?

These steps will shed a clothing size off you in about a month, for sure. Now, if this was too simple and you want even more results in less time, details can be found in Health 101 article, but just this alone will get you shedding weight.

So how do I drop that dress size?

Step one is eat, please. Aim for every 2-3 hours; and if you're afraid of heavy calories, then eat 3 square meals a day and graze on fresh veggies all day long. That will get your body feeling safe with a steady source of food so that it will release that weight. Step two, drink water. Aim for your average 4 water bottles of 16 oz. to keep your metabolism stable, and even more if you are active. Replenish what you use. Third is fitness at least 3 times a week in one way or another, as long as you get moving and sweating and go back for more. Remember to push hard enough to feel challenged, or else you won't get enough bang for your sweaty buck. Lastly, sleep your 6-8 hours, and pay your sleep debt if you cannot get those hours in during busy times. Your body needs the building and recovery time, or your engine will not be at its full potential. Be kind to yourself.

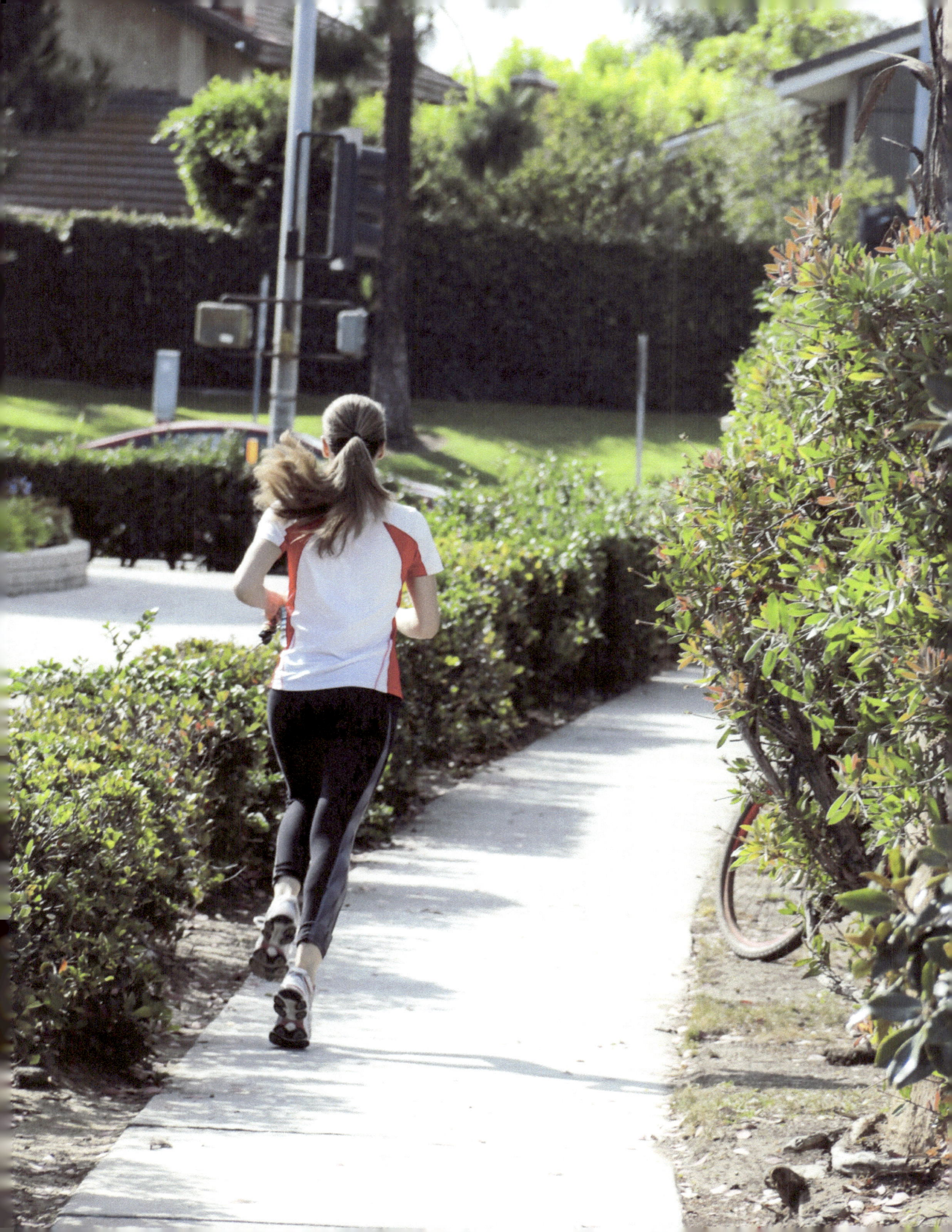

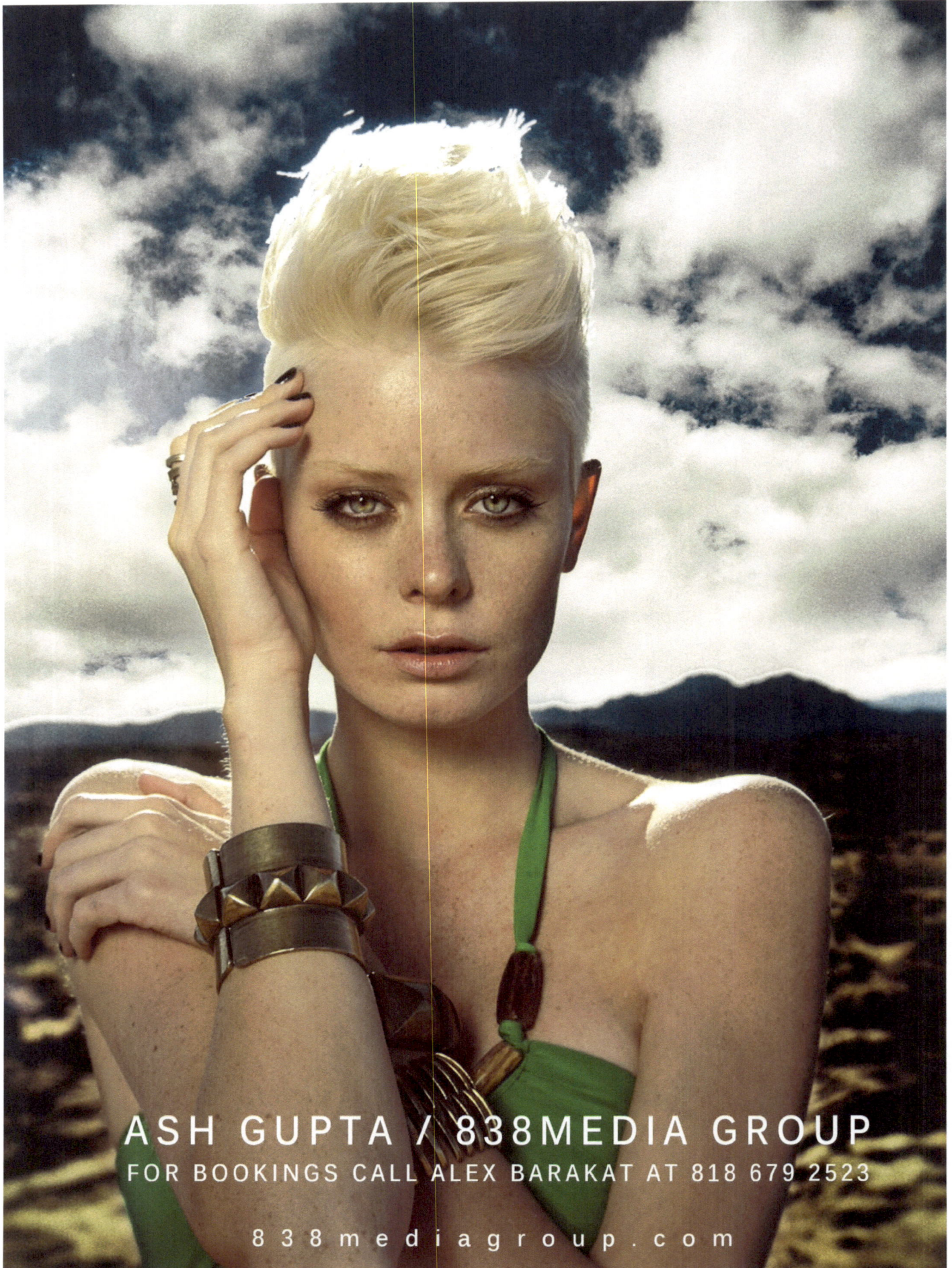

ASH GUPTA / 838MEDIA GROUP
FOR BOOKINGS CALL ALEX BARAKAT AT 818 679 2523

838mediagroup.com

Vitamin D

Naturally Enhances Mood

Regular sunlight exposure can naturally increase the serotonin levels in your body, making you more active and alert

Photographer/Stylist: Glenn Gordon
Model: Brad Bastian
Agency - AGordon Models - Manila
Written by Kaylene Peoples

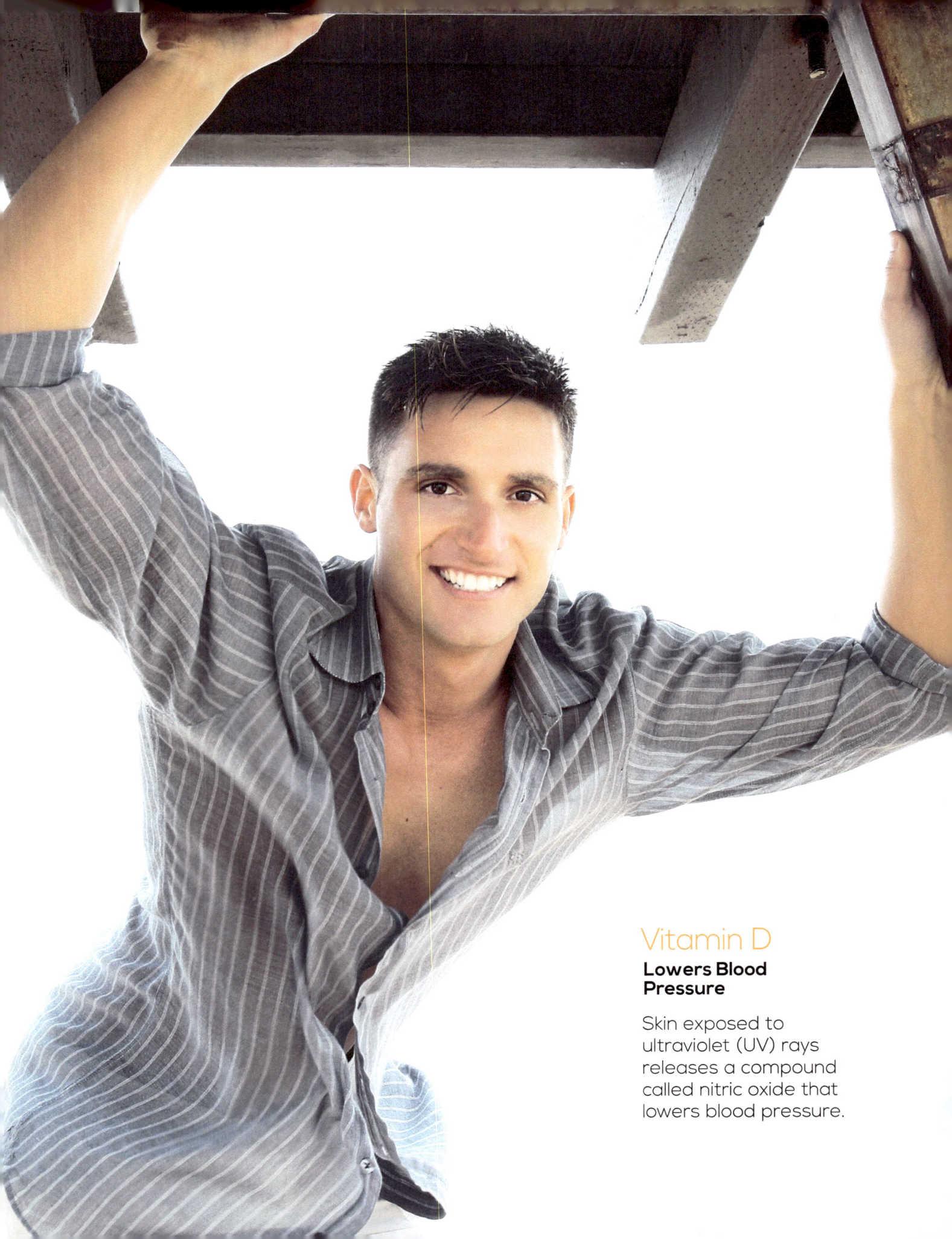

Vitamin D

Lowers Blood Pressure

Skin exposed to ultraviolet (UV) rays releases a compound called nitric oxide that lowers blood pressure.

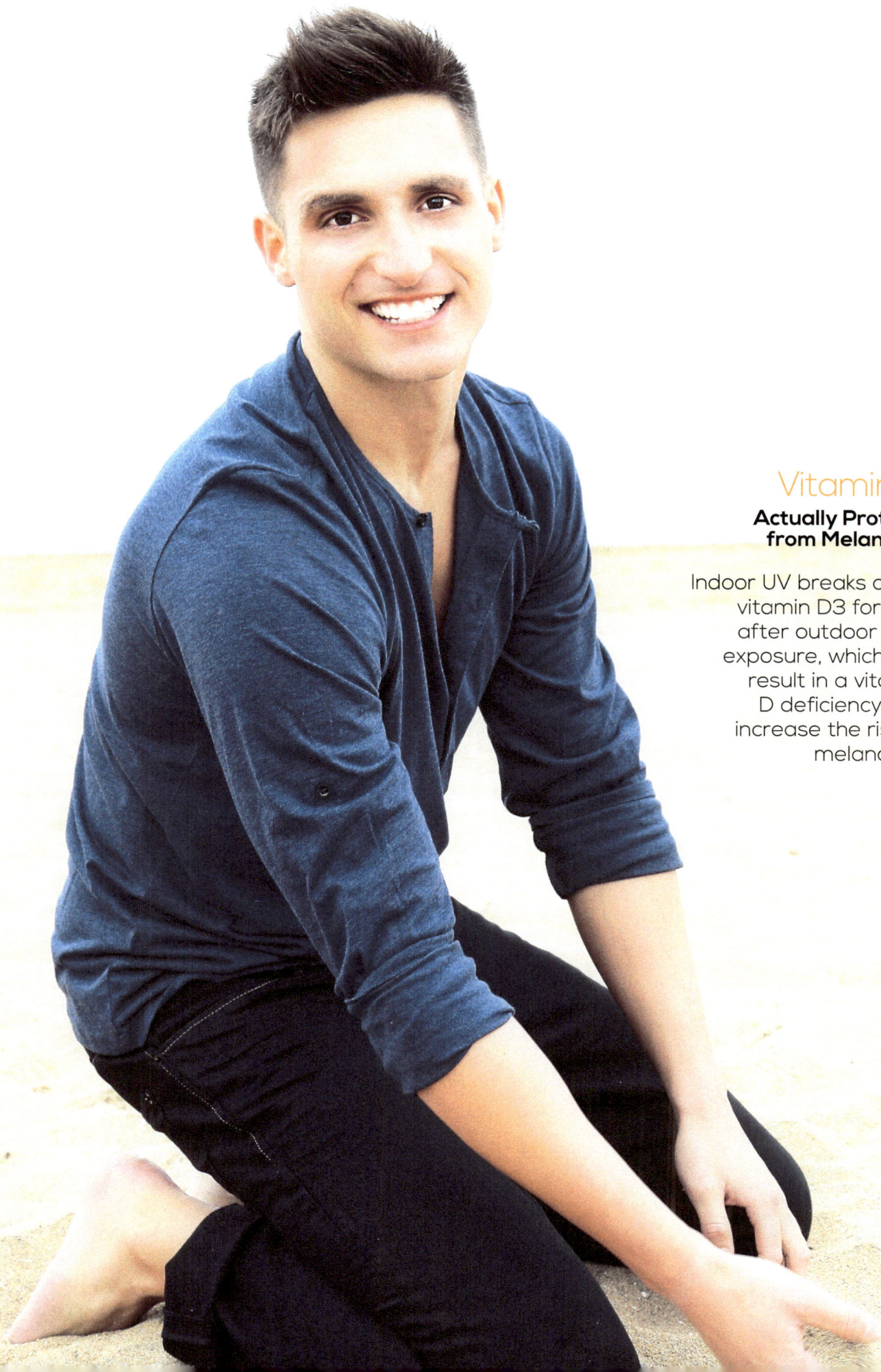

Vitamin D
Actually Protects from Melanoma

Indoor UV breaks down vitamin D3 formed after outdoor UVB exposure, which can result in a vitamin D deficiency and increase the risk of melanoma.

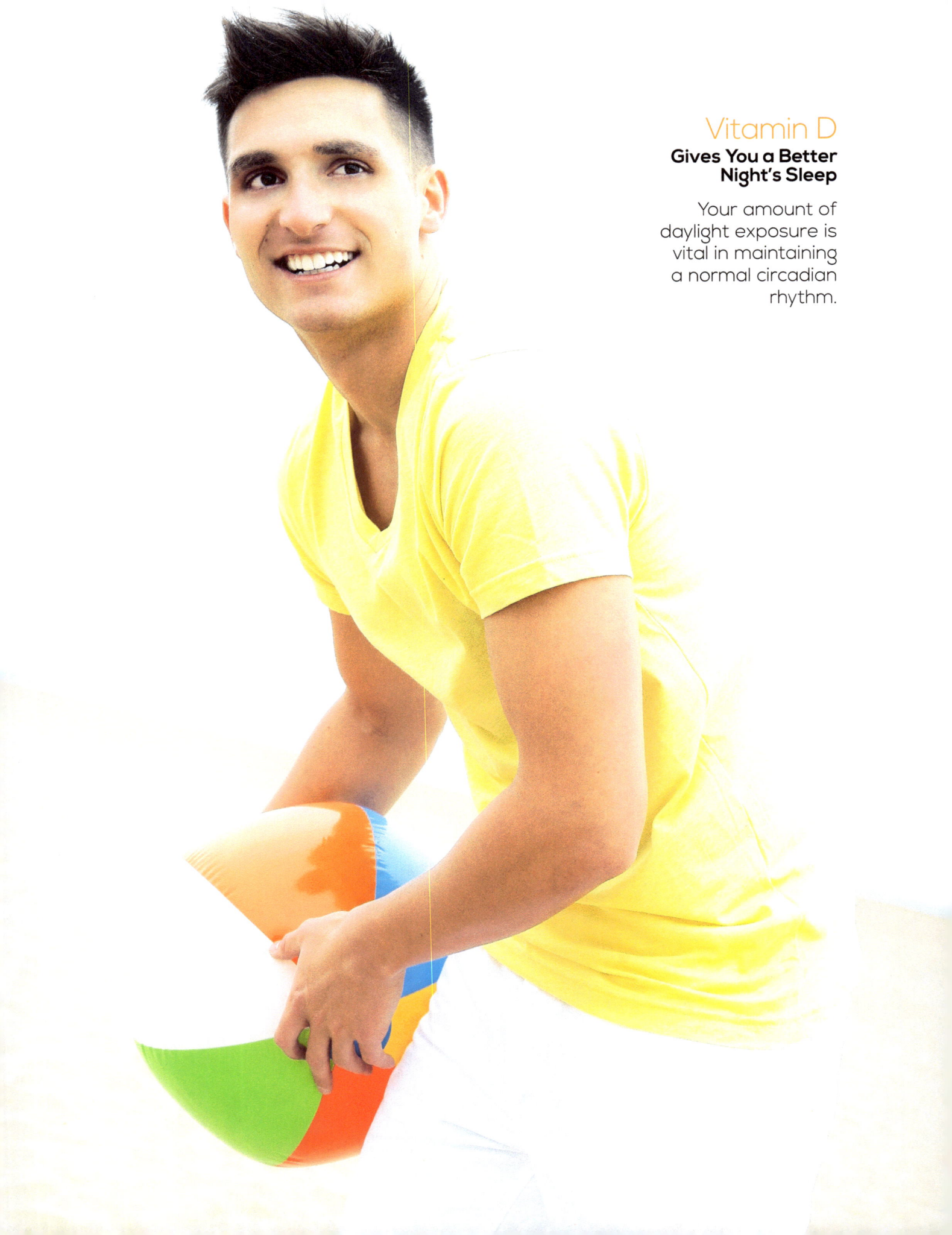

Vitamin D

Gives You a Better Night's Sleep

Your amount of daylight exposure is vital in maintaining a normal circadian rhythm.

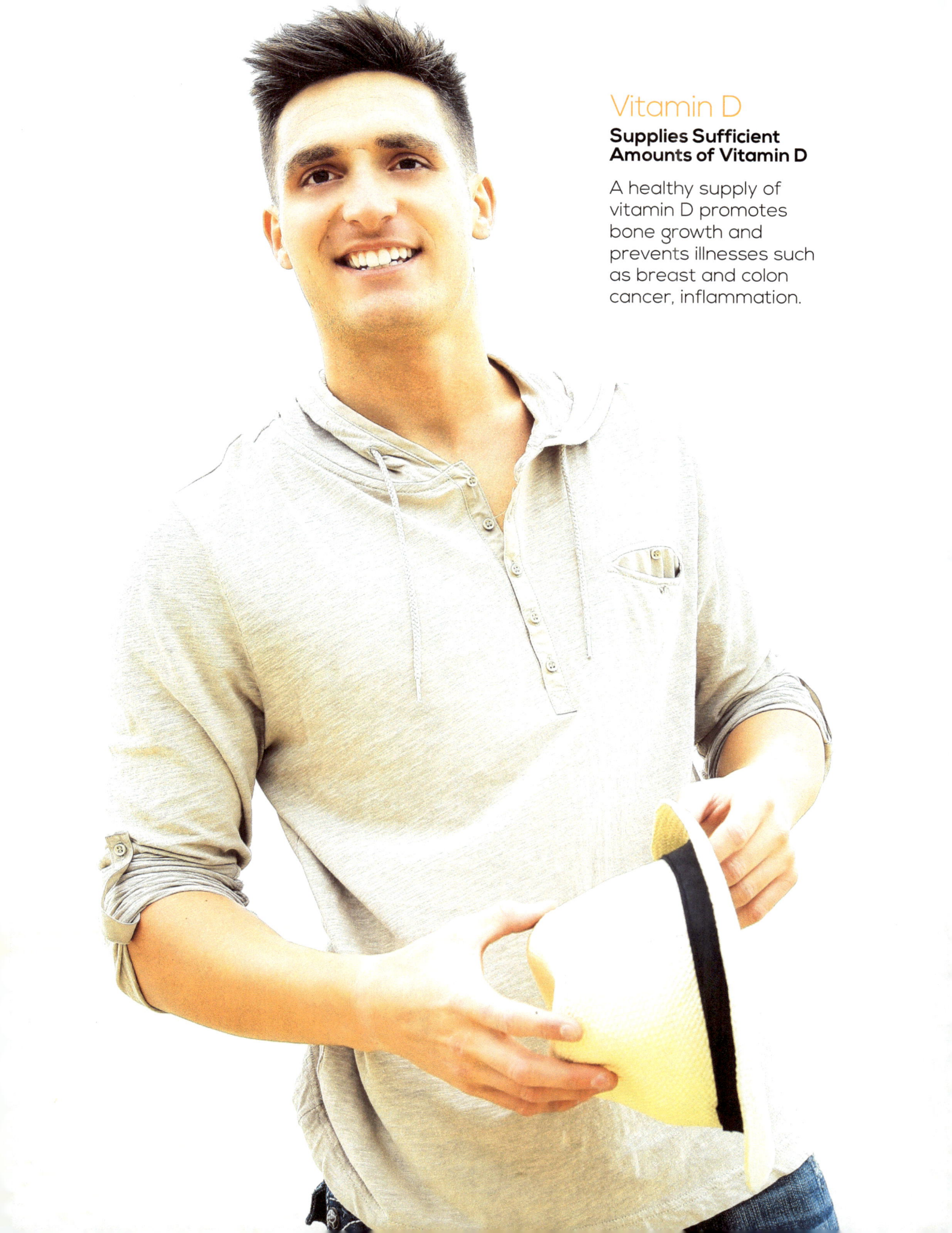

Vitamin D

Supplies Sufficient Amounts of Vitamin D

A healthy supply of vitamin D promotes bone growth and prevents illnesses such as breast and colon cancer, inflammation.

Fitness
Couture

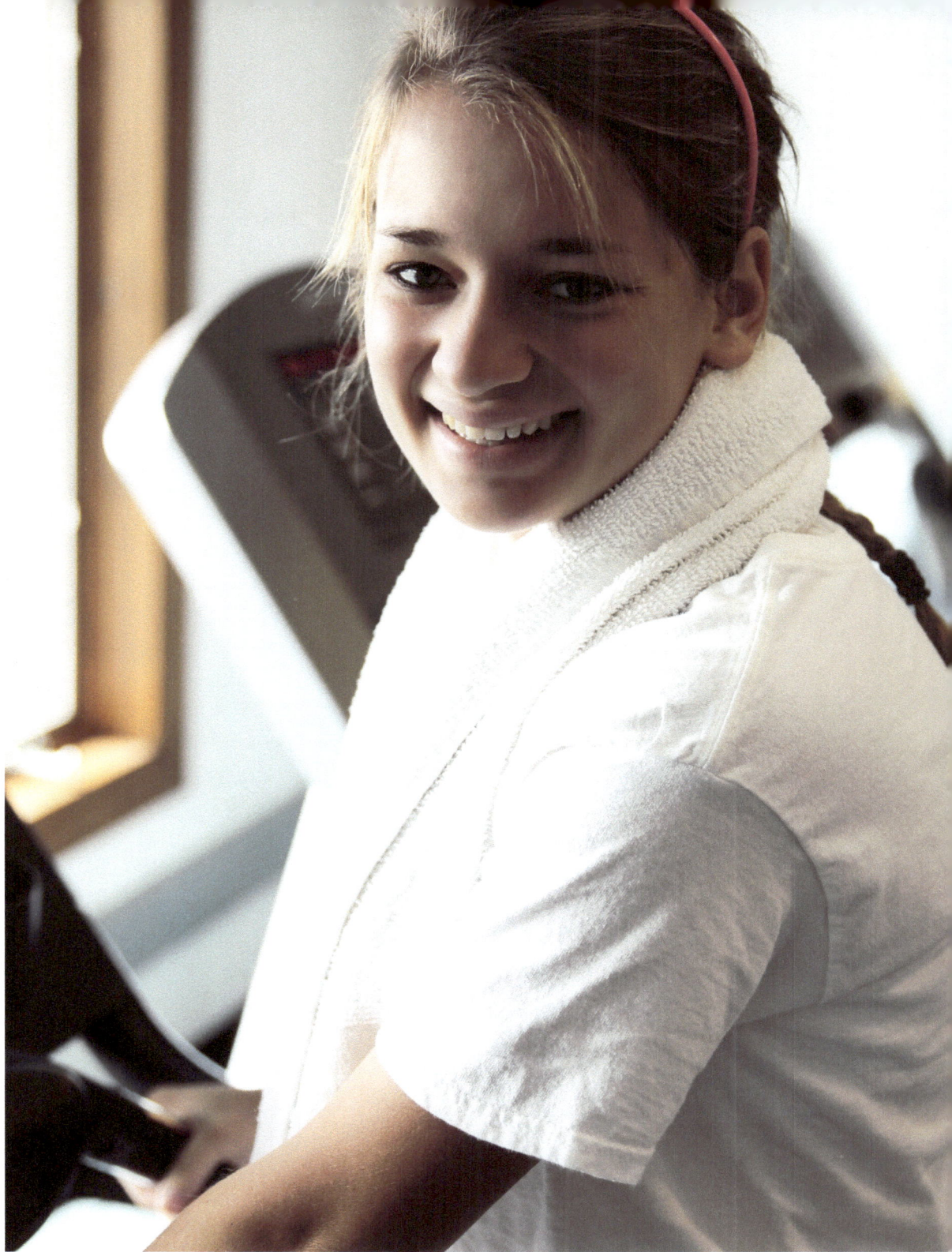

SOMETIMES WE JUST NEED A LITTLE
REMINDER OF WHAT HELPS US
SUCCEED. "FITNESS TIPS ANYONE?"

BY ANTHONY HEREDIA

FITNESS

Perfect Amount of Weight to Grow Muscle – To increase size/ shape of muscles you must have enough resistance to create micro tears, smart soreness. The tiny muscle fibers tear and then heal into stronger, larger muscle; hence the saying "no pain, no gain," but you definitely don't need to hurt yourself. If you don't feel soreness, then you simply strengthened the muscle for endurance and performance, but not really pushing the changing of its shape to its potential. The basic idea is to find a comfortable amount of resistance/weight for whatever it may be you are attempting, and then take it up by 10-30% above comfortable. Make sure the weight is challenging enough that you can only squeeze out about 10-12 repetitions. Once this weight gets to easily reaching those 12 reps, you simply increase again and watch the results roll in.

Sleep or Lose It – Who has time to sleep these days? Well, if you are concerned about your weight, fitness levels, or all-around health, then you had better find the time. During sleep the body repairs torn muscle for those trying to grow a larger body. It modifies and adjusts metabolism for increasing weight loss and does a lot of the neurological and nerve system repairs. You can be eating perfectly and working out daily; but without adequate sleep to recover from the day's toll, Olympians and soccer moms alike suffer dramatic compromises to their results. Low sleep is a top reason most of us gain weight regardless of how amazing we are during the day. Get some sleep.

Eat MORE – Now I know that sounds crazy; but when you cut your calories too low with too few meals, you train yourself not to favor a lean body but to prepare for rough times and store calories. You have heard it a thousand times before, but it's true: Eat three meals a day and two snacks for best results. The idea is to feed your body just enough of what it needs for the demands you put on it. As the body gets its needs met, it has no reason to hold onto excess fat if there is a steady stream of healthy calories coming in; so your fitness will reap much greater results. Keep in mind you gain weight only when you take in more calories than you put out. Therefore, you are safe to eat more and feed your metabolism as long as you don't overdo it. If you need more details, find yourself a calorie calculator through Google and see what your body needs in a day.

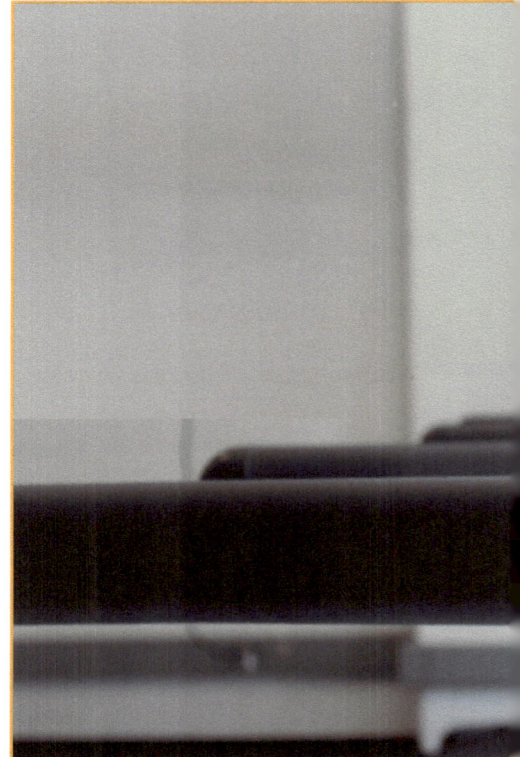

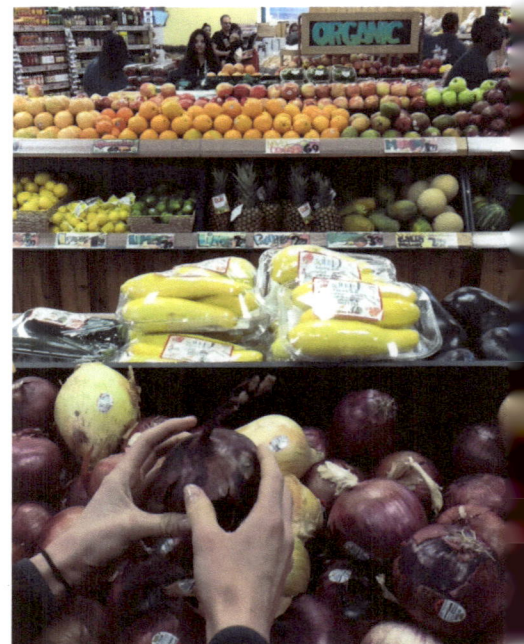

TIPS

Staying on Track with Nutrition – No matter who you are or what resources you do or don't have, you will always run into trouble staying on any form of diet. Forget the word "diet" and replace it with "balance journey." Now that may sound a bit cheesy, but it's true. Perfection is an illusion, and you will always slip on any program; so don't fear failure, but learn to plan ahead for bumps in the road to keep balance. We make our worst nutrition choices when we have fewer options. Prepare personally made trail mix, nut mixtures, granola snack bars, and whatever else you know is portable and doesn't melt easily. Place these items in all your high traffic areas. I cannot tell you how many times my stash of bars in my car have saved me on long days from pulling into a drive-through. Buy dried fruit or low sodium dried meat—or make your own—and keep them available in pre-portioned bags at work, in your car, and everywhere else you know you are weak. Planning ahead is trial and error, so just take it slow and forgive yourself when you trip; it's not about perfection but balance.

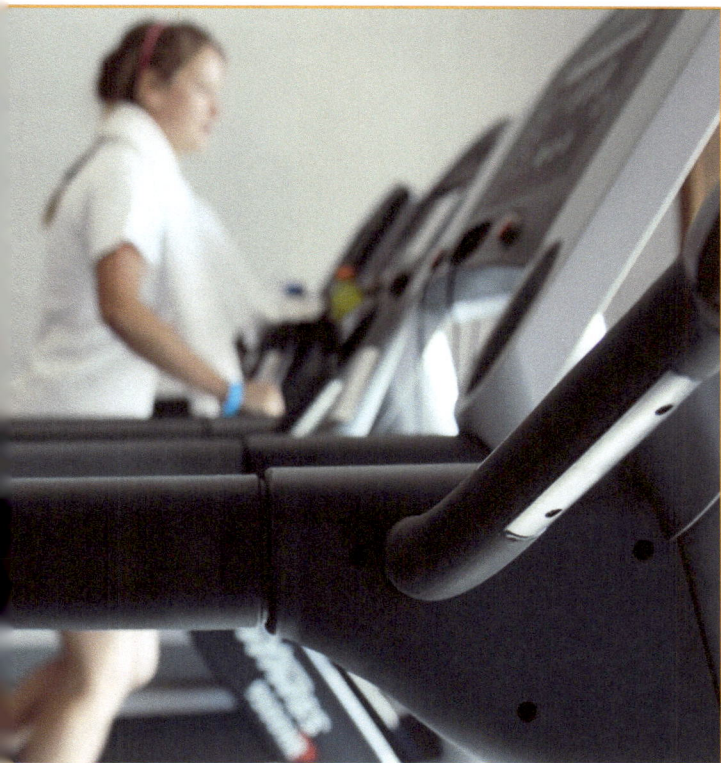

Use the Right Muscles – The most common mistake found in anyone's fitness regimen is his/her form, that is, bad form, which leads to wasted gym time and pain. Your body recruits stronger muscles when the weaker ones cannot do what you are asking them to do. This happens most commonly when you use too much weight, and the muscles you are trying to focus on can't handle it. Drop the resistance down until you only feel the exact muscle you are trying to use, and look in a mirror as you do this to make sure you aren't using any muscles you shouldn't. If you are curling weights in your hands, there is no reason your shoulders should be lifting up and squeezing toward your neck unless you're looking for trouble. Taking it slower with good form will get you results twice as fast without the hassle of injury.

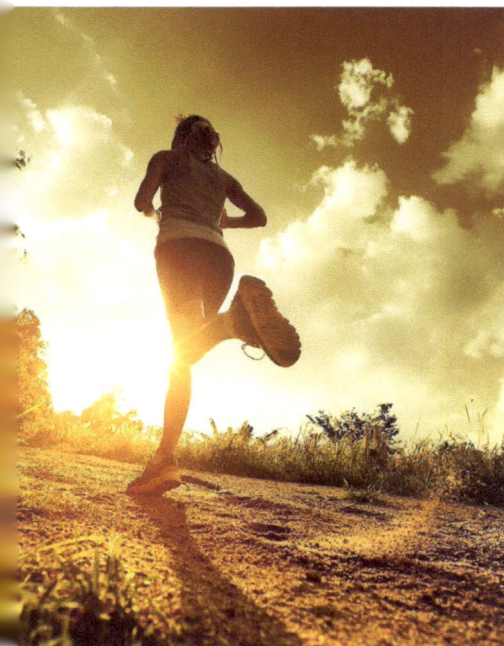

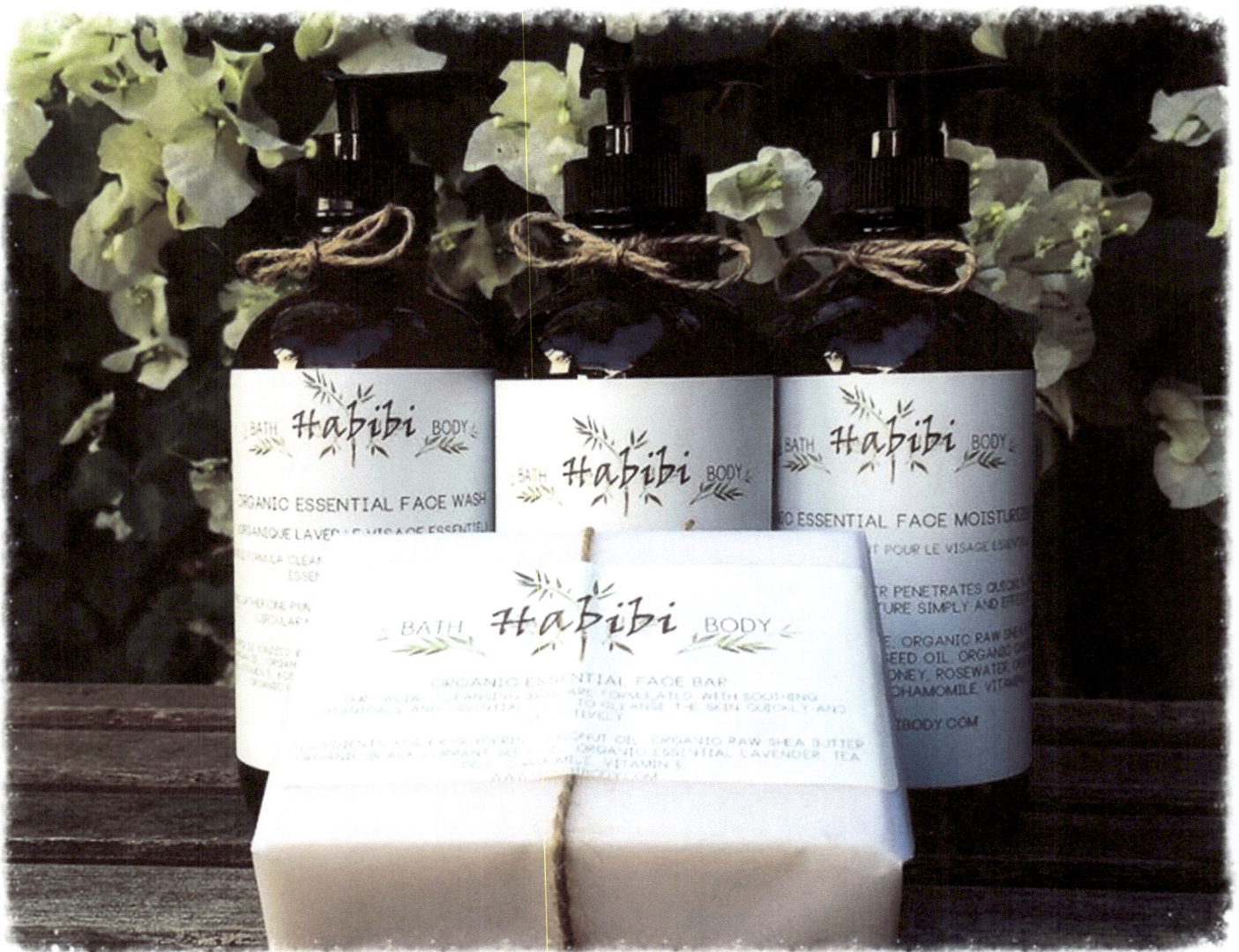

Habibi is the creation of indulgent body care... fusing pure organic ingredients with natural fragrance to create a collection of bath and body products. Organic shea butter, healing nut oils, and soothing botanicals are included in every Habibi product.

These recipies have been passed down through generations of my family, from grandmother, to mother, to me. Once classified as a series of "home remedies," those teachings have been expanded … mixing and matching pure ingredients to soothe the skin and promote healing. These methods can be described as "east meets west"; Habibi combines the basic teachings of ayurvedic healing with an expanded knowledge of essential oils, herbs, botanicals, nut butters and oils.

We present Habibi to you in the spirit of its creation with the hopes that you look and feel your very best from the first application to the last!

Available at www.habibibody.com

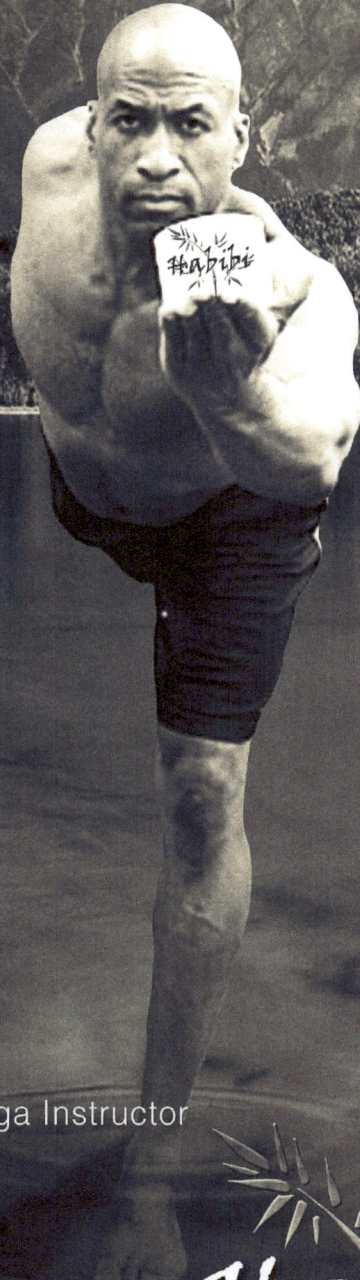

Tested on **power yogis**...not **animals**

Averill Kessee
Certified DDP Yoga Instructor

BATH *Habibi* BODY

Habibibody.com

Tanning Unveiled
SHOULD I?

BY ANTHONY HEREDIA

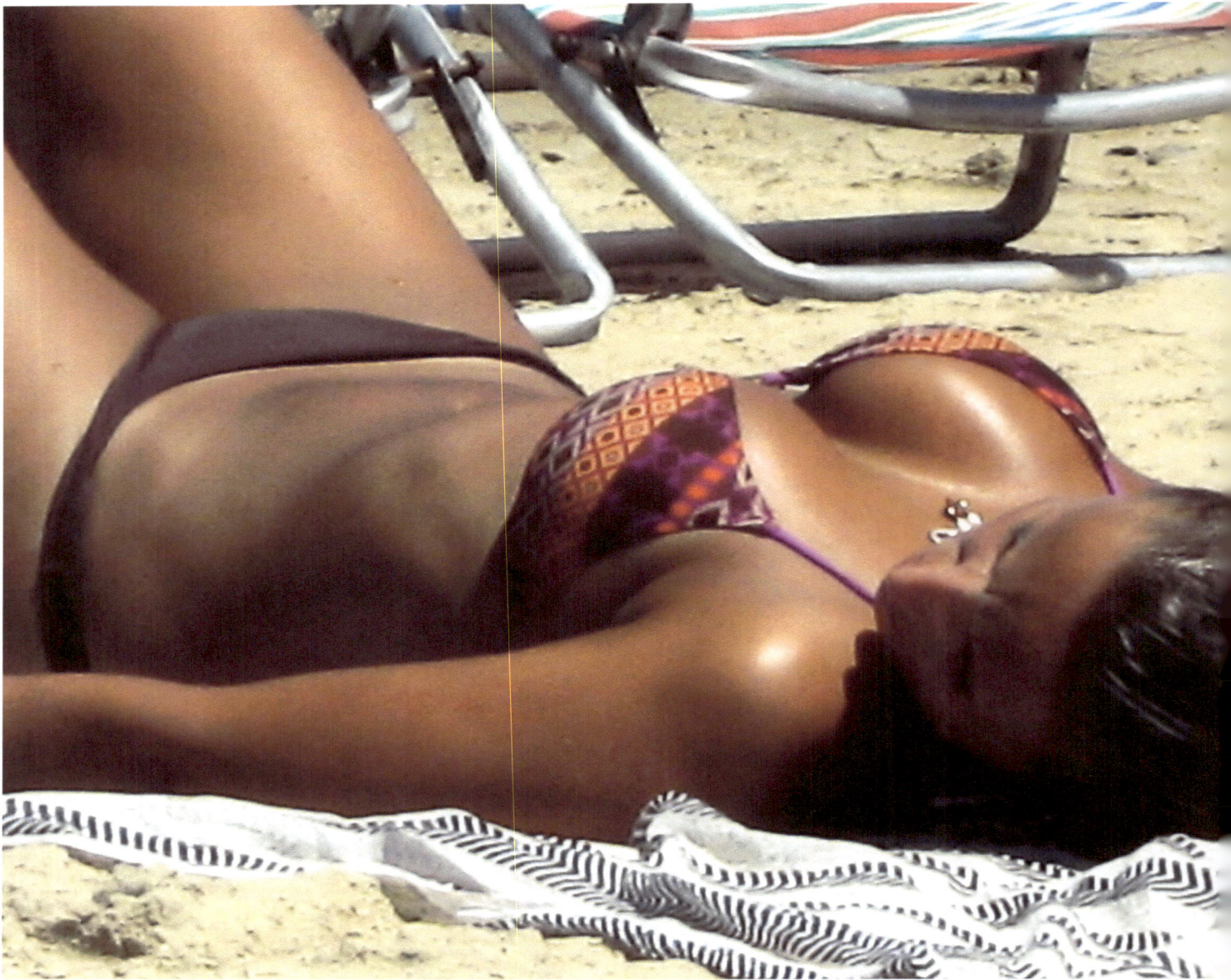

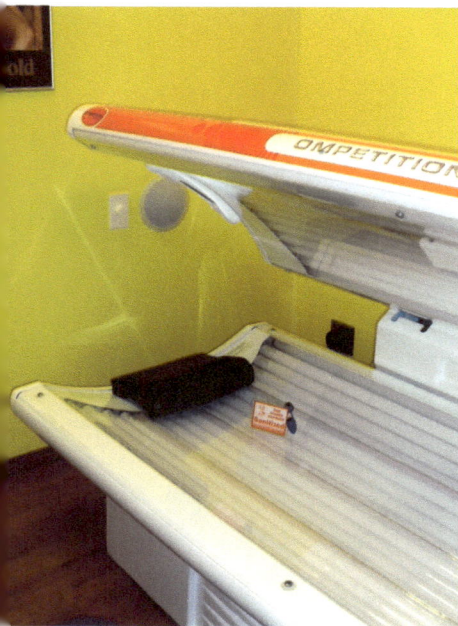

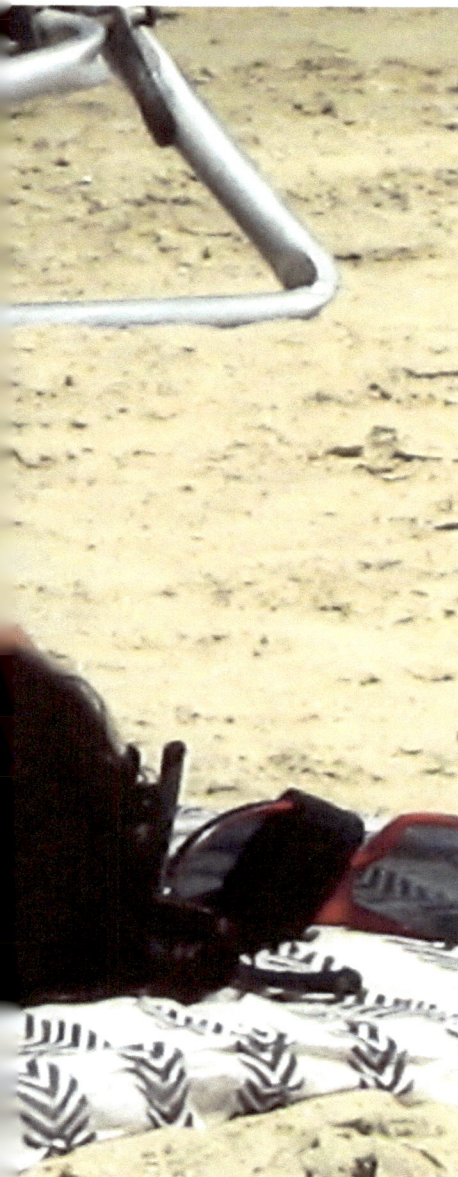

THE TOPIC USING A TANNING BED VS. NON UV METHODS HAS BEEN A HOT BUTTON FOR ALL TOO LONG, BUT THE VERDICT HAS ALWAYS BEEN THE SAME: YOUR SKIN WILL PAY THE PRICE.

Getting a beautiful bronze is attainable in a lotion or spray with your health intact as the bonus, but a surplus of UV will leave its mark. In modern days we are indoors so often and wrapped in suits and uniforms that no one has time to get much sun, let alone lie out for a tan; so it's easy to fall into the tanning booth trap. Don't get me wrong as I once tanned myself in a booth for convenience; but now knowing this, I am fine with a good spray tan and my health intact. Those who tan do so because of the confidence boost, the "healthy" glow they feel they attain from bronzed skin; but if you must tan, make it natural, or at least stay away from the indoor beds. You see, the actual process of your skin getting darker from tanning is a self defense mechanism to radiation from your skin, not a beauty mechanism. The UV rays cause your skin to release melanin (darkening you), which is designed to absorb radiation. This process is in response to damage. In other words, a forced tan is literally skin damaged, beautiful or not.

The International Agency for Research on Cancer branded tanning devices as being definite carcinogens which can increase the risk of skin cancer by 75% should someone tan regularly before the age of 30. The World Health Organization has classified UV tanning devices as among the most dangerous causes of human cancers, a very scary concept for an extra shade of brown, in my humble opinion. It seems that a golden brown is just so alluring because of what we see in the media; but even beauty director of *W Magazine*, Jane Larkworthy, said, "I can't remember the last time I saw a tanned model in my magazine or on the runway." The U.S. as a whole has taken notice of the damage and heavy risk from this and is trying hard to turn youth (16-28 yrs) away from this horrible pastime. Nearly 2.3 million teens tan indoors yearly, and they are the most vulnerable to damage they won't realize until it has been done. The U.S. Department of Health and Human Services intends to reduce the proportion of high school students who use tanning booths from the current 15.6% to 14% by 2020. Experts know that up to 90 percent of all visible changes in skin can be attributed to premature aging from the sun. UV damage is clinically documented to cause and accelerate skin sagging, wrinkles, discoloration, and roughness in skin texture as early as in your 20s.

In this battle the cons easily far outweigh the pros of stepping into a booth. Take this time to trade your booth membership for a spray membership and obtain the same results with your health intact. As usual, the time-tested advice of using sun block with an SPF of at least 30 and reapplied every two hours still holds true.

Moving Beyond Laser
FOR BEAUTIFUL SKIN

WHEN YOU THINK OF CLINICAL OR HEAVY DUTY SKIN REJUVENATION, YOU AUTOMATICALLY THINK OF LASERS; BUT AS TIME PROGRESSES, YOU WILL START TO THINK DIFFERENTLY.

BY ANTHONY HEREDIA

Technology moves lightning fast and thus has the ability to heal and rejuvenate just about every drop of the human body. Skin rejuvenation is just as common as dental work these days because of the myriad stressors to our bodies and skin, which makes our first impression. Regardless of who you are or where you come from, how nice or amazing a person you may be, your appearance will always speak for you first when meeting someone new for personal or business purposes. This is the reason so many invest in feeling their best when time, modern toxins, or Mother Nature has taken its toll on our skin. There is nothing wrong with wanting to get rid of acne scars that ruined your adolescence and are still with you through adulthood, or firming that drooping skin that the toll of gravity has taken. There are countless legitimate reasons to wanting to feel our best as we put our skin forward when we meet the world, so don't feel bad for considering something clinical as long as it is safe of course.

> Technology moves fast and has the ability to heal and rejuvenate the human body.

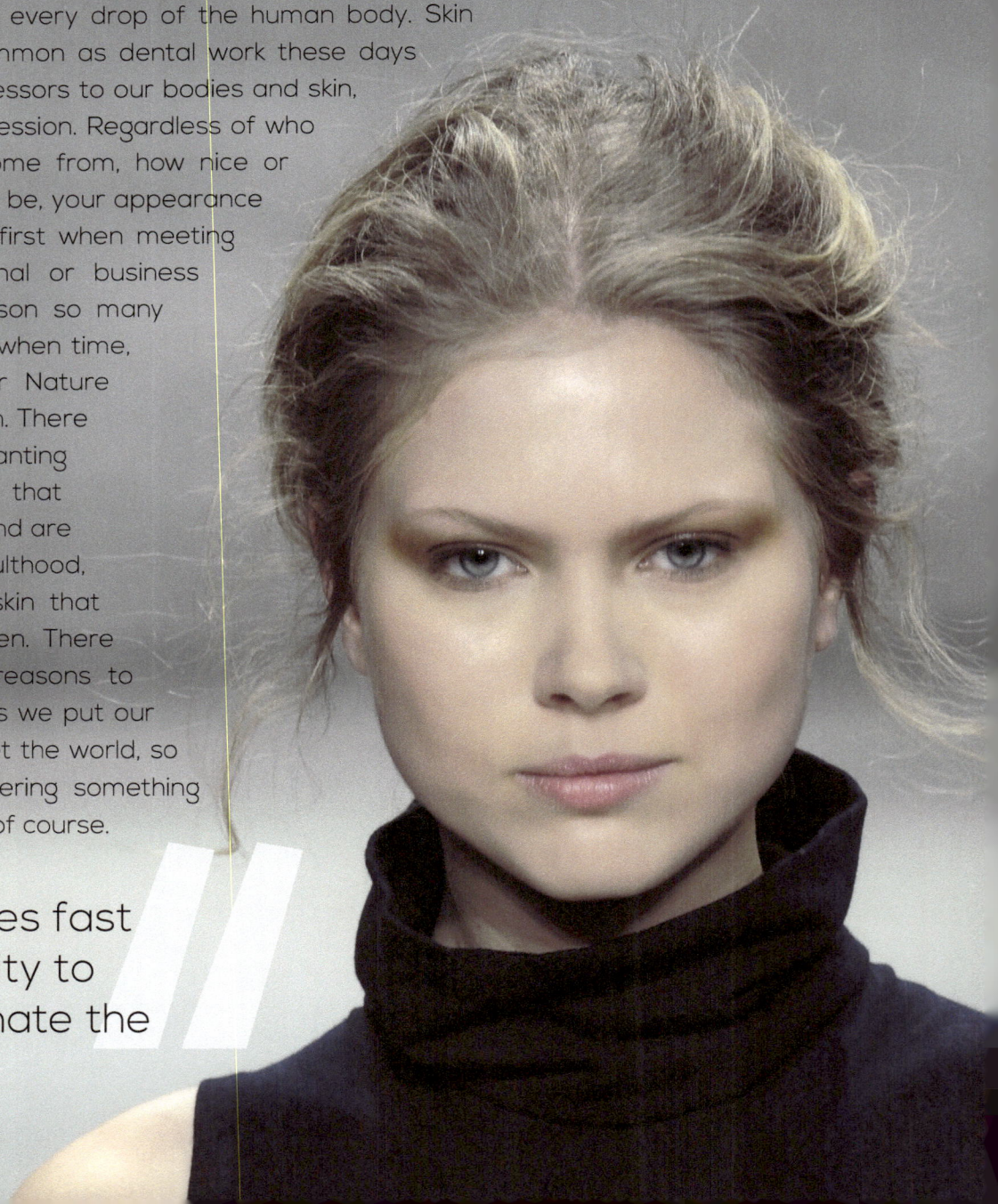

The market is saturated with topical over the counter and shelf stocked "miracles," promising you baby butt skin overnight, but buyer beware. This doesn't mean to say that not everything is ineffective, but if you aren't a dermatologist, then chances are you are taking a lot of shots in the dark and spending a lot of money on hope. My skin hasn't always been the best, thanks to wonderful acne teen years, so after trying every product on the shelves, I decided to go for the big guns. I visited Dr. Jacob Rispler at the Laser & Dermatology Institute of California in Los Angeles for heavy duty help. I did my research on dermatologists in LA, and this office ranked very high over all categories; so off I went. I went in thinking that lasers were going to be my best bet but was introduced to advancements in technology known as fractional radio-frequency treatments, fancy words for using heat and radio frequency below the skin with an array of micro pins rather than zapping above to heal from the inside out.

Laser technology is still amazing; but since lasers treat the complete outer surface of the skin, and there is more surface area that needs time to heal, this has been the norm until now. But science pushes on. The other technologies on the market are Fractionated co2 lasers and ultrasound devices which don't even come close to this new step. I have personally received two treatments of this so far and have seen for myself that science is awesome. As a science nerd I needed to understand the technical workings of course, and I appreciate technology helping me erase what years of teen hormones gifted me with and over the counter products failed in removing. This new technology uses heat that reaches the collagen layers below the skin to promote the collagen restructuring from the inside out. Dr Rispler explained, "It's not light based, so the treatment is colorblind," which allows this to work on just about any skin color and texture, whereas lasers have limits in this realm. Dr Rispler explained to me that "The effects continue to work in a linear fashion over 12 months"; so that even when I am done with it, all my skin will continue to get better, given I listen to all the other advice he gave me on caring for my skin. I had lots of bad habits that were making my skin worse when I came into the office, so this was very important to me to feel my best. I took every kind word they had for me to heart to ensure I keep my results. I still have another visit with this office, so I will post a follow-up article with my before and after pictures once I'm all done. I wouldn't be writing this if I didn't love the results so far. These types of procedures aren't miracles either, after all. They hit the reset button, but it is up to you to maintain your health.

Although Dr Rispler is treating me for deep acne scars, this treatment delivers improvement for a broad spectrum of symptoms, like texture, pigmentation irregularities, blood vessels, redness, deep lines; but the biggest focus is on reversing the appearance of aging. There is nothing wrong with wanting to fight time through healthy means. We are allowed to feel and look our best but not to try to look like anyone else.

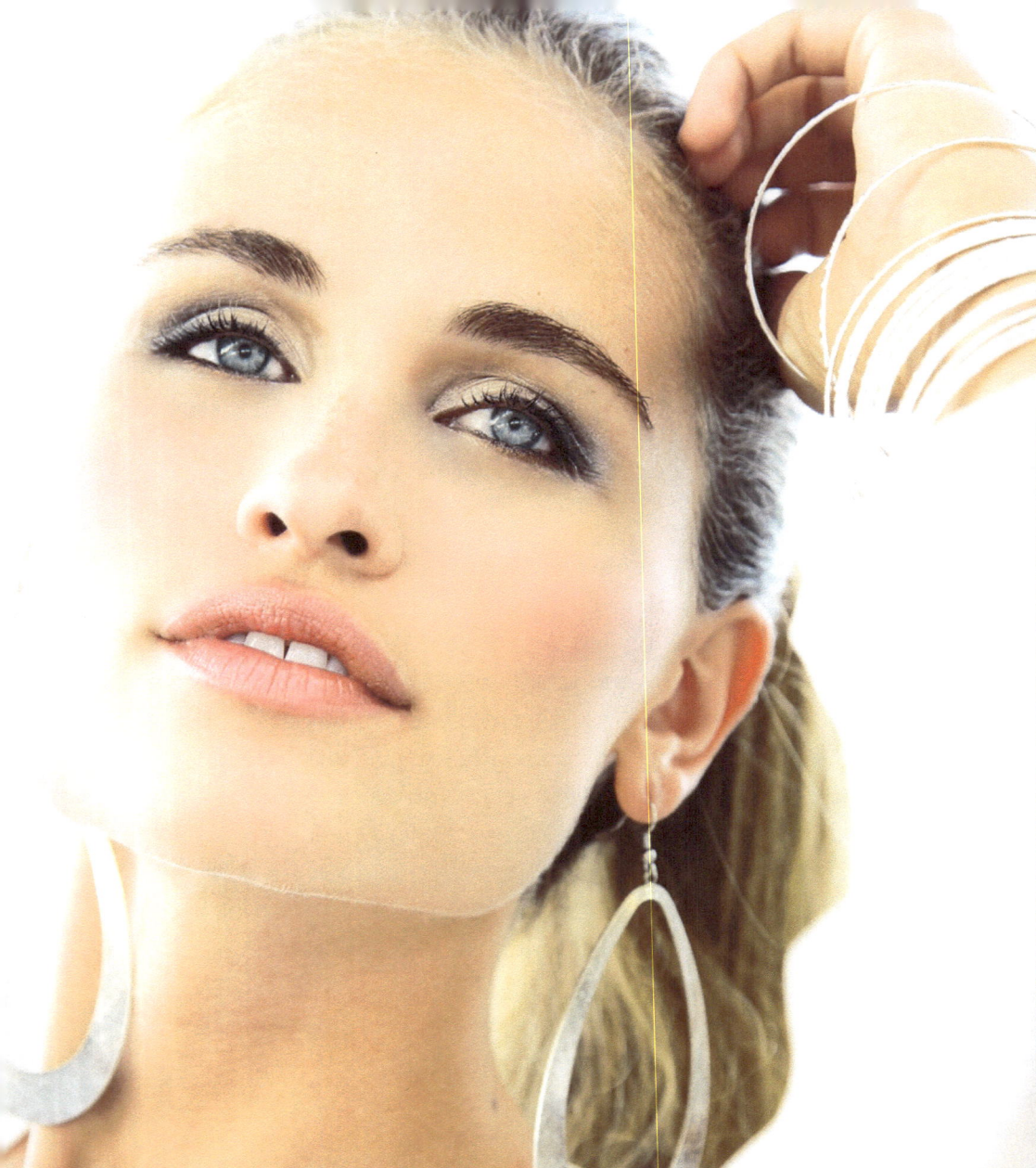
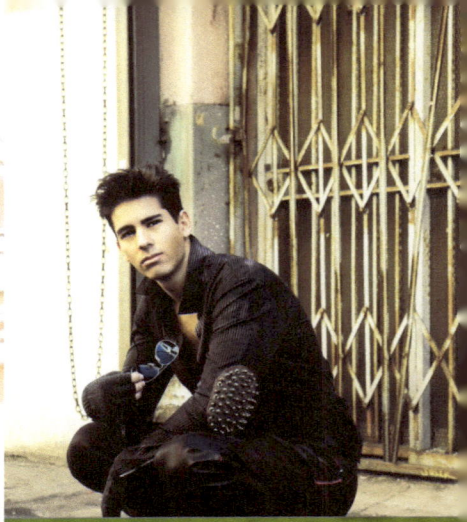
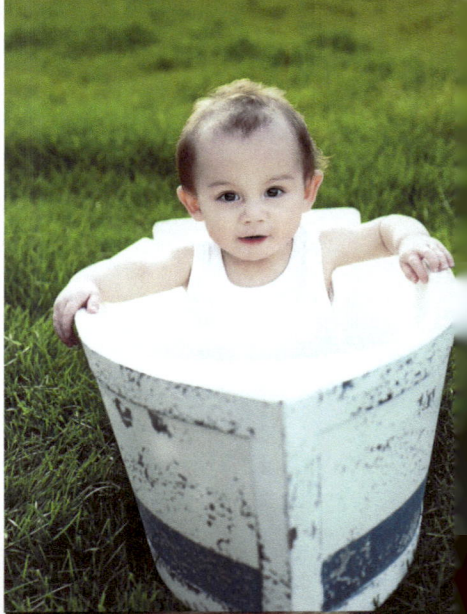
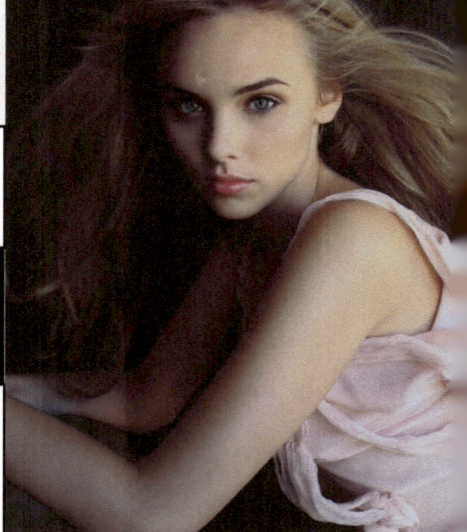
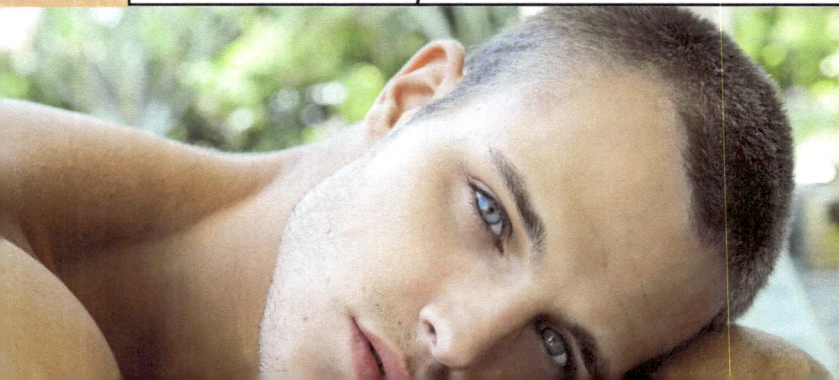
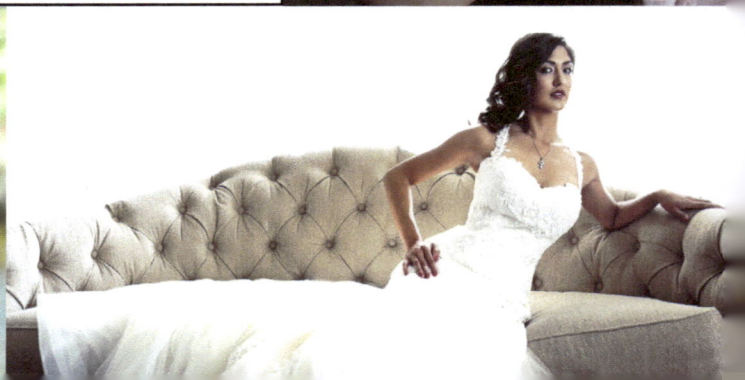

WORKOUT HAIR

BY SHAHADA KARIM

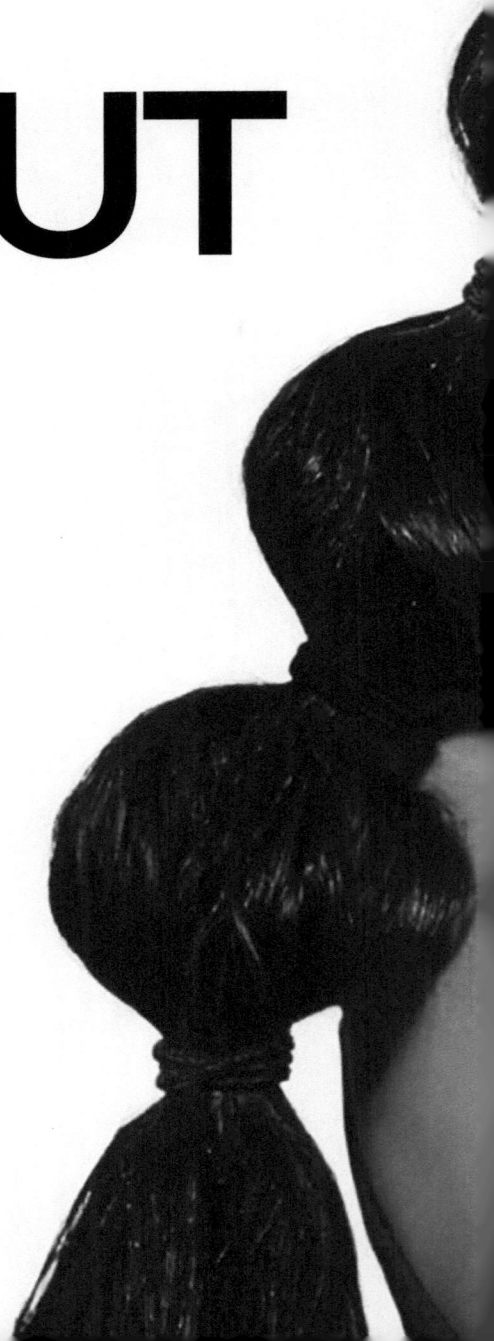

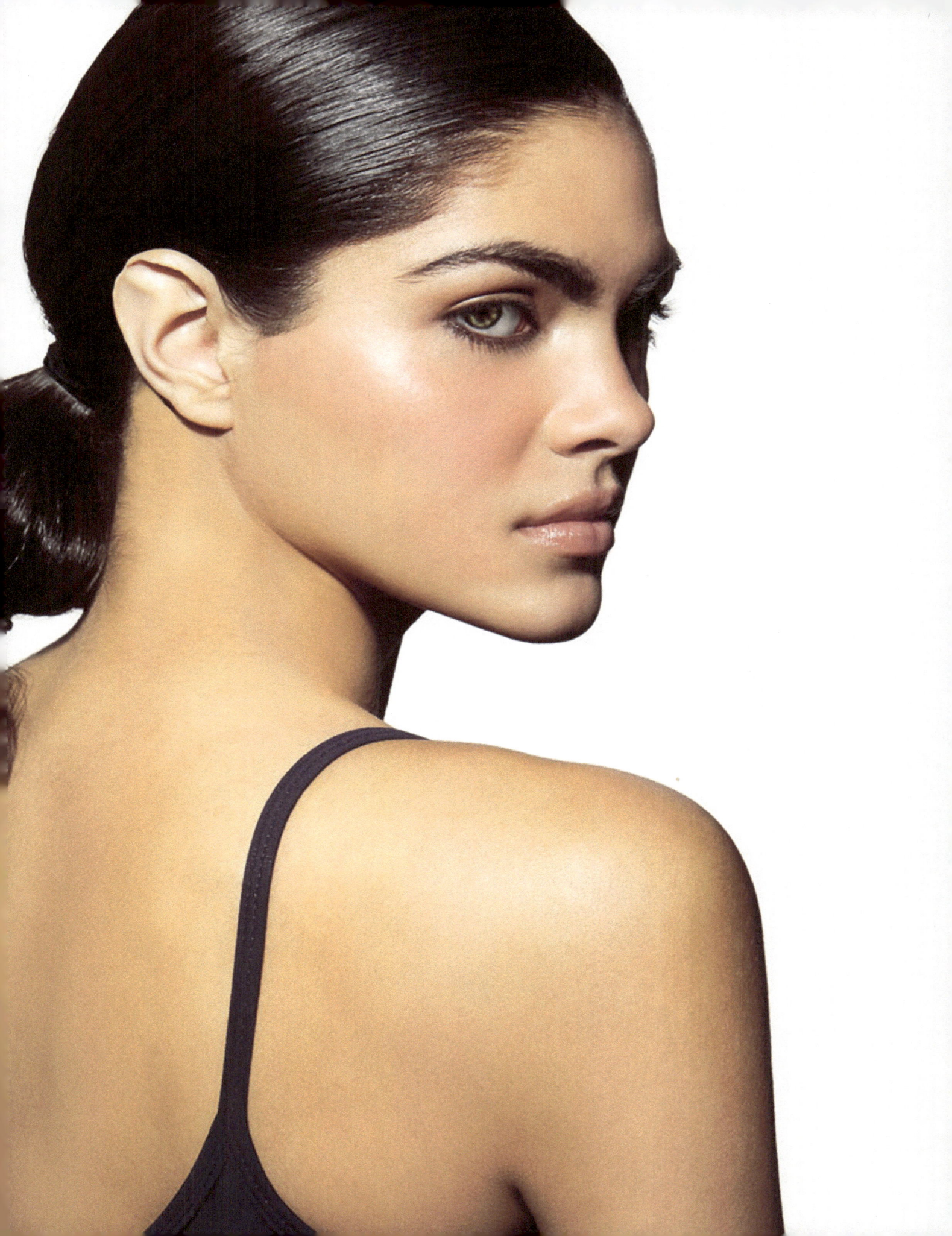

Save my hair!

Millions of people are packing gyms, parks, tracks, streets . . . you name it . . . all in the name of getting the perfect summer body. But all that activity wreaks havoc on your hair. So if you're trying to truly look good from head to toe (and not just from the neck down), we've got a few hair-saving tips to keep you together.

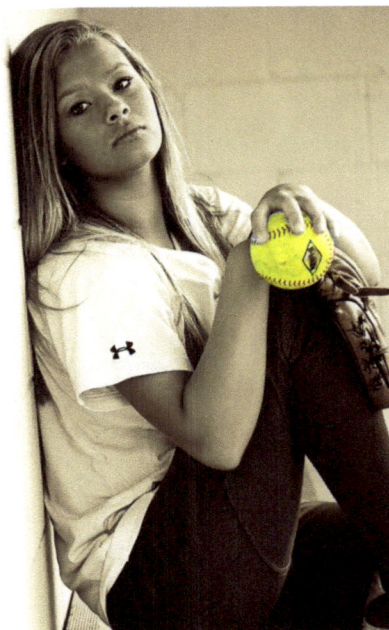

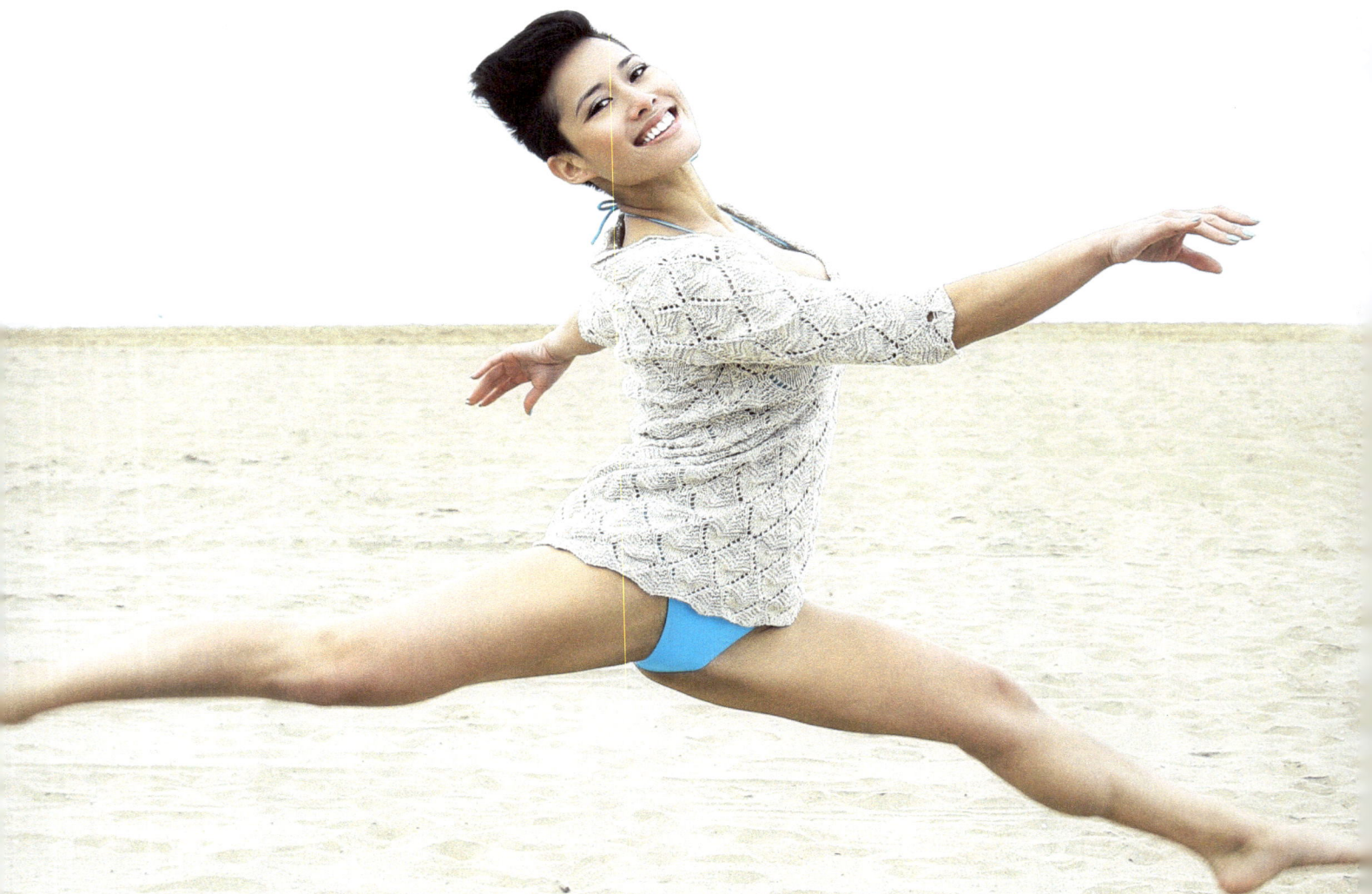

Put in a ponytail. One of the simplest ways to preserve your hair is to put it up. Besides being in the way of a good workout, letting your hair flow free during exercise can also be unsanitary. Gyms are notorious hubs for millions of organisms. The less you get in your hair, and possibly carry home with you, the better.

Wrap it up. You can go one step farther and put on a scarf or bandana to keep hair in place during a workout. The cotton fabric also helps to absorb excess oils or sweat and can help you preserve that blowout just a little bit longer.

Invest in a good conditioner. Sweating it out during the workout can wreak havoc on even the most resilient strands. Keep them in top shape with a good deep conditioner at least once a week.

Give it a rest. Just as you take rest days during a workout week, give your hair a styling rest. Opt for a few low maintenance styles like the ponytail (still a great post workout in a sleek style at the nape of the neck), a chignon, or a braid. If you want to wear it loose, give the blow dryer and flat iron a rest and opt for natural curls or waves instead.

BEST FACE FORWARD

BY SHAHADA KARIM

It's tough to look good while working out. We'd all like to think that we look like Victoria's Secret Angels with a light sheen of sweat on our bronzed skin, but the truth is probably closer to last night leftovers from a pretty wild party. While we don't advocate heading into the gym in a full face of makeup, there are a few tricks to help you look your best while getting in that daily dose of exercise.

▶ Sunscreen and Moisturize

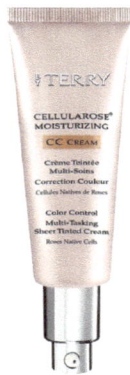

Protect yourself. Even on cloudy days, you need to use sunscreen. Never leave the house without it. Even if you're dipping in and out of the car on the way to and from the gym, use sunscreen. And we shouldn't need to emphasize how important it is if you're going to go walking or running outdoors. Remember that SPF (sun protection factor) numbers tell you how long you've got before you need to reapply. There's no such thing as layering SPFs for a stronger result, so opt for something higher than 15 that works with your skin type and tone.

Go easy on your skin. Rather than trying to cover it up with foundation, try a tinted moisturizer that will smooth imperfections without clogging your pores. We're huge fans of By Terry's Cellularose CC Cream. The sheer coverage is just enough to give your skin a healthy glow.

▶ Go Waterproof

Waterproof Mascara is your friend. You can maintain the illusion of long, lush lashes without worrying about raccoon eyes halfway through your run. Our favorite is Volume de Chanel Waterproof Formula. If you're a fan of another mascara, not to worry. Anastasia's Lash Genius adds a waterproof coat to any mascara formula. Just use it as a final step to seal in your favorite formula.

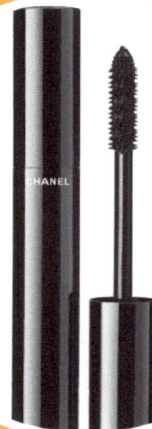

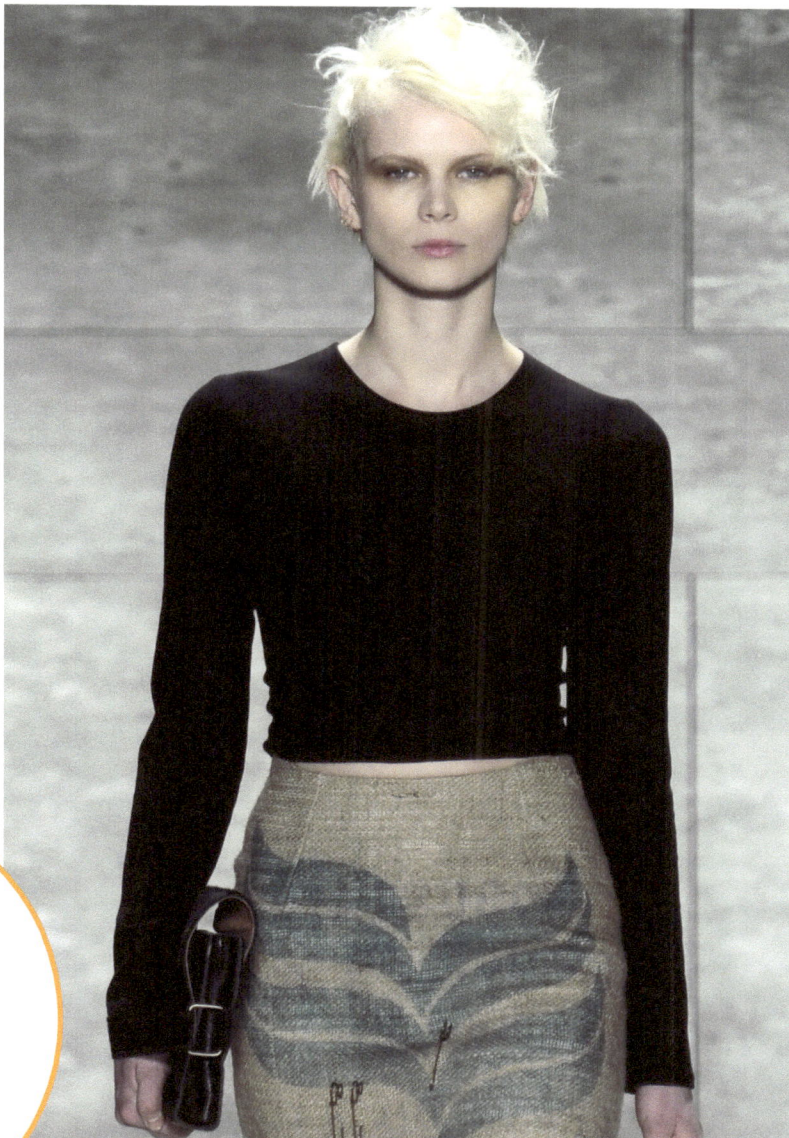

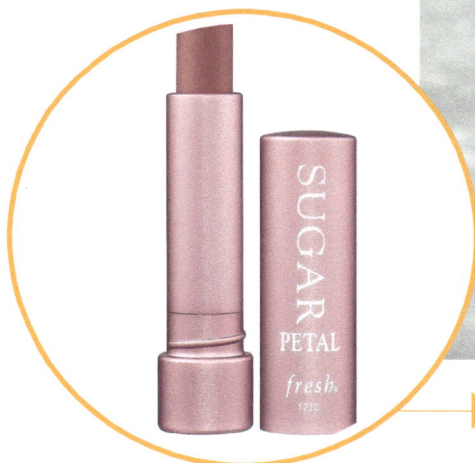

Love Your Lips

Love your lips. Do yourself a favor and invest in a really good lip balm. Chap Stick is cute, but all that wax just ends up leaving your lips coated, not to mention that nasty ring you end up with inside your lips—don't pretend you don't know what we're talking about—instead of moisturized. Instead, invest in a Fresh Lip Treatment. Whether you go clear or opt for a tinted variety, the combination of soothing oils and butters will leave your lips looking their best even as you sweat it out.

Mind Over
Muscle

You don't have to be a body builder to have a bit of definition. With just a few minor tweaks to your routine, you can show some muscle in no time at all!

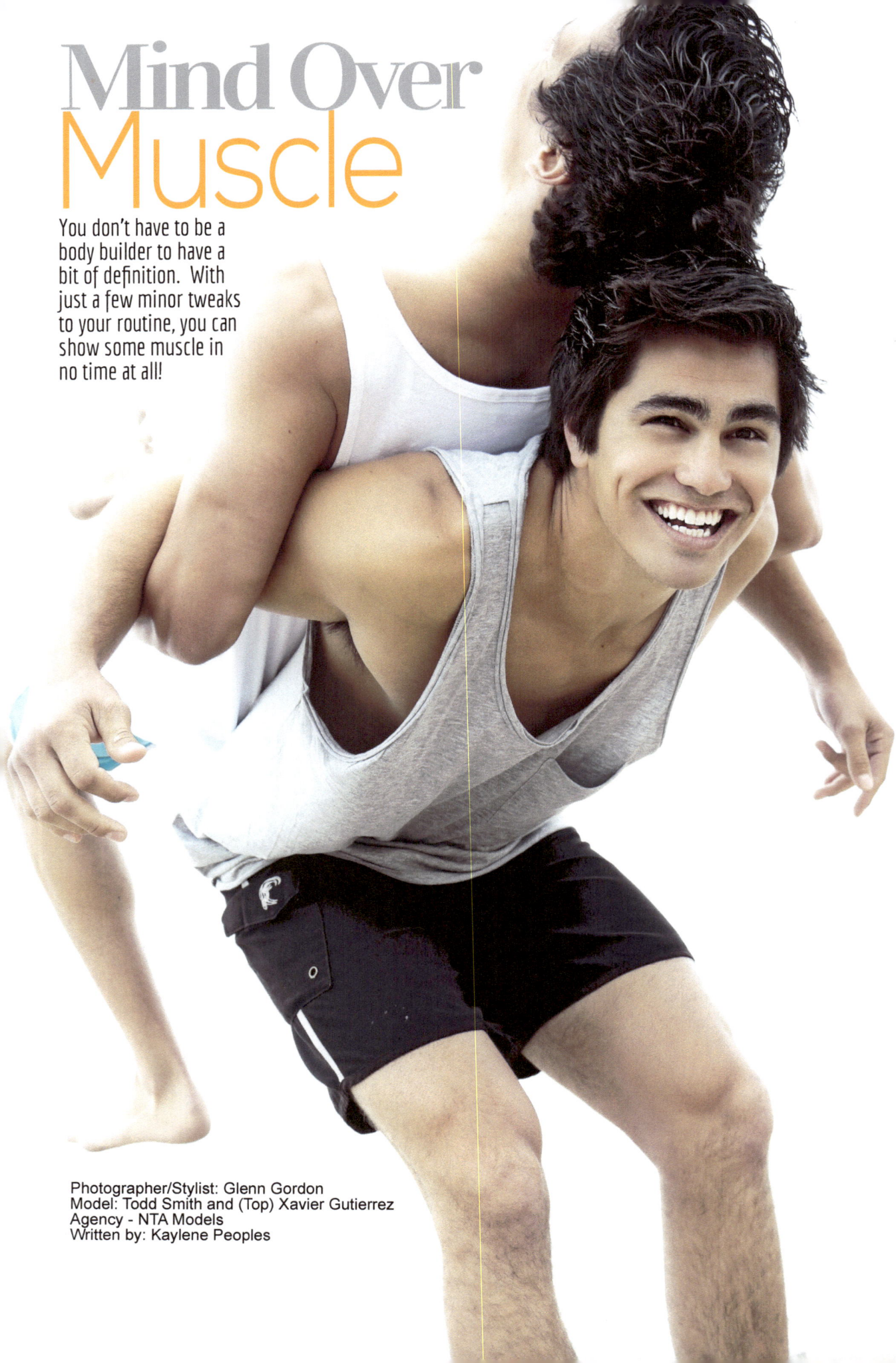

Photographer/Stylist: Glenn Gordon
Model: Todd Smith and (Top) Xavier Gutierrez
Agency - NTA Models
Written by: Kaylene Peoples

Mind Over
Muscle

Proteins Over Carbs

More protein, less carbohydrates will do the trick. Nobody's telling you to go "Atkins," but do your muscles a favor and feed them what they want. Eat a piece of fish with broccoli.

(Model: Xavi Corte)
Montemar Resort

Mind Over
Muscle

Power-Based Exercises

Do a power-based resistence exercise like an incline bench press or a weighted pullup; increase the weight and decrease your reps to build mass.

(Model: Xavi Corte)

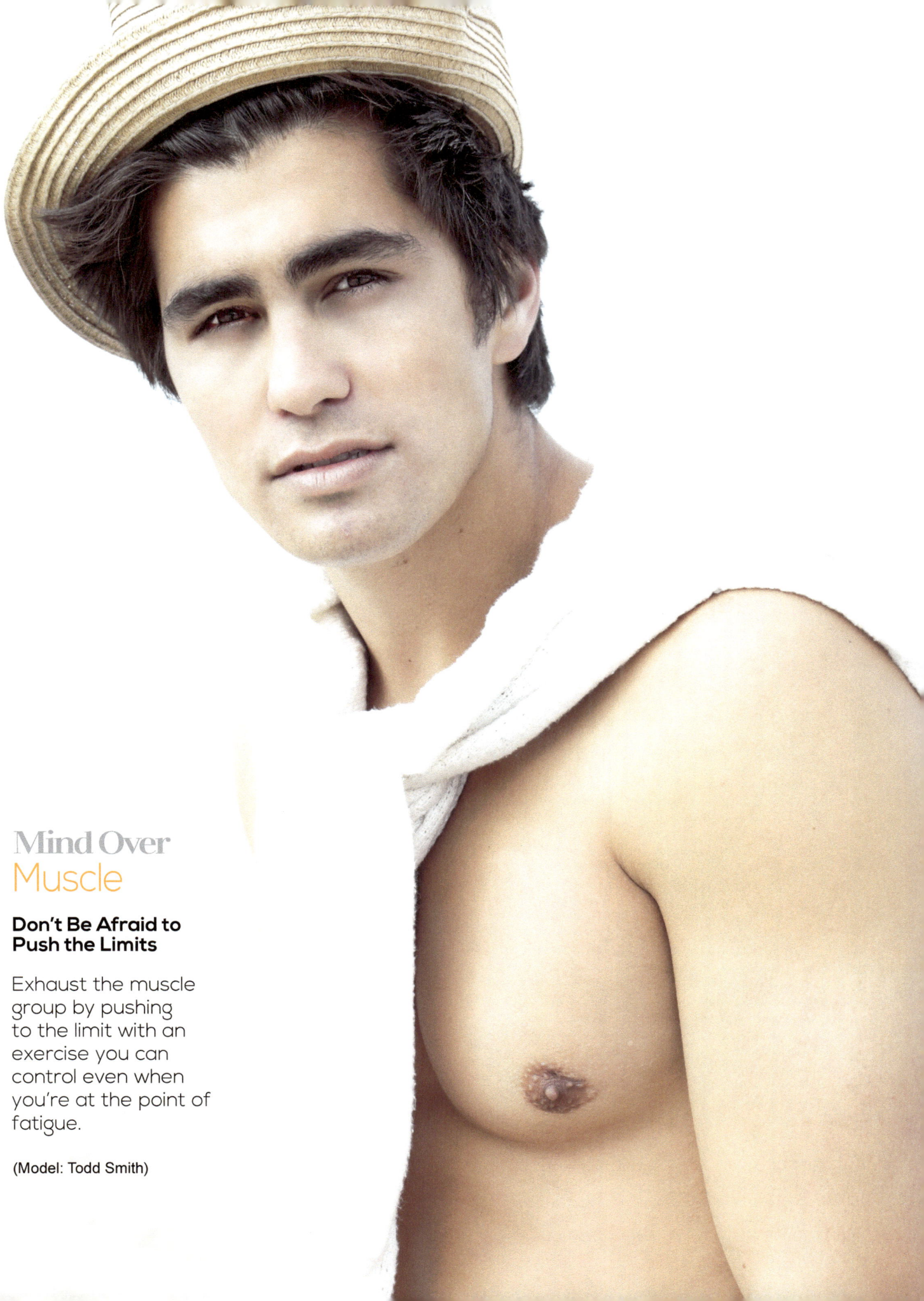

Mind Over
Muscle

Don't Be Afraid to Push the Limits

Exhaust the muscle group by pushing to the limit with an exercise you can control even when you're at the point of fatigue.

(Model: Todd Smith)

Mind Over
Muscle

Tear Down then Repair

Use exhaustive supersets to tear leftover muscle fiber, forcing your body to repair it and make you stronger.

(Model: Todd Smith and (Top) Xavier Gutierrez)

Mind Over
Muscle

Repair Muscles While You Sleep

Make sure to rest for a minimum of seven to nine hours a night. Give your muscles a day off. While your goal is to get lean, you don't want to hit the gym twice. You'll burn so many calories that you can't build muscle.

(Model: Todd Smith)

THE ART OF WELLNESS

SIMPLIFYING HOLISTIC HEALTH

Available at www.dahlhousenutrition.com/

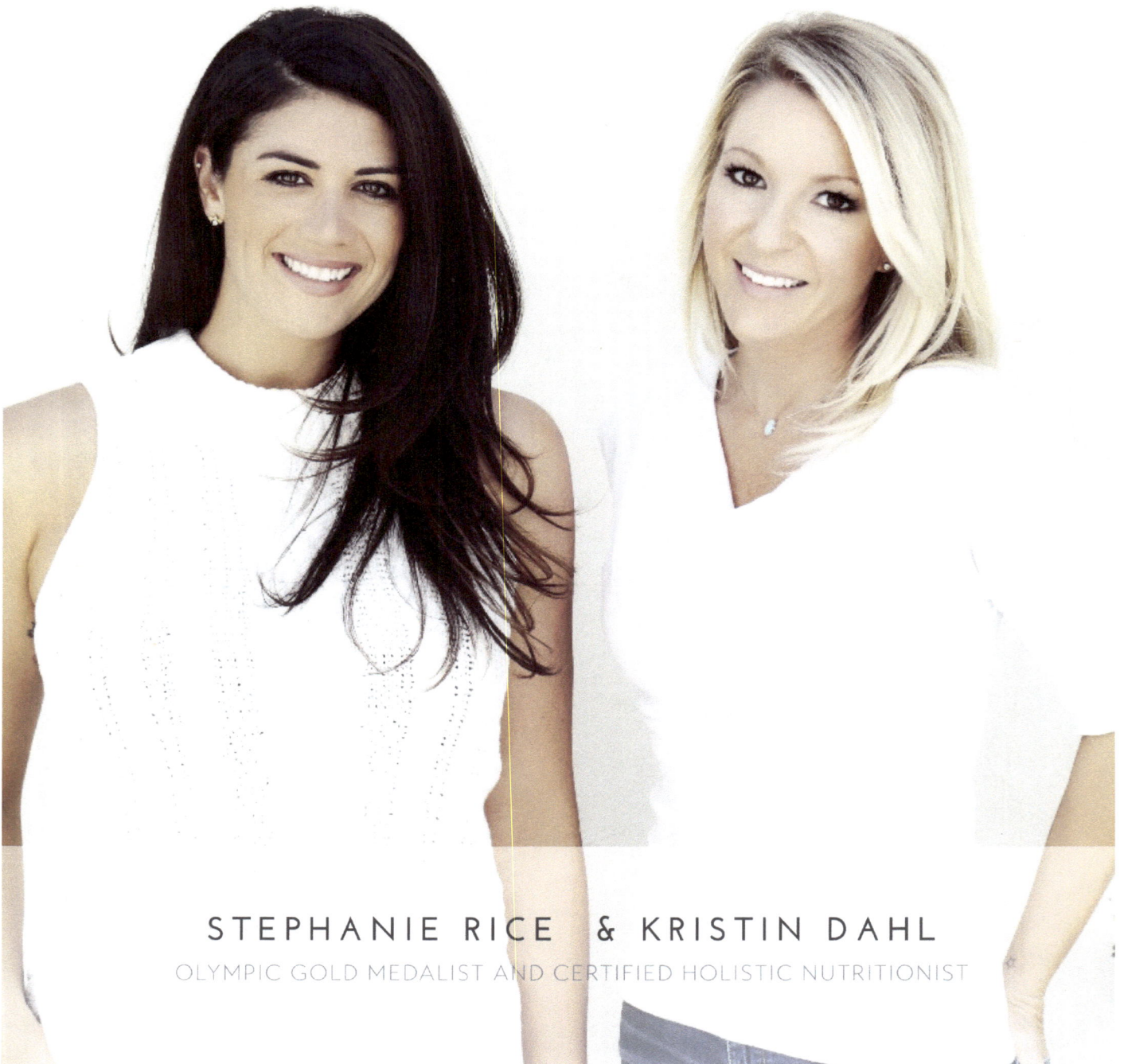

STEPHANIE RICE & KRISTIN DAHL

OLYMPIC GOLD MEDALIST AND CERTIFIED HOLISTIC NUTRITIONIST

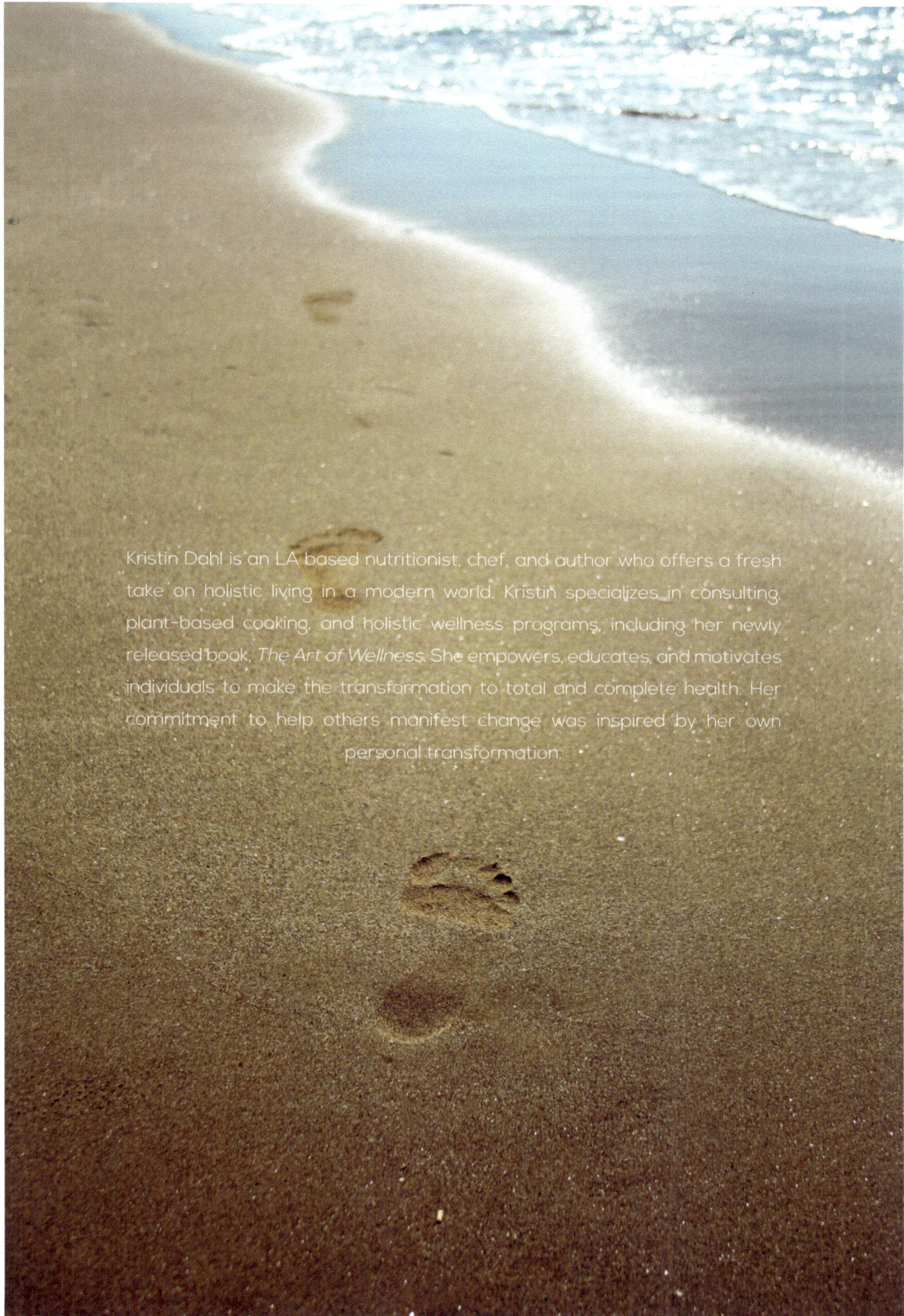

Kristin Dahl is an LA based nutritionist, chef, and author who offers a fresh take on holistic living in a modern world. Kristin specializes in consulting, plant-based cooking, and holistic wellness programs, including her newly released book, *The Art of Wellness*. She empowers, educates, and motivates individuals to make the transformation to total and complete health. Her commitment to help others manifest change was inspired by her own personal transformation.

DAHLHOUSE
NUTRITION

INTERVIEW WITH HOLISTIC NUTRITIONIST KRISTIN DAHL

BY ANTHONY HEREDIA

(Photo of Kristin Dahl
Taken by Kelsey Combe)

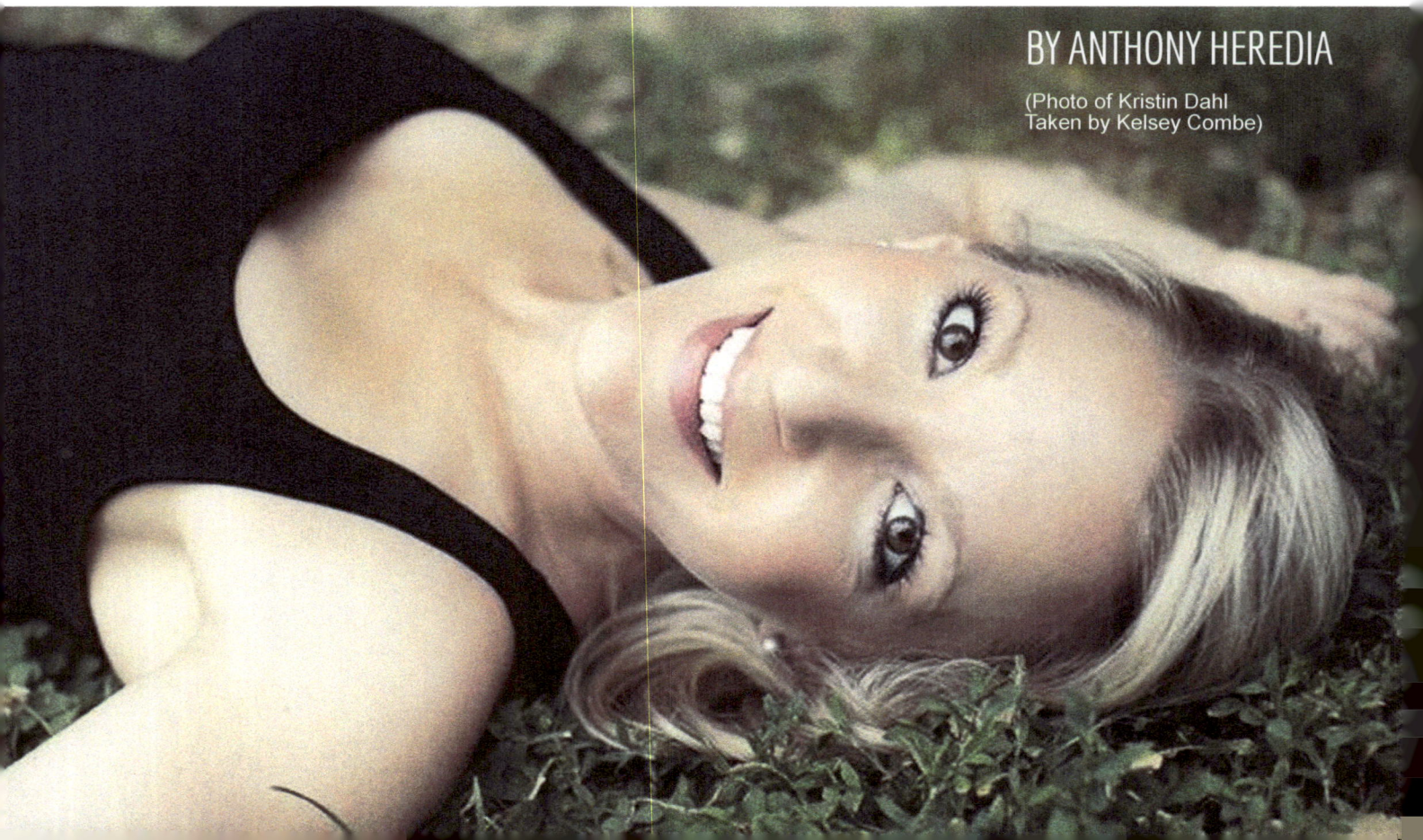

Kristin Dahl has become a contributor to *Agenda* magazine, so we wanted to take the time to pick her "healthy" mind on how to improve the nutritional lives of our readers. Kristin is an established provider of holistic health services as a certified holistic nutritionist. She is a natural healer and life coach. Her specialties range from private cooking, kitchen clean-outs, grocery store tours to one-on-one nutritional consults. Kristin's education is from The Institute for Holistic Nutrition, The Natural Gourmet, The Omega Institute, Strala NYC, and The New York Open Center. Now Kristin spends her time invested in her thriving private practice, based in Santa Monica, CA. I am taking this opportunity to share her passion and ask her opinion on some strong health topics in which we all share curiosity.

So what inspired you to grow a career in nutrition, Kristin?

All of my life I have been interested in wellness, nutrition, and healing. I also LOVE helping people. About 10 years ago, I started getting more and more interested in cooking, nutrition, and holistic living. I started seeing healers of various backgrounds and met with homeopaths, naturopaths, acupuncturists, Ayurvedic doctors, and massage therapists. I devoured wellness, self help, and spiritual literature.

I visited the spa regularly, shopped at the Farmers Market, and made most of my meals at home. The more I dove in, the better I felt. I wanted to share my transformational journey with people and learn the science and mechanics behind it all. I decided it was time to devote my life to wellness and went back to school. This was a radical career change for me, but one of the most rewarding experiences of my life. This change not only inspired a career in nutrition but also inspired me to support my friends and family in theirs.

Do you have a memorable moment in your career of you helping your clients through nutrition?

I had a client in New York who was going through a major life transition. She reached out to me for nutritional support, and we ended up working together one-on-one for several months. Through this experience she was able to make a radical life shift. She dropped weight, gained energy, and felt physically and psychologically better than ever. She was one of my first clients, so this was a tremendous growing experience for me as well. She really dug deep and was committed to manifesting change. In turn, this invigorated me and made me more passionate than ever. Our work together made me believe that what I am doing truly makes a difference, and I am infinitely grateful that she came into my life.

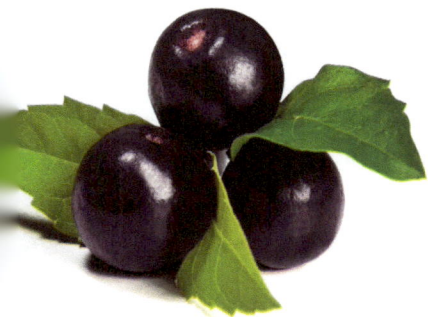

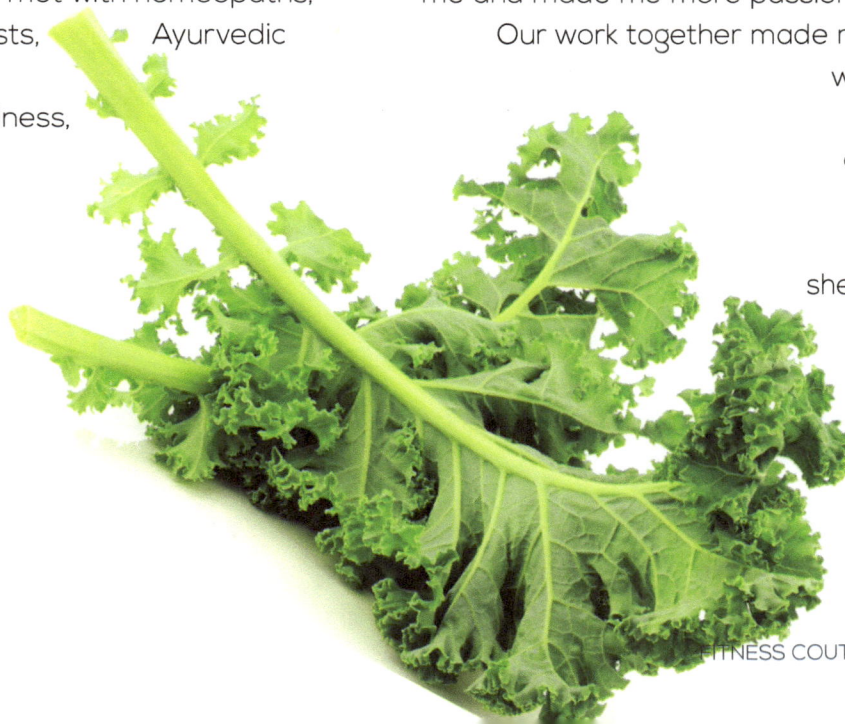

> All of my life I have been interested in wellness, nutrition, and healing. I also LOVE helping people.

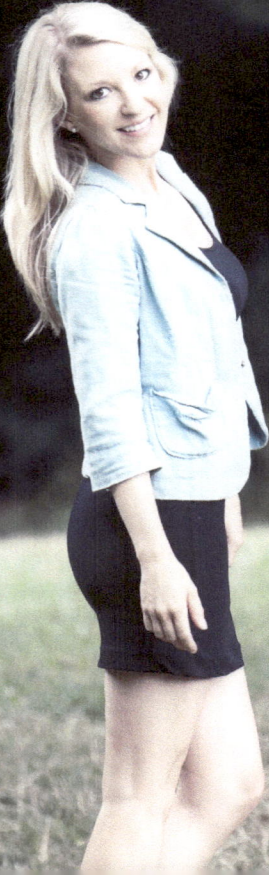

The simplist way to start feeling better ASAP is to ALKALIZE your body.

What are some simple steps our readers can take today to clean themselves inside out and boost their metabolism and feel their best?

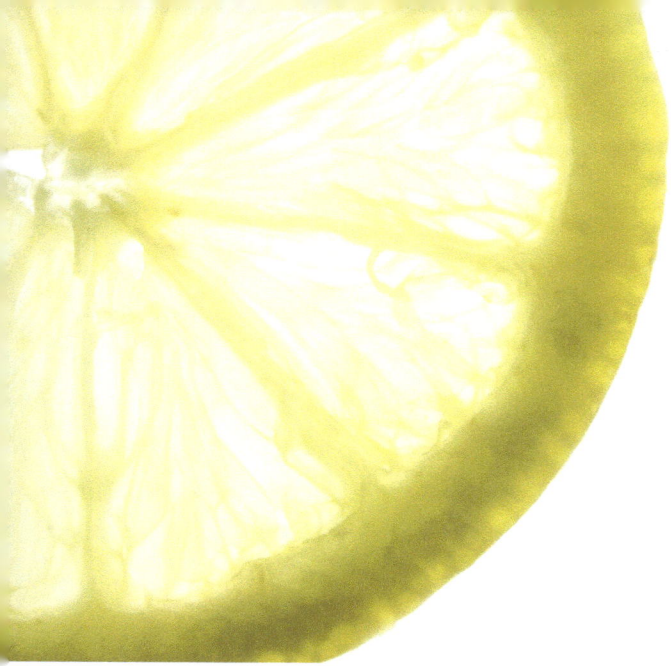

The simplest way to start feeling better ASAP is to ALKALIZE your body. Most of the standard American diet is acidic; coffee, alcohol, and sugar are among the top offenders. All of these foods create an acidic environment in your body, leading to weight gain, skin issues, low energy, and a slowed metabolism. The fastest way to boost your metabolism and get your body on the fast track to health is to start alkalizing your body every day! Here are a few tips to start rebalancing your body and start looking and feeling your very BEST.

-Start every day with lemon water. This will not only alkalize your system but will stimulate your digestion and start cleansing your body.

-Swap your morning cup of Joe for herbal tea or green tea. Both are alkaline and help detox the body and boost metabolism. If you simply can't break the habit, scale back to just a few times a week or less than once a day. Look for low acid coffee or cleaner brands, such as bulletproof coffee.

-Get moving and don't forget to breathe deeply! Exercise and deep breathing are both incredibly alkalizing to the body. Did you ever notice that people who exercise regularly have a certain glow about them? Getting your heart rate up and breathing deeply send oxygen (alkalinity) to your blood stream. Work out as often as possible for glowing skin, regulated digestion, and a speedy metabolism!

What do you feel is a simple change we can all do to make the biggest difference in the way we eat now?

Cook at home! This is probably the single most important change you can make when it comes to eating clean. When you dine out regularly, you are eating twice the salt, sugar, and fat than you would at home. KNOW YOUR FOOD. Shop for the ingredients, buy from local farmers, and try to limit the amount of processed foods you are having. The more you do this, the better you will feel, guaranteed. Your waistline will thank you, too. Over the past few years, more and more people are developing food allergies, sensitivities, and autoimmune conditions. If we start taking charge of what is going into our bodies, these problems will be less likely to occur. If you do plan a special night out, research healthy restaurants that are committed to serving only the cleanest cuisine. Look for farm-to-table, vegan, and organic restaurants. Most of these places will offer gluten- and dairy-free.

KNOW YOUR FOOD.
Shop for the ingredients,
buy from local farmers,
and try to limit the
amount of processed
foods you are having.
The more you do this,
the better you will feel.

La Boqueria
Photo: Brett Bixby

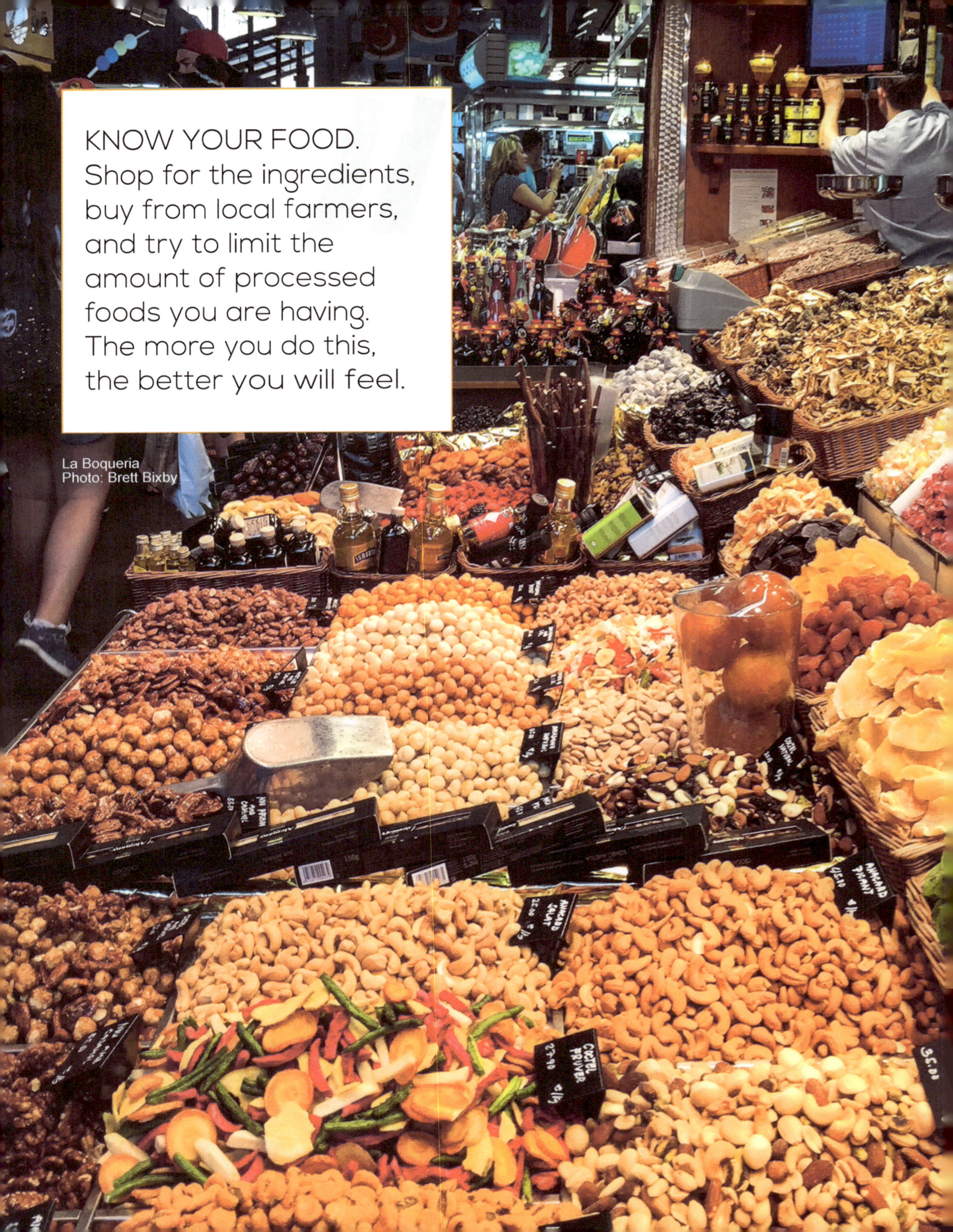

What about current health topics and trends; are there any that alarm you or excite you?

One trend that both alarms and excites me is the juice craze. Did you notice that there are juiceries popping up all over town. Maybe your favorite market even started carrying pressed juice, or you noticed a juice cooler at the gym or yoga studio? It's wonderful that the general public is starting to become more aware and that people want to cleanse and get healthy. Juice cleansing is a powerful way to cleanse your body, seasonally or whenever your system is feeling overloaded. Juice is alkalizing to the body, gives your digestive system a break, and is a healthy snack option. This trend is exciting for many reasons, but I will also let you in on why this alarms me. The one thing that alarms me the most is the amount of sugar that some of these juices contain. Even though it comes from natural sources, you have to be careful not to drink juice with too many sweet fruits or added sweeteners. Without the fiber intact, you might as well consider your juice cleanse a sugar cleanse, if every juice you drink is loaded with fruits and sweeteners. The concept of a juice cleanse is to clean your body, eliminate Candida and give you more energy. Make sure at least 80-90% of the juice you are drinking contains little to no fruit or sugar additives. Another thing that alarms me is that some people are approaching juice cleansing as a diet. It's important that juice cleansing is used to detox, as a diet transition, or to break away from food addictions. Juice should not be a permanent food replacement. It's imperative that we eat a well balanced diet, with plenty of fiber and a variety of foods. Know your body and do what feels best. That could be a 3-day juice cleanse once a month, seasonal cleansing, or the occasional 1-day cleanse if your body is feeling overwhelmed.

Well, what do you personally do to stay feeling your very best (nutrition and fitness wise)?

I've always been an active person. Doing some form of exercise everyday keeps me feeling my best. I love hiking, yoga, and dancing. I've tried every workout under the sun, but I stick to what makes me feel most balanced. I spend a lot of my time working out in the great outdoors, which is a double reward because it ends up nourishing my body and my soul at the same time! When I can't get outdoors for a workout, I'll head to the gym, a fitness class, or run through a yoga sequence at home. I also love going for long walks, and I'm known for randomly dancing my ass off at home. As far as nutrition is concerned, I always try to keep things as clean as possible, while maintaining balance. I find that I have the most energy and vitality that way. I like to make healthy treats in moderation and am a sucker for raw chocolate. I've been dairy- and gluten-free for several years. Though this is not the best for everyone, I found that eliminating these foods made me look and feel my best. Not only physically but also psychologically, I noticed a radical shift in my digestion and mood. I cook 90% of my meals at home, using local, farm-fresh, and organic ingredients. I hardly eat any processed foods, and I cleanse seasonally to refresh and recharge.

Lastly, what is something you do or have personally struggled with (nutrition/fitness wise) that you have been able to take control of and how?

Several years back, I struggled with overeating and emotional eating (even if it was healthy food). Instead of facing my fears or working on whatever was bothering me, I would overindulge or eat to the point of sickness. I was able to take control of this by becoming more connected to myself. I started seeing a therapist, read self-help books, and took yoga classes, which drew me closer to my center. Now, when dark feelings come up, I give myself time to sort through them. I ask a friend for support or head to a yoga class to go inward and sweat it out.

Spa Massage Etiquette

WHAT TO DO AND WHAT NOT TO DO FOR STAR QUALITY

BY ANTHONY HEREDIA

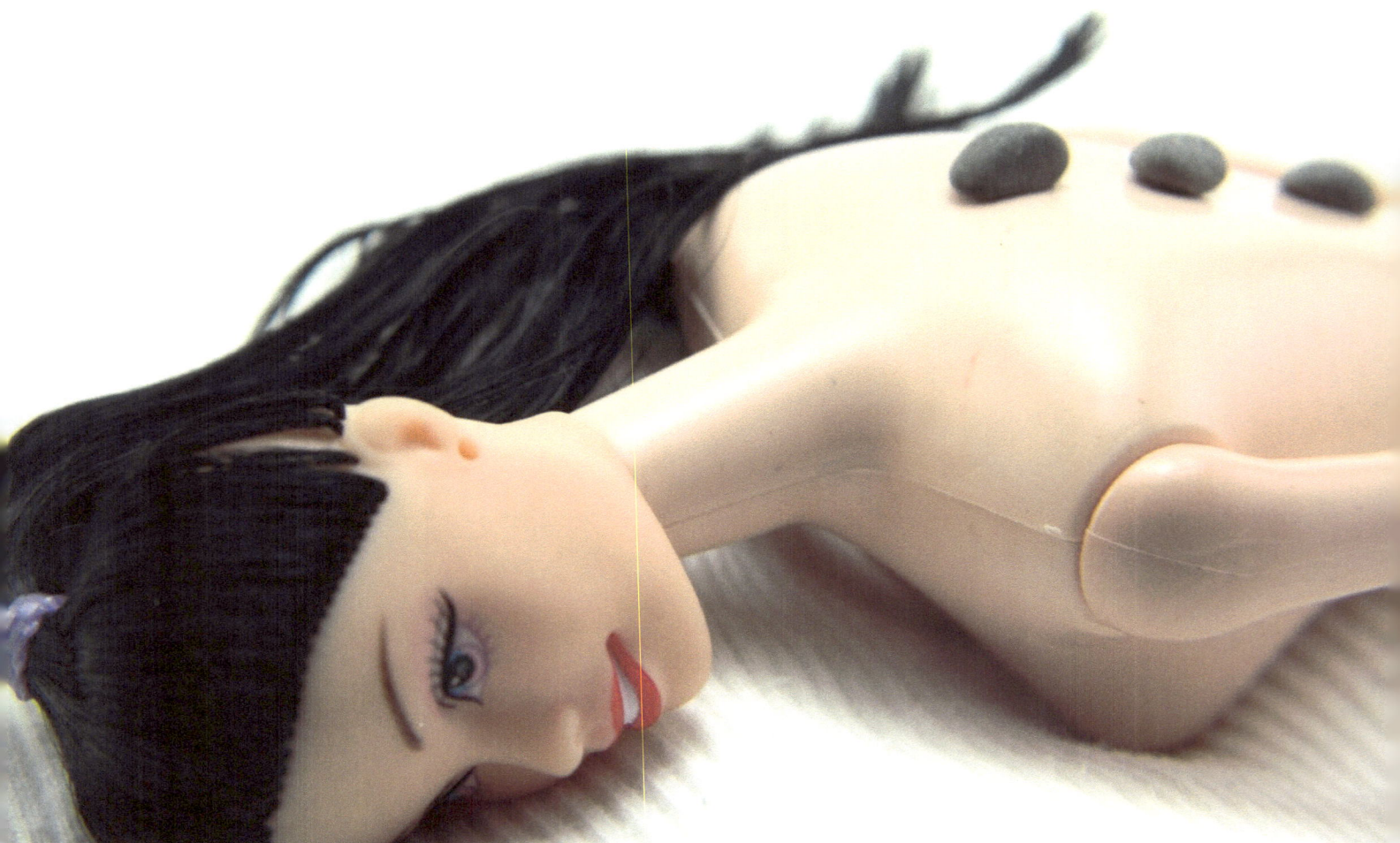

DO

Shower: Getting a massage does not count as your shower, and it will really not help you get a great treatment not being fresh. If you don't respect your body, it is hard for your therapist to do the same when harsh odors may be coming from you because of a long day, a gym session, or just not cleaning properly in the bathroom. A professional therapist will never say anything, but don't expect him/her to give the odor-rich area much detail, if any at all. If you want foot work, please make sure your feet are clean and have no odor. So goes the rule for the full body. When an area is dirty, the therapist drags that dirt throughout the rest of your body; not good for either person. It is also important for your enjoyment since you are less likely to be able to relax, knowing you are probably emitting not so fresh scents due to bad planning. If you smell good and are clean from head to toe, I promise your treatment will be a thousand times better than if you skipped the shower.

BE ON TIME: Be on time: Most spas and treatments have multiple clients that are booked back-to-back, which means if you are late by 10 minutes and expect your full time, you have just made everyone else for the rest of the day late by your time. There are opportunities where your therapist might not have someone right after you and be kind enough to give you extra time, but please do return the favor and tip handsomely as it is their time and they don't get paid any more for staying later for you.

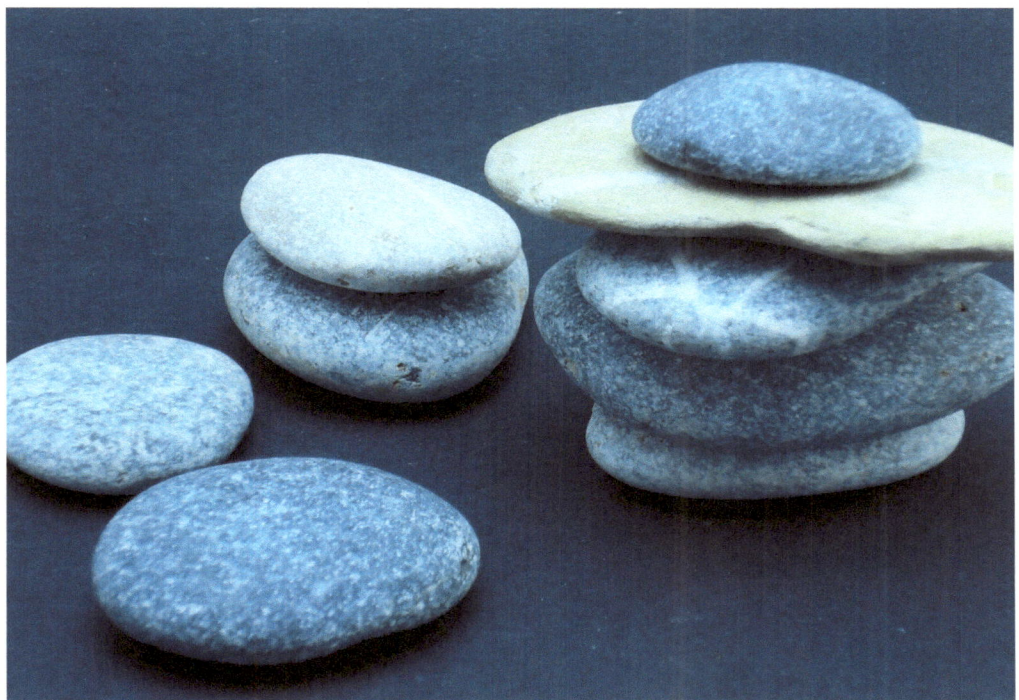

Improve your visit by doing this.

Be Honest:

Within the first few minutes of meeting your therapist you will be in your treatment room discussing your health, and you really do need to be honest for your own health. Therapists need to know about major surgeries and important medications for your safety. If you lie about not taking blood pressure medication, your therapist can send you to the hospital, never being the wiser. If you have an embarrassing skin problem, you run the risk of contaminating your therapist and every client he/she sees afterward; so please just be honest. Most respectable veteran therapists know a way around just about everything for you to be honest and still enjoy an amazing treatment; so there is no need to endanger multiple lives by withholding important information. Trust me, just give full disclosure.

Speak Up:

This is your massage, so if something just doesn't feel right, please feel confident to say so. Experienced therapists will ask about every single component of your session at least once if not twice, but don't assume they will. If you want the room dimmer or the table warmer, you should feel free to ask. If you want detail work on your hips but prefer no work on your feet, speak up to enjoy yourself.

Dress Down to Comfort:

Full nude is the norm nowadays and makes for the best massage at respectable upscale spas since it gives full access for your therapist to reach all the areas that are bothering you. Always make sure you are comfortable, though. If you don't want to have your hips touched, then you are fine keeping shorts on. Feel comfortable to keep underwear on should you need to, but the main idea is that a therapist will assume that if you do wear underwear, you don't want the area covered to be touched, so don't expect. Even nude you will be covered at all times, and only the area that is being worked on will be revealed one at a time and recovered afterwards, so relax and enjoy yourself.

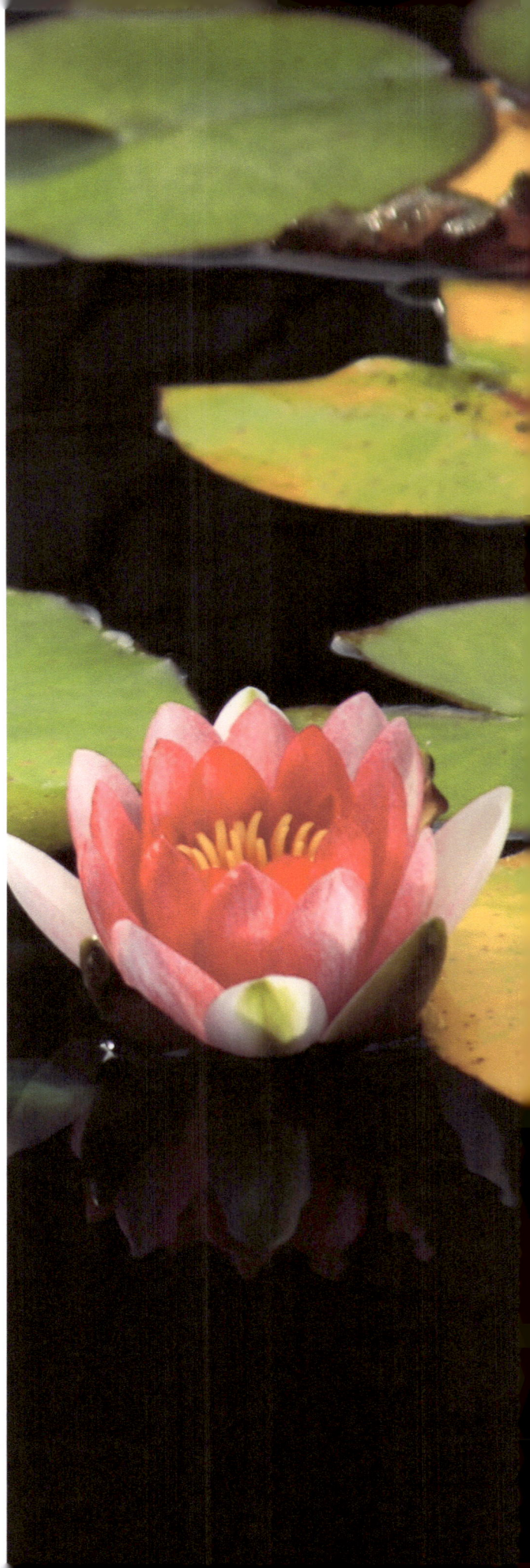

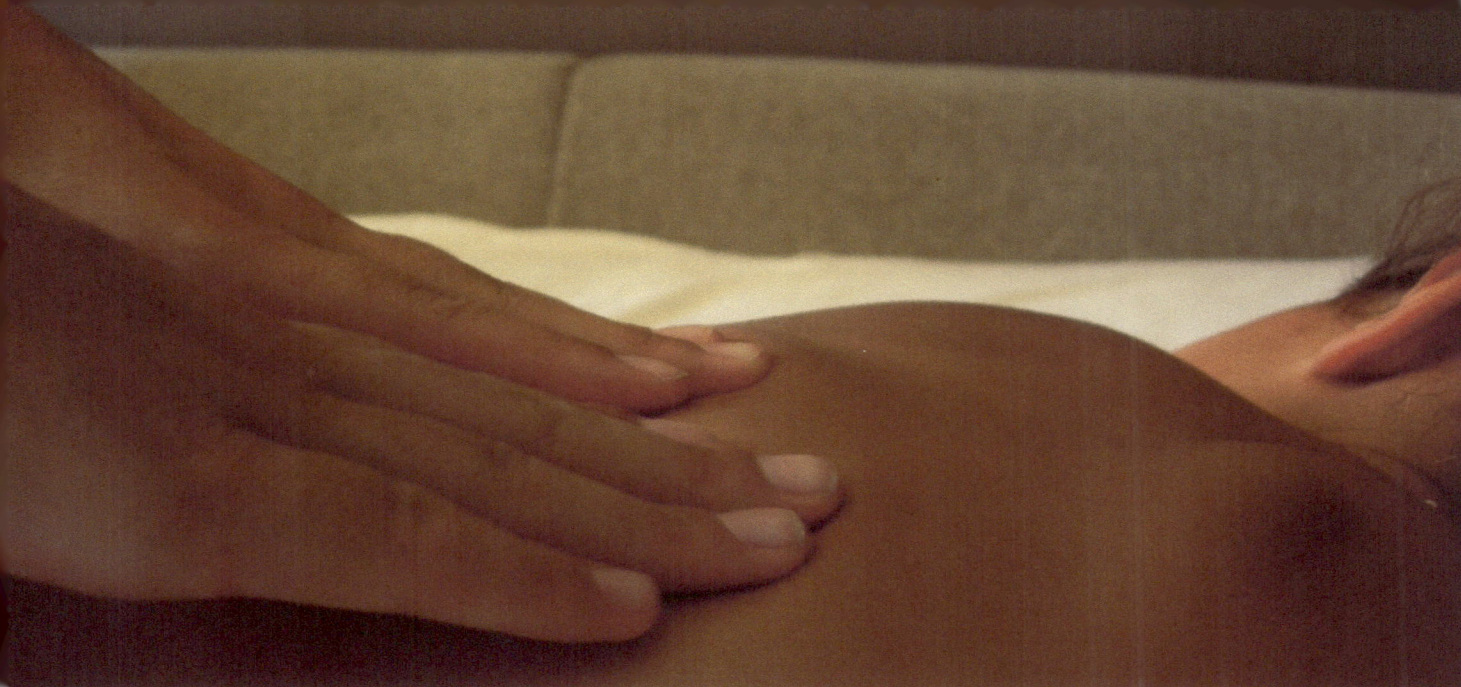

Feel Free to Talk But Expect Time to Fly:

The idea of talking during your massage should always be left up to you as a therapist is not being quiet to be rude but to let you relax. Sometimes the therapist needs to force you to relax, but it's always up to you whether you want to talk. The catch with talking is that your time flies so much faster, and not all therapists are great at multitasking; so you might lose some quality on your Zen time. This is totally up to you, but I suggest you just enjoy some "you" time and stay quiet in your head.

Tip Generously:

Your therapist will always see how much you tip and although most aren't trying to buy a new car with your tip, the amount is basically a sign of gratuity and respect for how they treated you. This small token of your appreciation can double their flexibility with you and even shoot up the quality because they feel valued and appreciated. Typical tip is 20% for a great job and 15% should it not be everything you wanted but were still happy. Any less will say you just weren't happy or didn't care for the service. In that same breath, they will know if you just didn't care for them; so avoid the same therapist if you just don't respect him/her enough to tip properly.

Give Plenty of Notice When You Cancel:

Sometimes your therapist will be called in just for you, and if you cancel right before, the therapist is stuck at the spa without getting paid (not to mention all the fees you may incur as a result). Spas are very nice about rescheduling you, but if you cancel too often, you will get a reputation, so be considerate. Aim for 24 hours if you need to cancel.

Use the Bathroom:

DON'T

Get Hurt:

It does not need to hurt to work. This is HUGE! A therapist causing excruciating pain is compensating for a lack of experience or education, and you should not suffer. It is very true that the deeper tissue treatments can be uncomfortable, but it should always be tolerable. On your personal scale of 1-10 with 1 being "are you even there?" and 10 being "get me off this table!" the deeper pressure session should range at heaviest a 6,7, or 8 at the very max; but 6-7 is best. Pressure of 9 or 10 will only hurt you and make things worse as it makes your body defend itself; and if your therapist doesn't know that, run out the room. The only type of massage that is supposed to be the extreme levels of pain is called Rolfing, but that is a whole other word for professional athlete-type people, not your everyday spa goer. Every part of you is different. If something needs less or more pressure, speak up to enjoy yourself to the fullest. A good therapist will be happy that you did so they can give you their best.

Try to Get Freebies:

It doesn't feel great as a therapist having a client booked with a relaxing Swedish treatment who is clearly trying to get a freebie deep tissue to avoid the measly price difference. Usually the price difference is anywhere from $10-$20 for moving over to deep tissue land, and you may not see the big deal; but a therapist feels crummy and unvalued when someone tries to cheat him/her into working harder for free. You will likely get more pressure; but it won't be the best session you can have as your therapist, first of all, has to hold back to avoid getting in trouble; and secondly, I'm sure the therapist feels resentful and taken for granted. The small price difference will affect the quality of your session if you truly have those freebie intentions. Don't forget, though, that if you really just want to have a firm pressured Swedish massage, you are more than welcome to enjoy one; but don't ask for a knot or two to get worked out.

Get Intoxicated:

A drink or two is fine, but drinking too much before your massage can actually make you ill and extremely dehydrated to a dangerous degree.

No excuse for a spa faux pas!

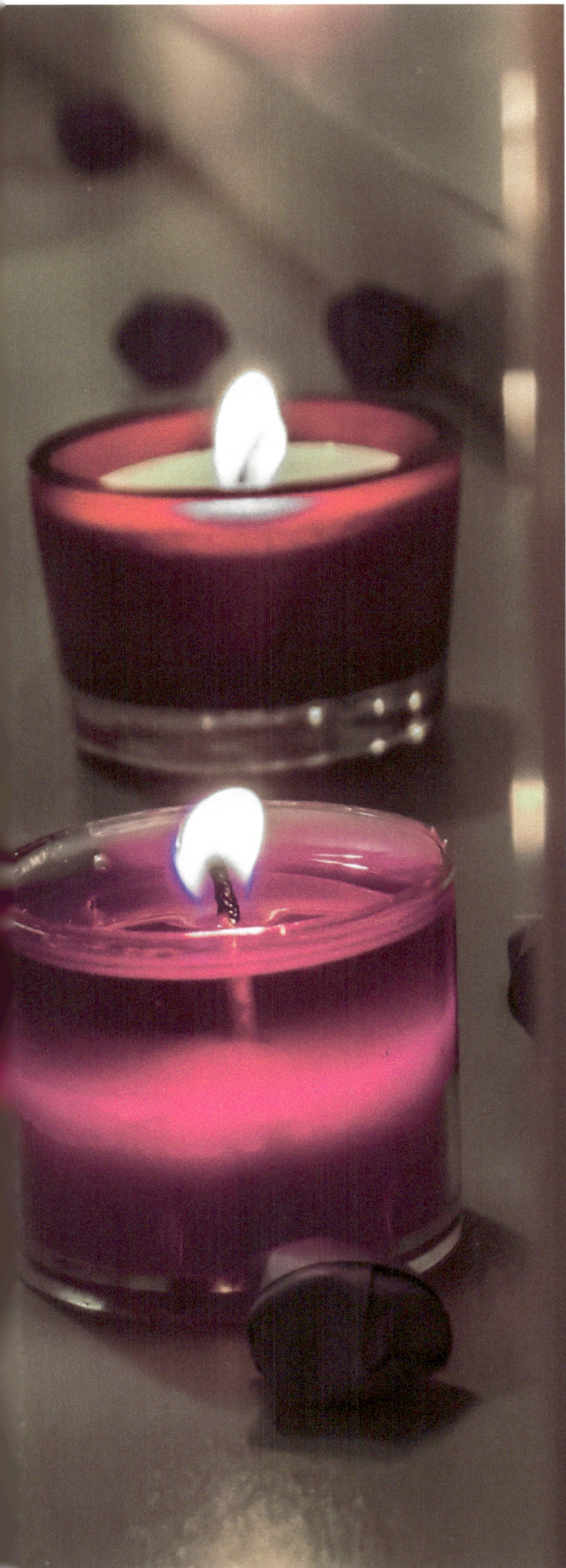

& Never

Duh . . . Pass Gas on Purpose:

If you subscribe to *Agenda*, you have a level of class, but for anyone who hasn't been schooled in social etiquette, continue reading. This should be an obvious one: Bodily functions happen, and if they do and are unavoidable, don't worry about it. Your therapist is a professional.

Worry About Body Hair:

Ladies, don't feel bad about not shaving. A therapist works on very grizzly men, so you are more like silk to them. You will feel better if you do shave; but if you don't, don't stress it and apologize for it. Just enjoy yourself.

Worry About Your Body:

Seasoned therapists have seen the human form in every shape, color, and size; and guess what. They just about all have the same parts (give or take). Don't worry about that scar or a few extra pounds; don't think about the tattoo or anything else for that matter. Just mentally let go and enjoy your body being rejuvenated.

Get Massaged When You're Sick:

You will not be able to fully enjoy your treatment, and there is the possibility that you will pass on your illness to the therapist and other guests. Stay home, rest, and come back when you are feeling wonderful and ready to feel amazing from your pamper session.

Linger Too Long After Done:

Keep in mind that your therapist has fewer than 10 minutes to walk you back and reset for the next guest.

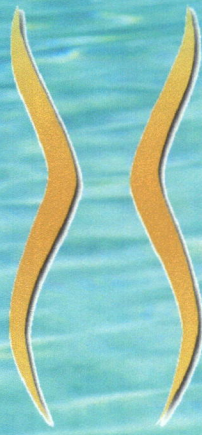

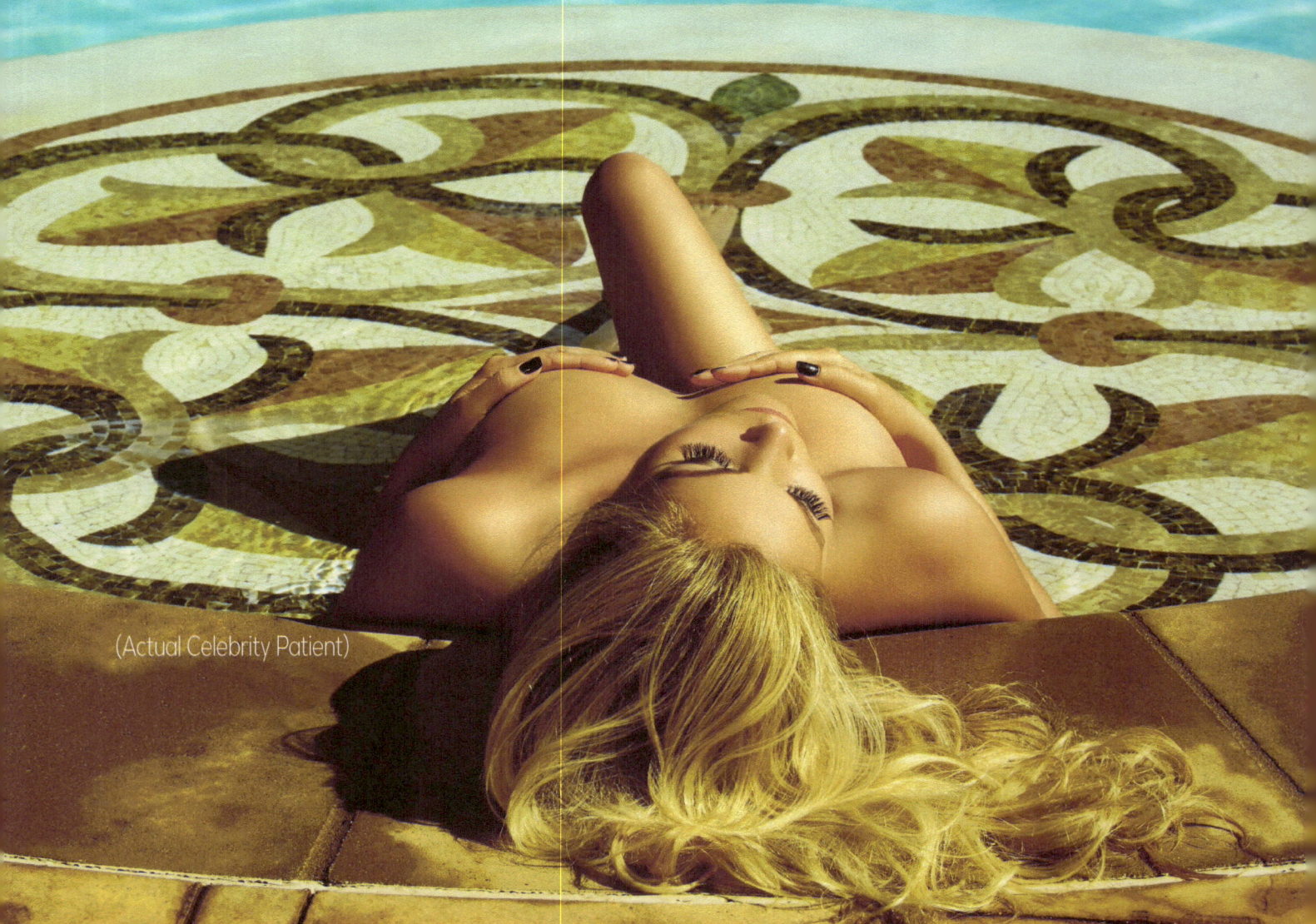

ELITE
BODY SCULPTURE

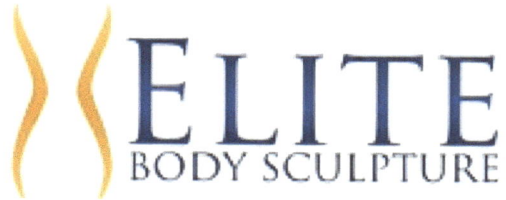

Specializing in
Removing Unwanted Fat

AirSculpt
Laser Liposculpture™

Up a Cup ™
(Natural Breast
Enhancement)

Brazilian Butt Lift
(Natural Buttock
Enhancement)

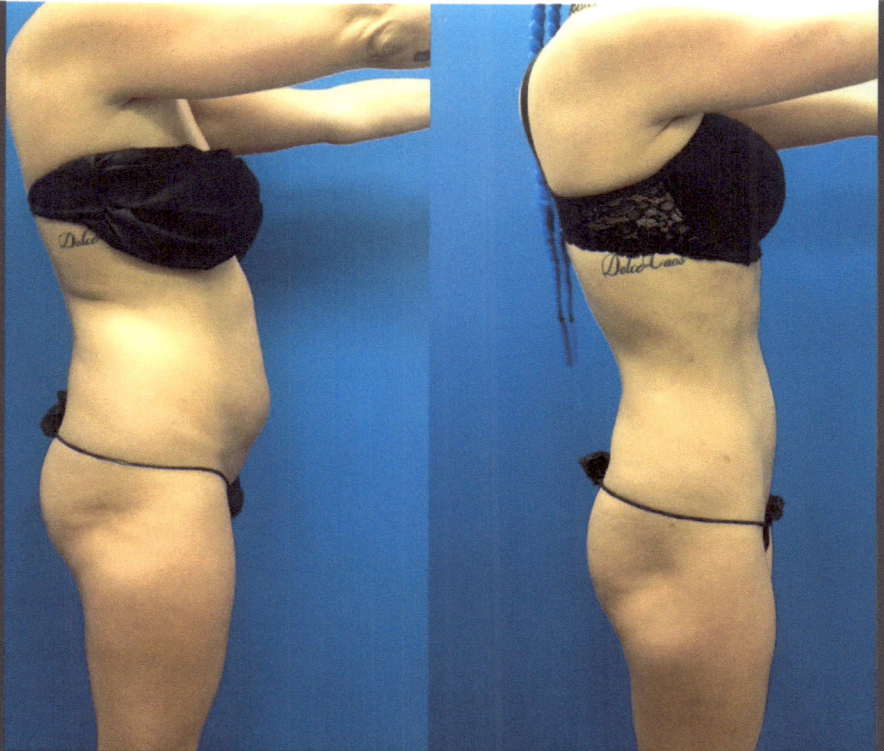

We offer minimally invasive laser procedures to give you a smoother result much faster than you ever imagined possible. Most patients are back at work in less than 48 hours!

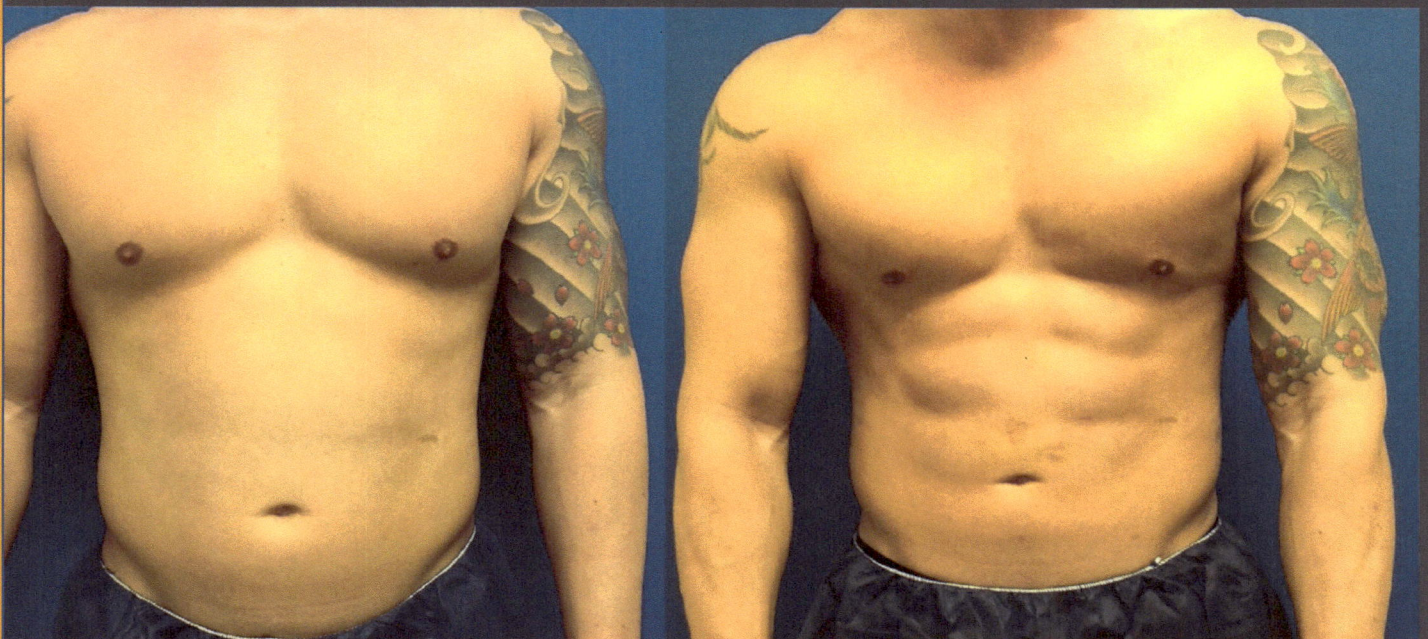

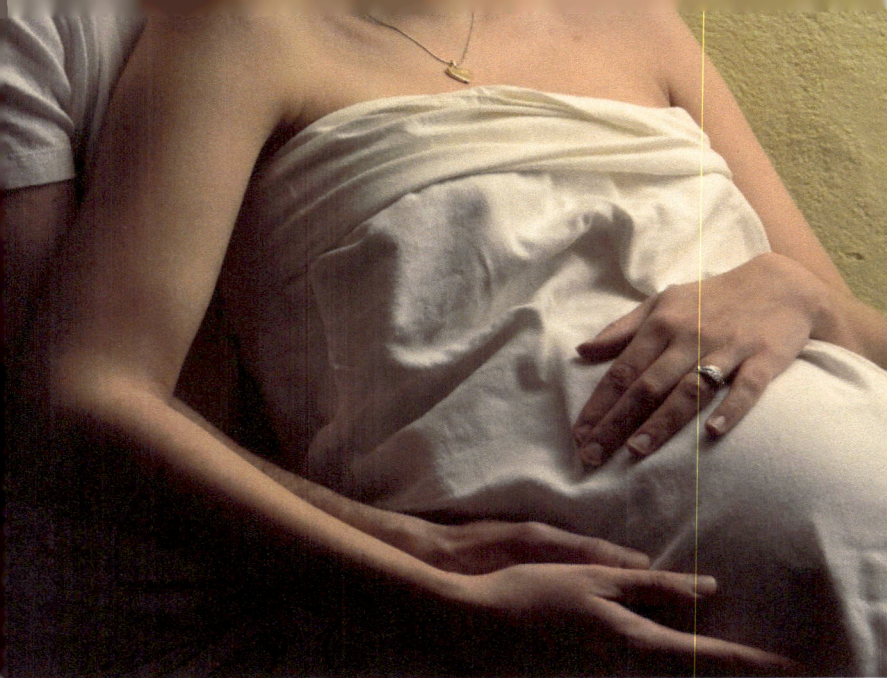

Fact 1

Obese youth are more likely to have risk factors for cardiovascular disease, such as high cholesterol or high blood pressure. In a population-based sample of 5- to 17-year-olds, 70% of obese youth had at least one risk factor for cardiovascular disease. Obese adolescents are more likely to have prediabetes, a condition in which blood glucose levels indicate a high risk for development of diabetes. (Facts 1-4 from Center for Disease Control)

CHILDHOOD

DON'T LET THIS HAPPEN TO YOUR LITTLE ONE.

BY KAYLENE PEOPLES

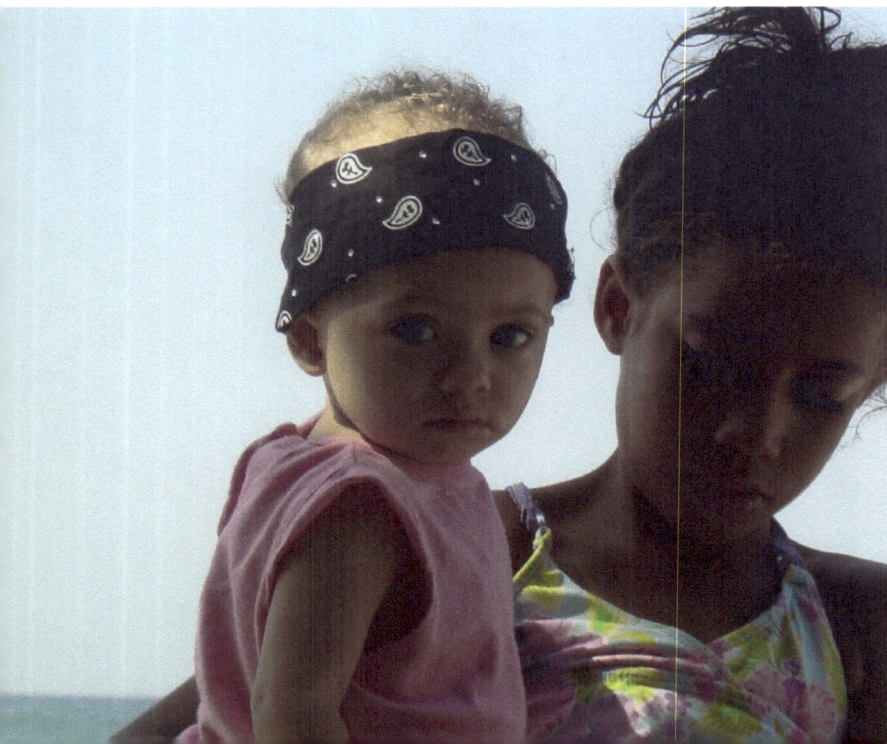

Fact 2

Children and adolescents who are obese are at greater risk for bone and joint problems, sleep apnea, and social and psychological problems such as stigmatization and poor self-esteem. Children and adolescents who are obese are likely to be obese as adults and are therefore more at risk for adult health problems such as heart disease, type 2 diabetes, stroke, several types of cancer, and osteoarthritis.

Fact 3

Overweight and obesity are associated with increased risk for many types of cancer, including cancer of the breast, colon, endometrium, esophagus, kidney, pancreas, gall bladder, thyroid, ovary, cervix, and prostate, as well as multiple myeloma and Hodgkin's lymphoma. Healthy lifestyle habits, including healthy eating and physical activity, can lower the risk of becoming obese and developing related diseases.

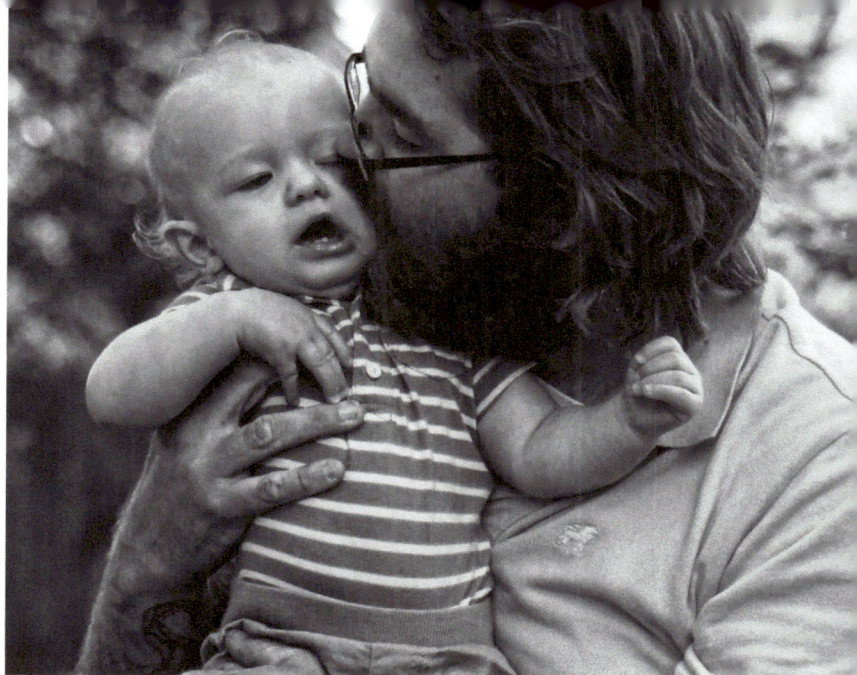

OBESITY

A PROBLEM OF EPIDEMIC PROPORTIONS IN THE 21ST CENTURY.

Fact 4

The dietary and physical activity behaviors of children and adolescents are influenced by many sectors of society, including families, communities, schools, child care settings, medical care providers, faith-based institutions, government agencies, the media, and the food and beverage industries and entertainment industries. Schools play a critical role by establishing a safe and supportive environment with policies and practices.

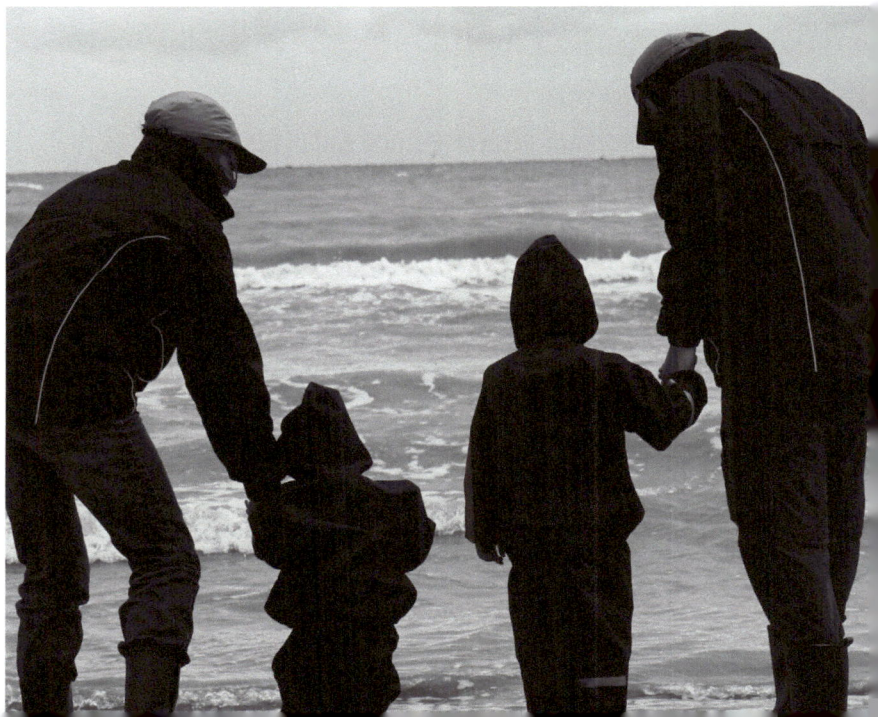

So you are working out. With regular visits to the gym, yoga classes in the evenings, and plenty of leafy greens, proteins, and grains, it surely looks as if you're taking the proper steps to ensure a long, productive, life. Congratulations! Let's jump ahead . . . you're married. You have two perfect kids. You and your spouse live an active lifestyle. There's only one problem, offspring number two is not as fit and doesn't want to join in when you go on your family hikes, jogs, ski trips, dog walks, etc. Nowadays children are at risk for all sorts of adult diseases. Childhood obesity is now common, and diabetes quickly follows, not to mention other weight-related health issues your child could acquire. Jeffrey, who is only 10 years old is flunking P.E. and is wearing the same size as Mark, his 14-year-old brother. You are concerned but don't know what to do about it. According to the Center for Disease Control, childhood obesity is a serious problem in the United States. For children and adolescents between 2-19 years of age, 12.7 million have been affected. There are many controversial views as to what's causing this epidemic of children growing up unhealthily. Sedentary lifestyles are the norm for a lot of kids these days, with computers, video games, and television, coupled with homework and cell phones. If your child is not naturally active, what motivation does he or she have to exercise or eat properly? Unfortunately, you cannot monitor your child at all times. After all, you have to go to work! Negative influences are everywhere, and you can't pick your child's friends all the time. So where do you start?

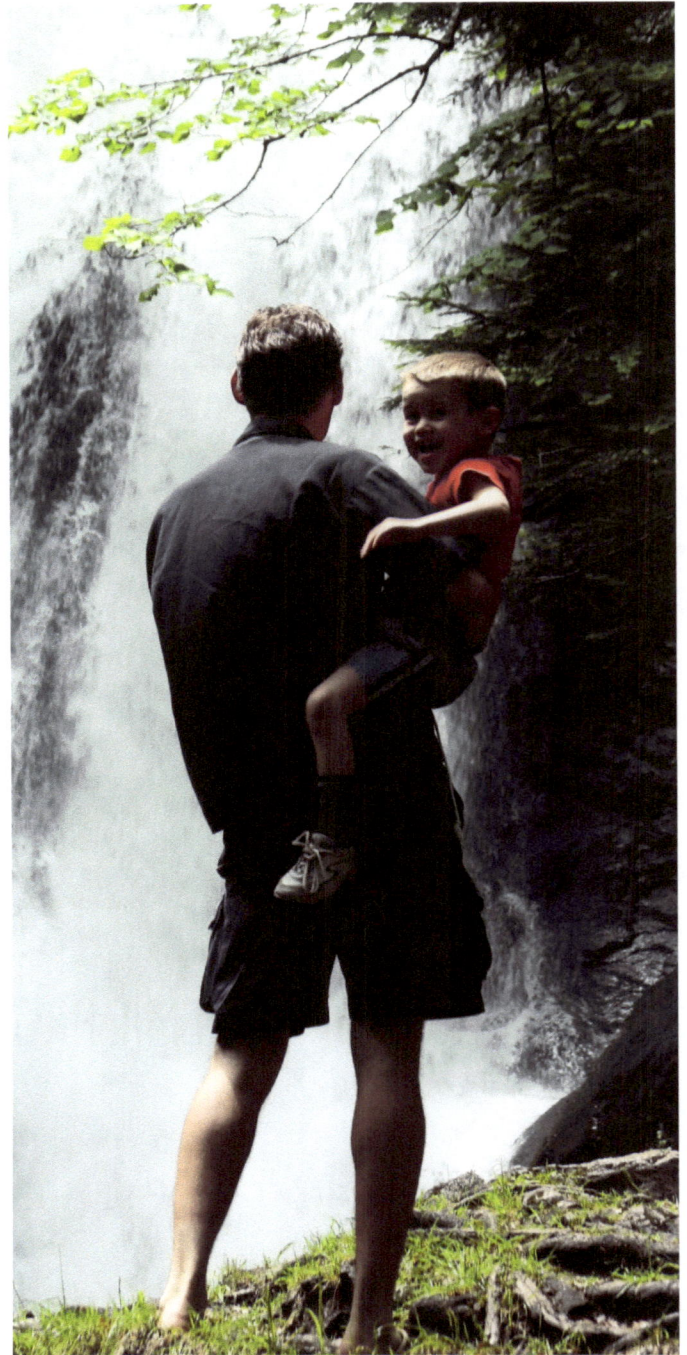

Practice Good Nutrition

Fast food chains are the biggest contributors when it comes to childhood obesity. This is a bad choice for nutrition. In fact there is very little nutritional value provided at most fast food chains. Instead of a Happy Meal, cook something your child will enjoy at home, and don't forget to offer a healthy sweet treat at the end of the meal. If your children grow up with healthy eating habits and a working knowledge of what to eat and what not to eat, they will be less likely to overeat and gain unhealthy weight. Knowledge is everything, and your kids will learn from your example. It's up to you to teach them how to eat the right way. (For nutritional advice, visit kidshealth.org.)

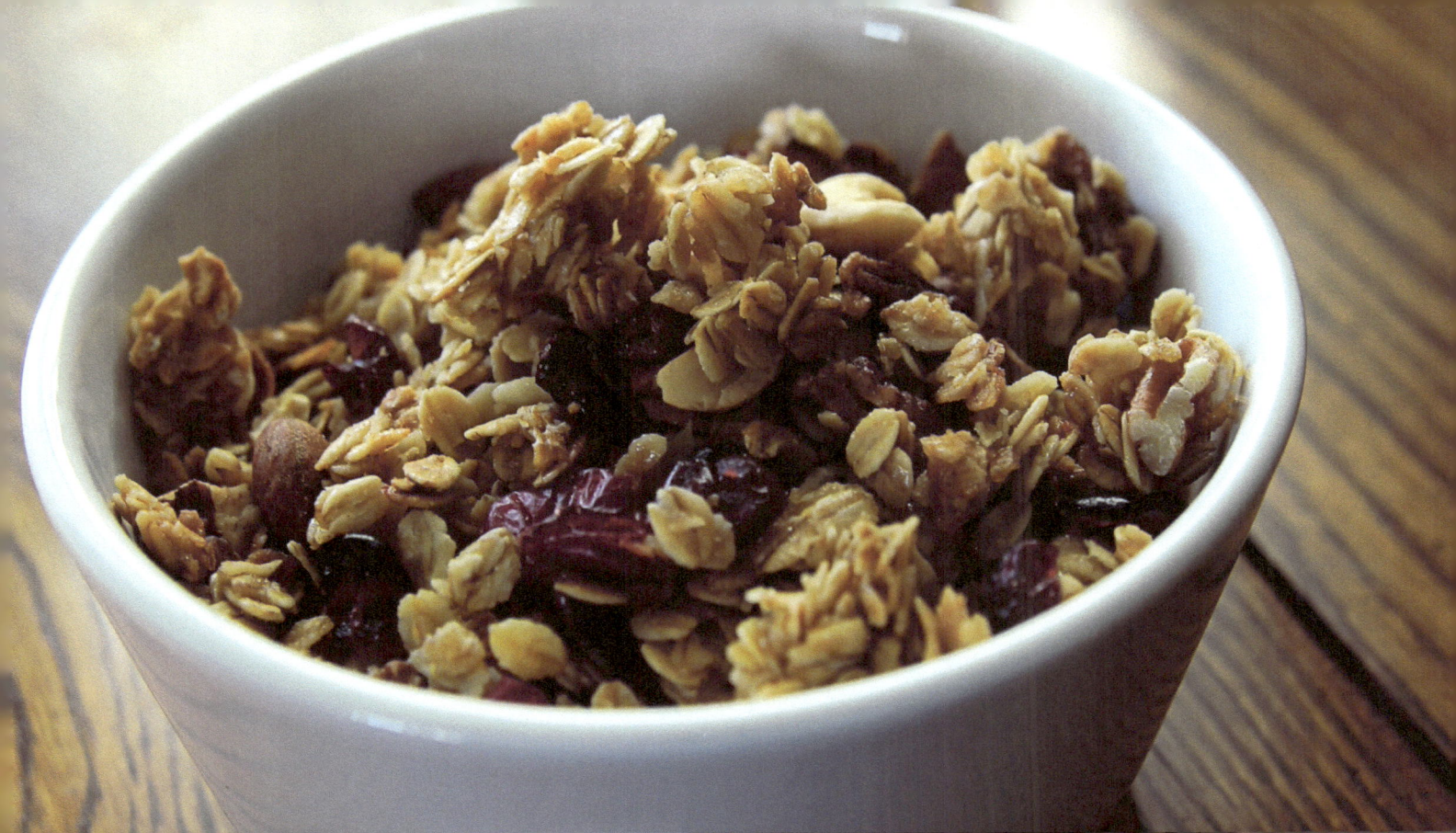

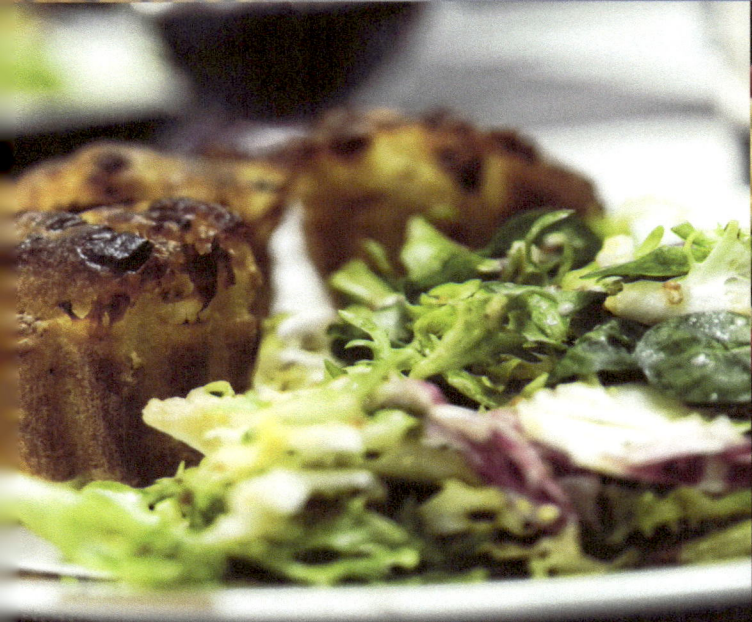

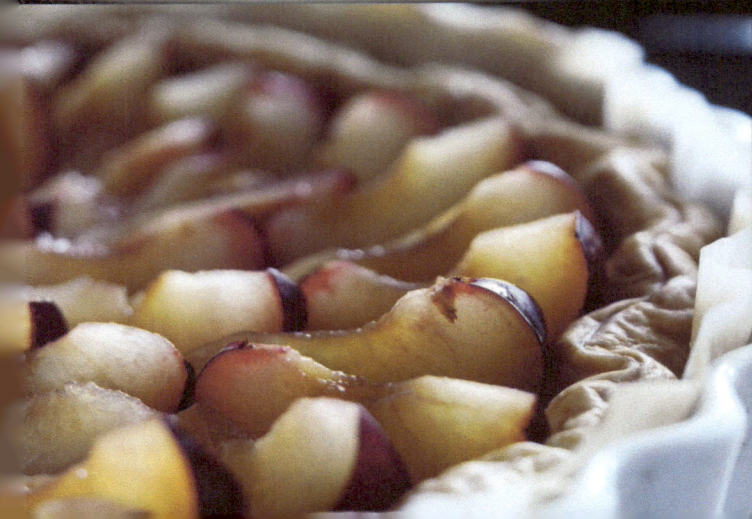

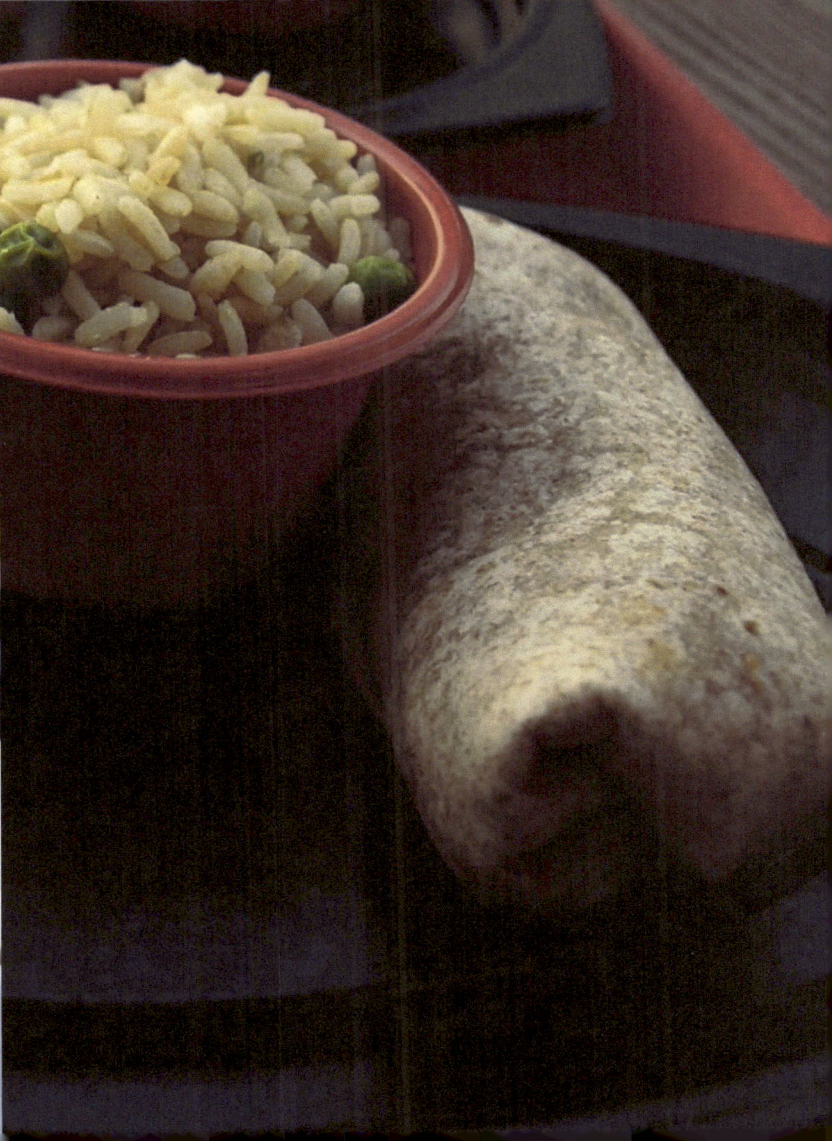

Choose an activity your child likes.

First of all, finding an age-appropriate activity or sport can be challenging if all your child does is play with electronics. But there are electronic-based activities the entire family can enjoy. So let's start with those.

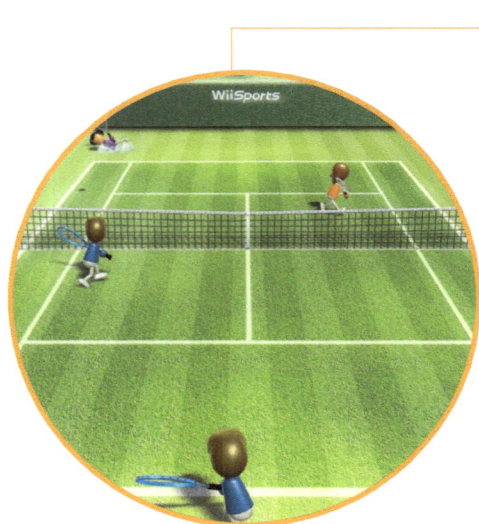

01

Nintendo Wii Sports - According to Nintendo, "This is what video games should be: fun for everyone. Wii Sports offers five distinct sport experiences, each using the Wii remote controller to provide a natural, intuitive and realistic feel. To play a Wii Sports game, all you need to do is pick up a controller and get ready for the pitch, serve, or that right hook. If you've played, watched, or read about any of these sports before, you're ready for fun!" These games retail for $19.99 each. The games are tennis, baseball, golf, and boxing. Other Wii products also offer other games with the following sports: basketball, wrestling, soccer, NASCAR, roller-skating, bowling, and so much more.

As an avid bowler, I enjoy a good game with Wii with my friends. You are still using the muscles that you would when actually playing the sport of your choice. Wii provides great cardio, and most importantly, it gets your body moving! Wii doesn't replace the actual sport, but it serves as a great substitute for healthy activity when there is no alternative to exercise available.

02

Organized Sports – Did you know that being involved in an organized sport has been proven to raise children's IQ levels? According to sports psychology author Jim Taylor, PHD, "Endurance sports have been found to enhance brain development and raise IQ. Sports build confidence, develop focus, and teach kids about emotional control. Kids learn essential life skills, such as hard work, patience, persistence, and how to respond positively to setbacks and failure."

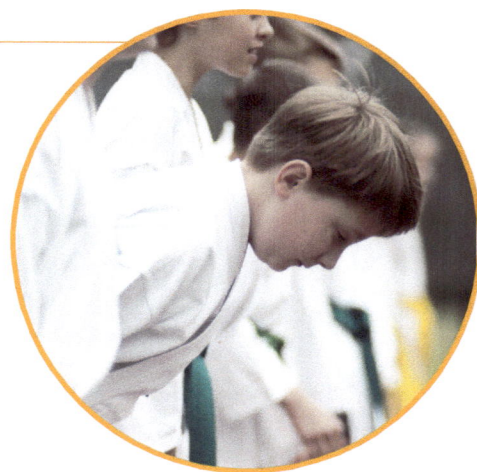

My 12-year-old nephew's self-esteem skyrocketed after his involvement on his school's swim team. I remember asking him last year when he first joined how he felt about doing a sport in school. He was nervous and timid about his involvement. Now, just a short year later, he has won so many ribbons, and he is more self-confident. He has also trimmed down quite a bit, and he is well on his way to enjoying fitness. The added benefits include learning how to be on a team, accepting defeat, experiencing victory, learning discipline, taking direction, maintaining a certain G.P.A. to keep the privilege of competing, and so many more benefits.

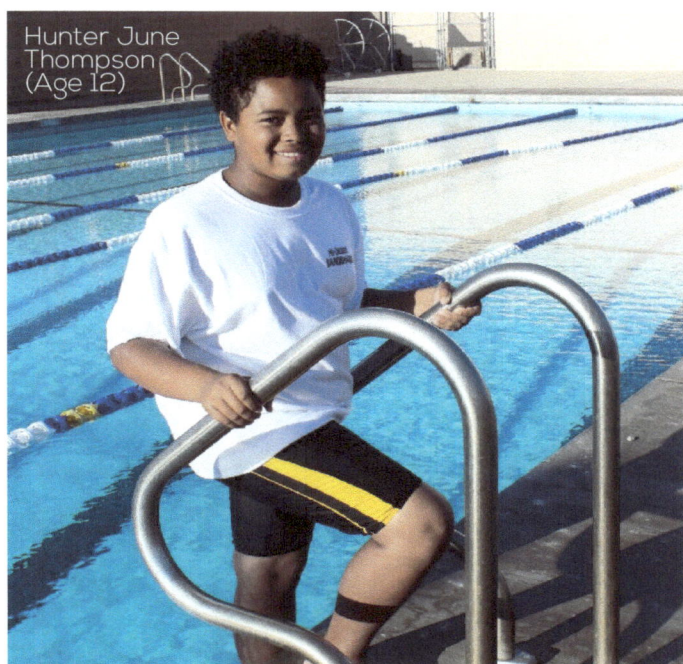

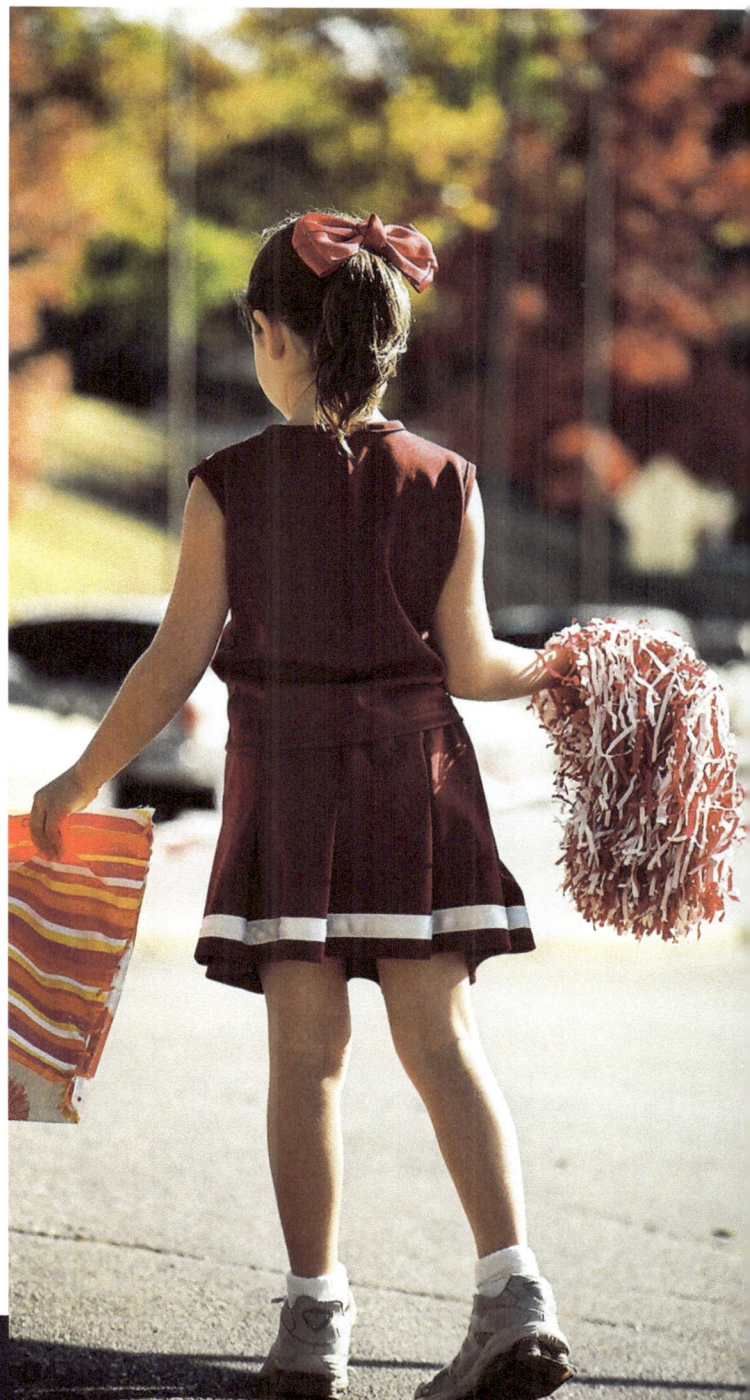

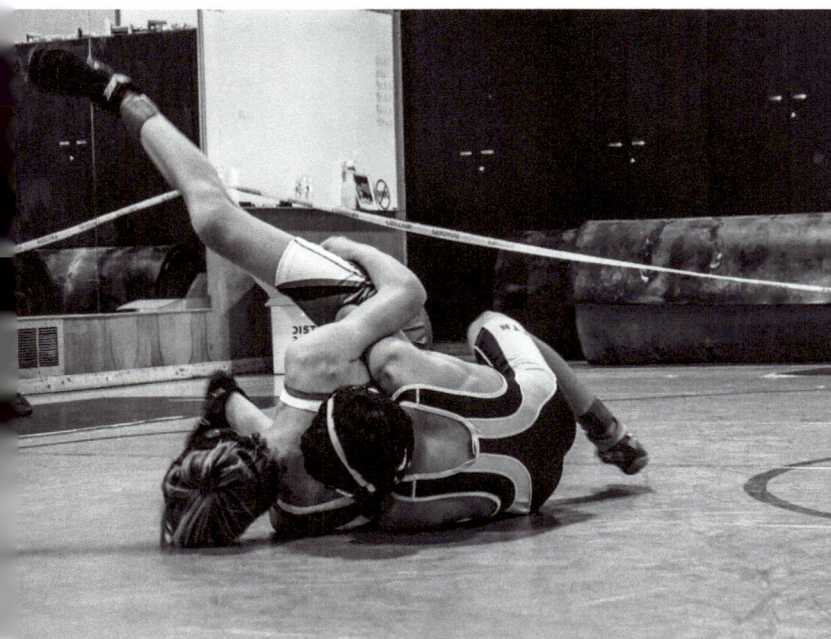

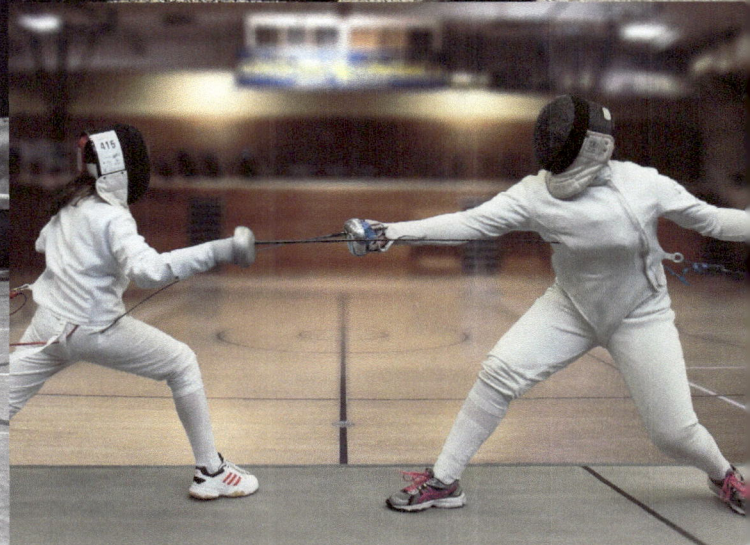

Hunter June Thompson (Age 12)

A HAPPY CHILD IS AN ACTIVE CHILD!

Whether your child is at risk of becoming overweight or currently at a healthy weight, you can take pro-active measures to get or keep things on the right track. Here are some key points to remember:

1. Limit your child's consumption of sugar-sweetened beverages

2. Provide plenty of fruits and vegetables

3. Eat meals together as a family as often as possible

4. Limit eating out, especially at fast food restaurants

5. Adjust portion sizes appropriately for age

6. Limit TV and other "screen time" to less than 2 hours a day

(The Mayo Clinic)

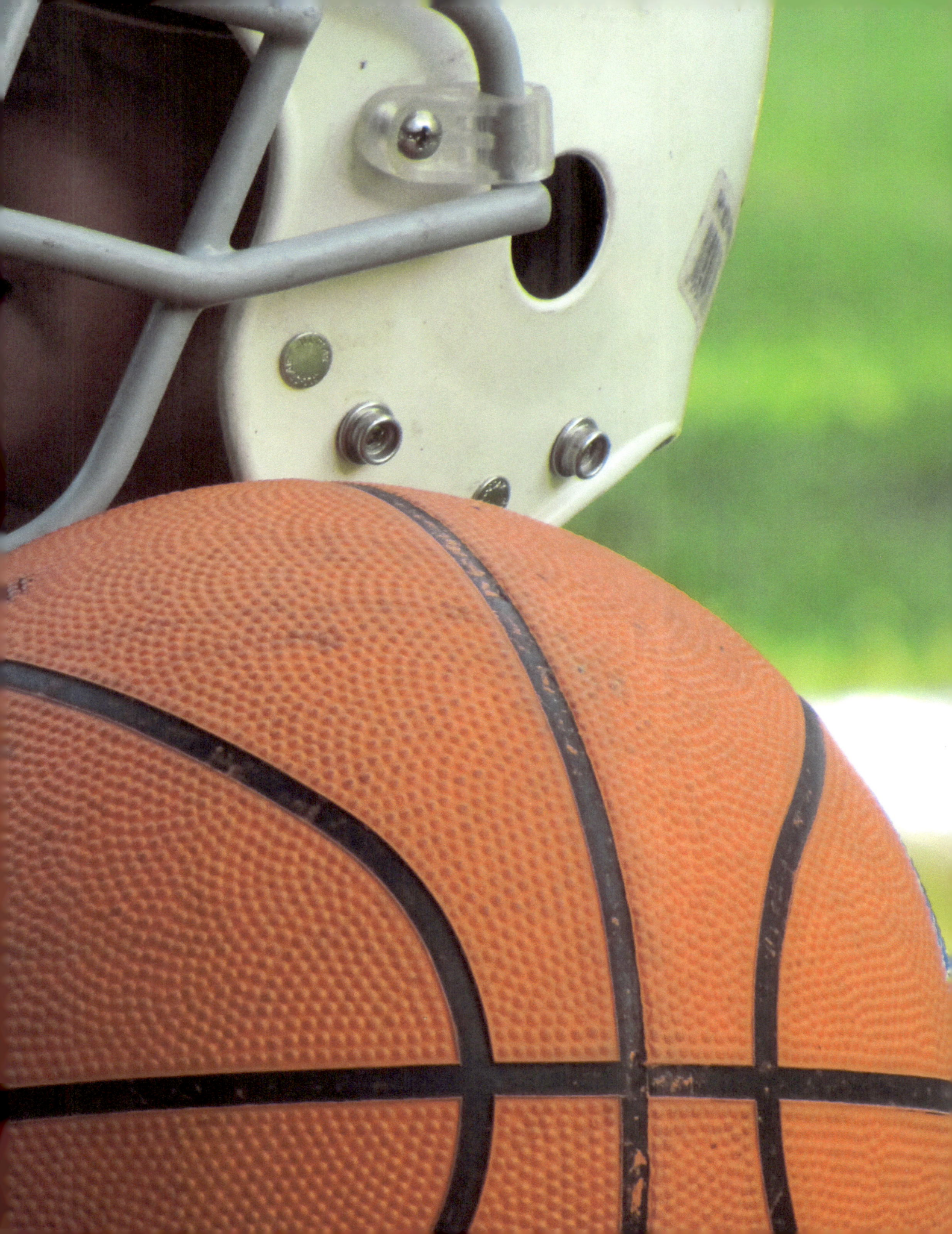

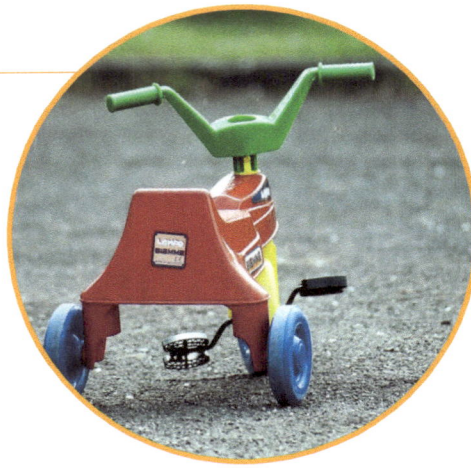

03

Get Things with Wheels! – As early as 2 years old, your child can be riding his/her tricycle and building muscles. What is great about a bike, or rollerblades, or even traditional roller skates is the whole family can partake in this activity. Did you know that one hour of bike riding can burn up to 600 calories? The same goes for rollerblading. So what are you waiting for? Just remember to practice safety. Always wear a helmet and kneepads. Make sure your child's bike has reflectors, a light, and that your tires are always filled with enough air.

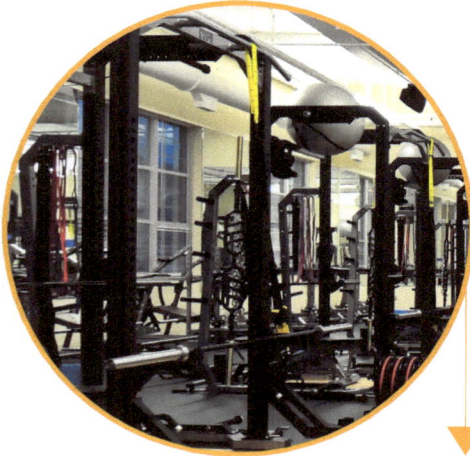

04

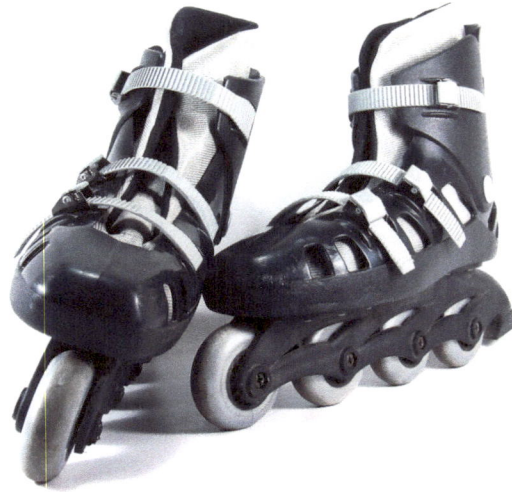

The Dreaded Exercise DVDs and Indoor Sports Machines – This is my least favorite, but could work for your sedentary child if done right. Depending on your budget and the size of your rooms, you may be able to furnish a gym in your home. My recommendation for motivation is to get a flat screen TV and strong Internet, and start building your home gym with an elliptical machine or a treadmill; some weights, yoga mats, and a killer stereo system. Make the room off-limits unless your child promises to work out in it. This is a very expensive way to stay fit, but it's worth it to get your child moving. The children can listen to their mp3s while exercising on a machine. They can be on the bike watching a movie, or get involved in an exercise DVD. They can do this as often or as little as they like. They can invite their friends to work out with them at home, also. This beats having to go to practice, suit up for a game, or even leave the house if the weather is bad. This is not a bad way to go. I strongly suggest you make this room as enticing as possible. Set limits, rules, and guidelines. Offer rewards for progress. Always keep a scale in your home gym.

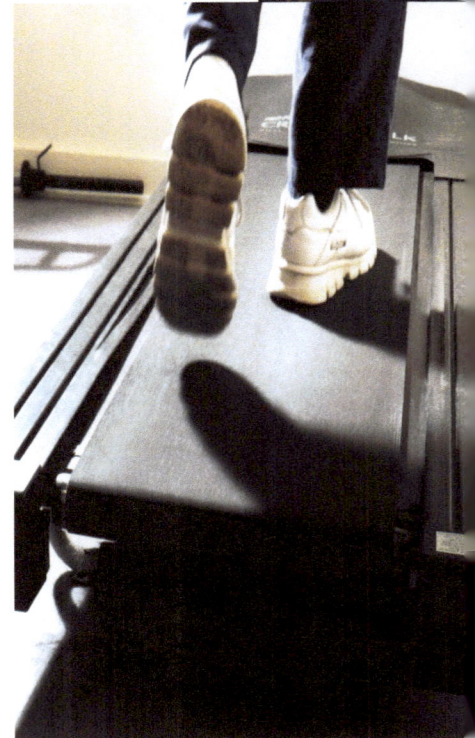

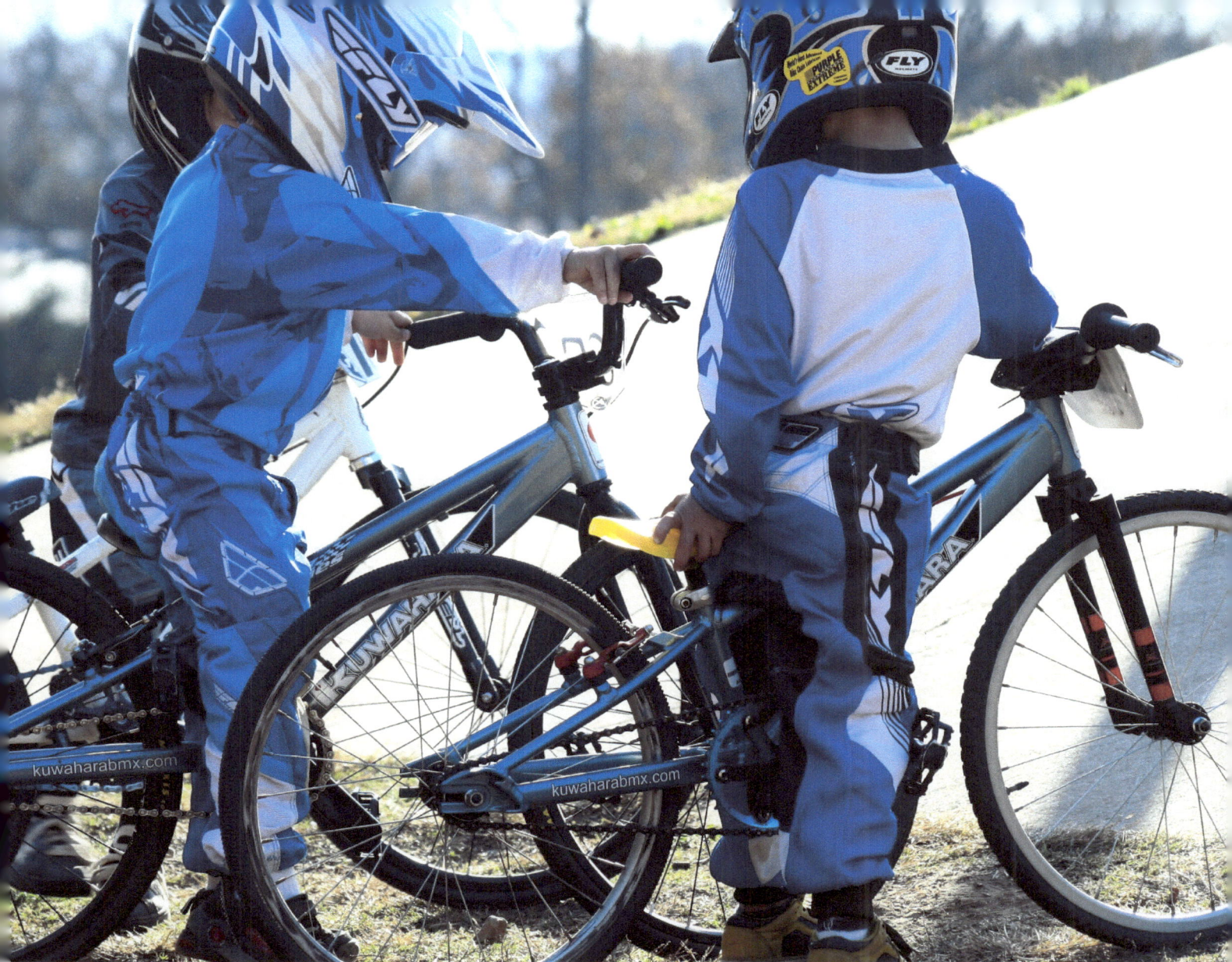

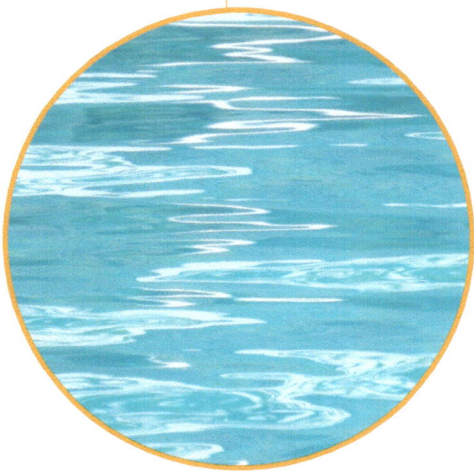

05

Get a Pool – Having a pool in the backyard has kept many children physically active just out of the sheer joy of hanging out with their friends, playing Marco Polo, diving off the board, racing together. The children who swim together remain friends forever! Plus it's a whole lot of fun. There are other outdoor options in your home, depending on your lot size: tennis court, basketball court, trampoline . . . The list is endless.

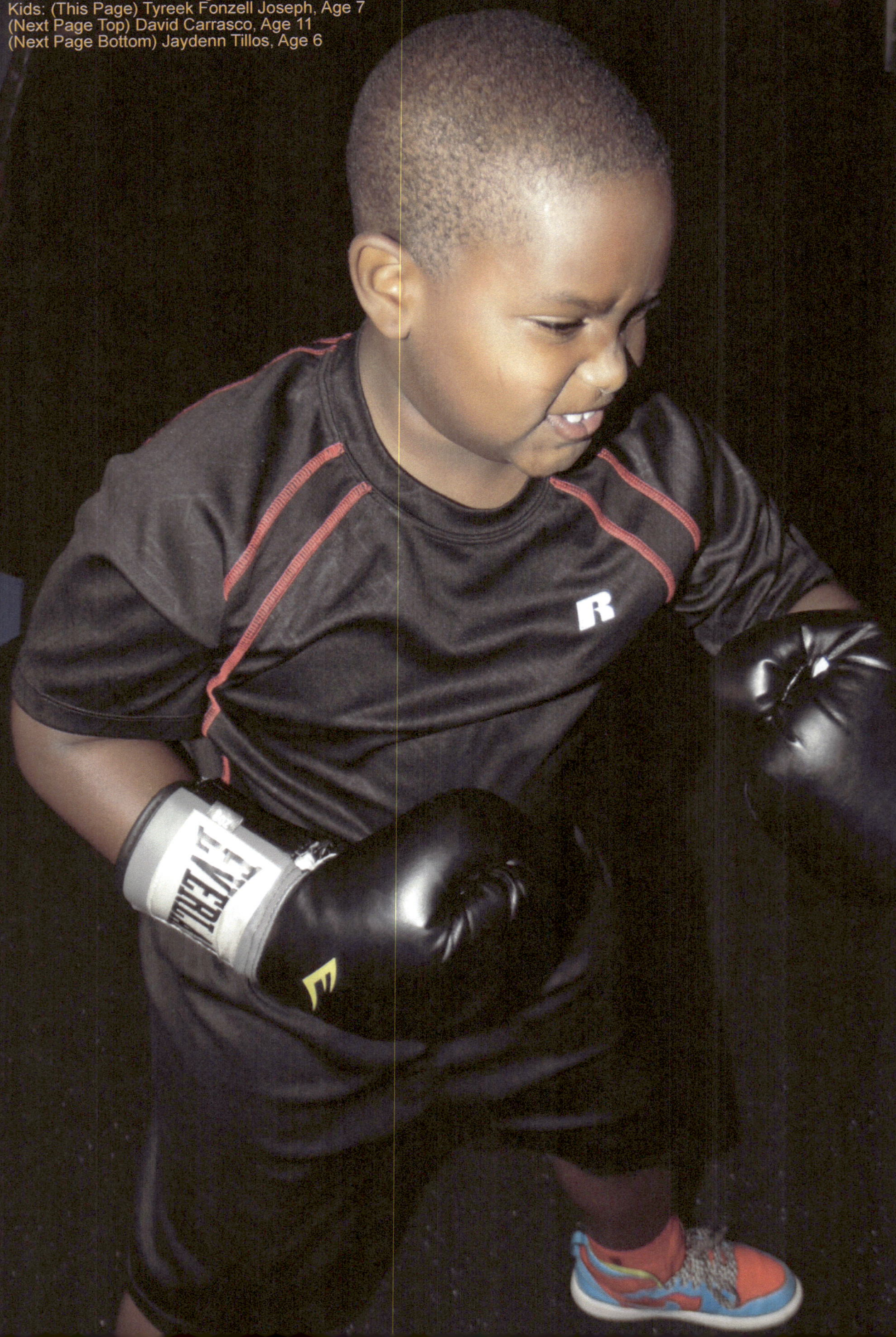

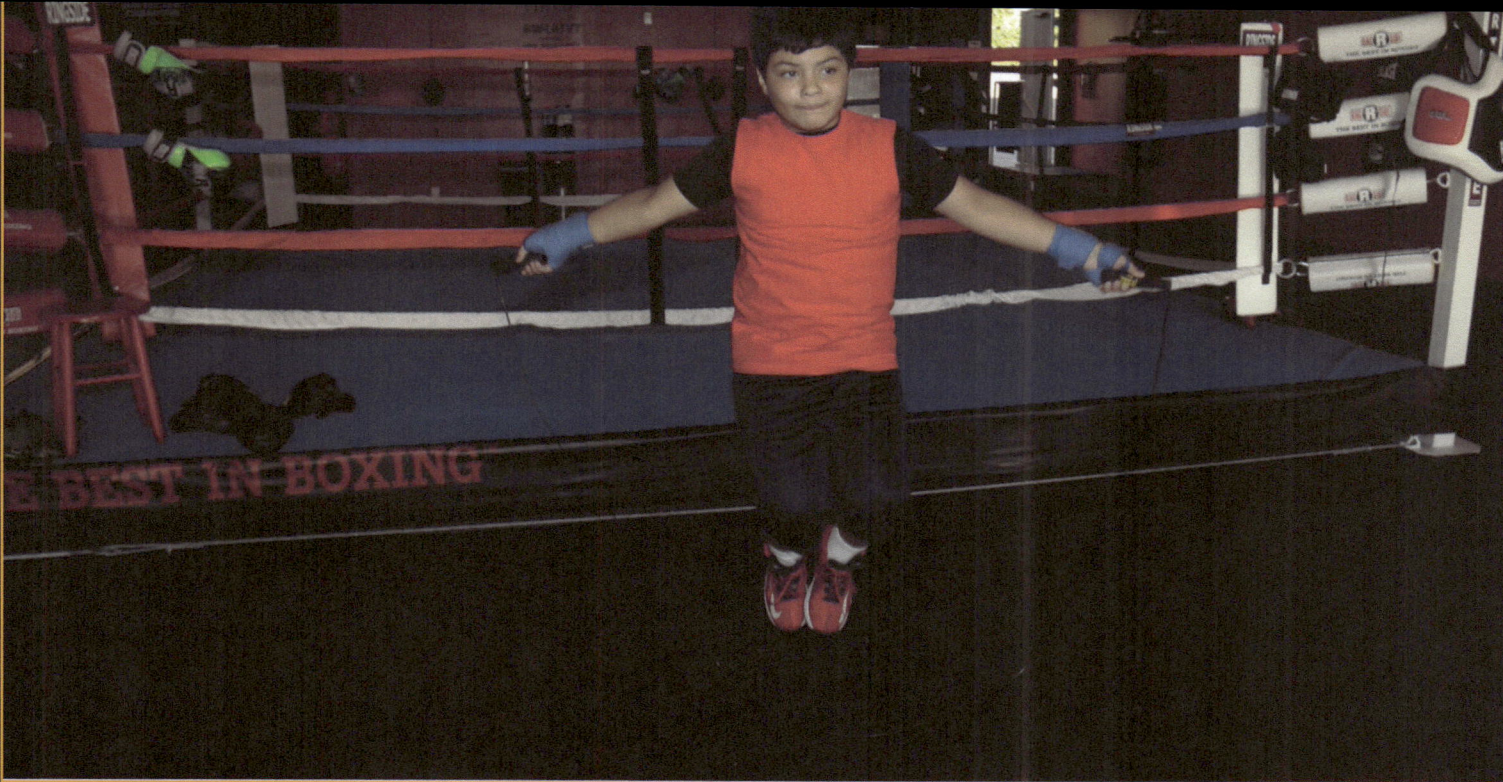

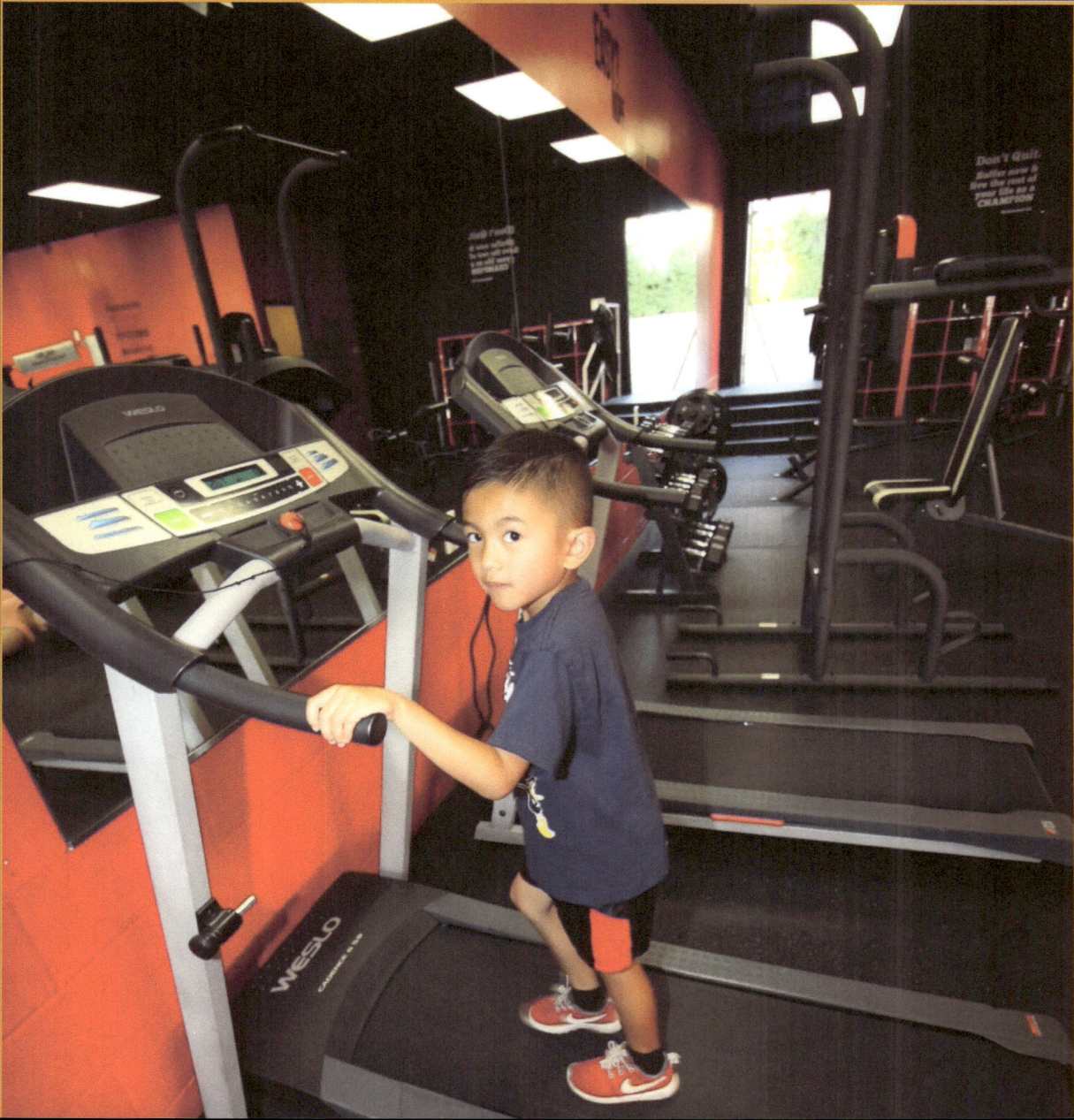

Kids love to move!

There are so many sports and activities in which your child can excel while having a great time.

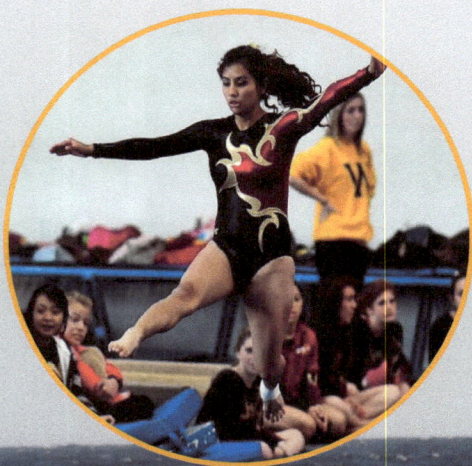

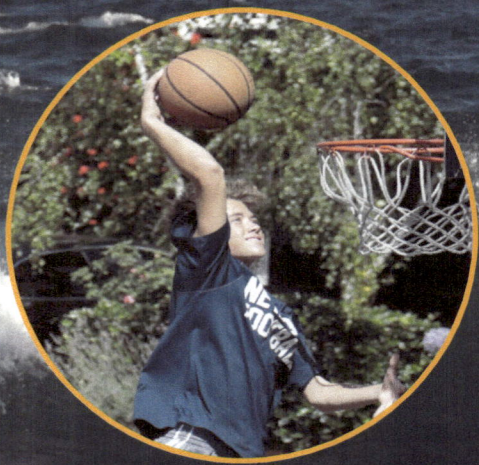

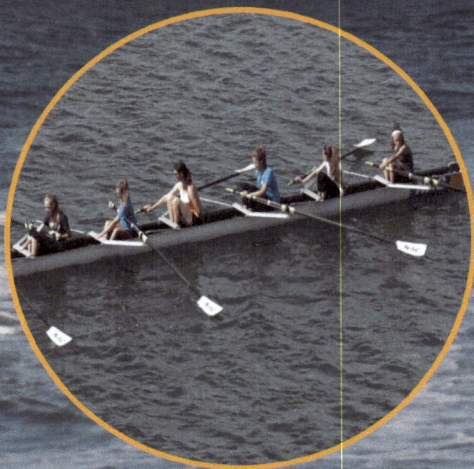

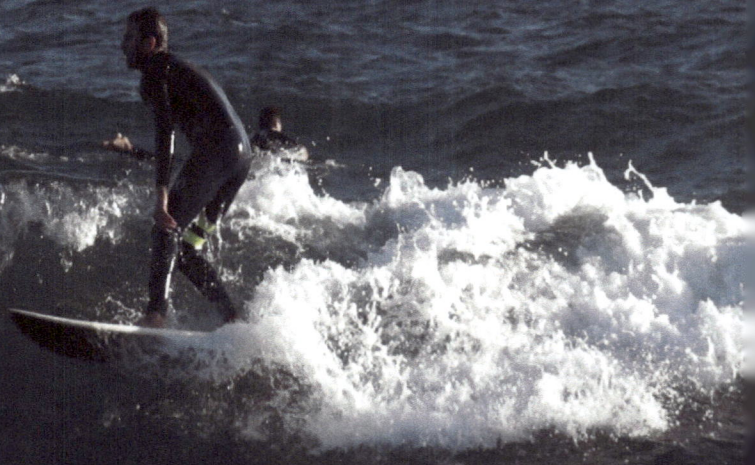

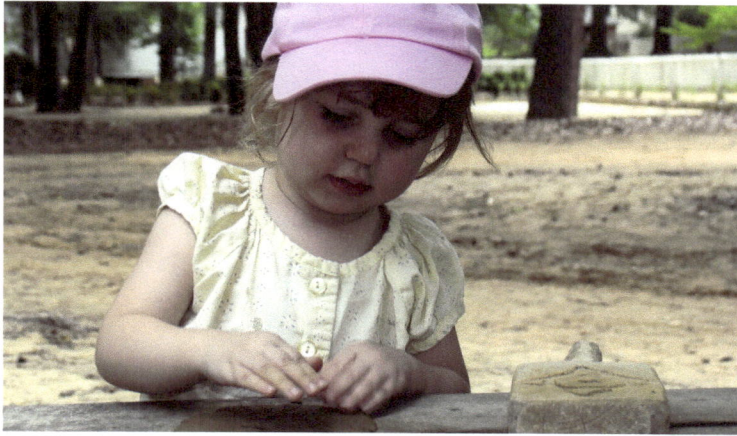

06

Community Centers, Day Camps – Most neighborhoods offer activities for children at their community centers. If your child is shy, this may be a good alternative, giving him/her a chance to meet other kids and share similar interests, while being active. The prices for activities vary, but they are usually very reasonably priced. Day Camps usually are offered during the summer, and are similar to community centers. Your child can be involved in a fun activity such as kayaking, volley-ball at the beach, hiking, and more. Day camps provide lunch, and there is adult supervision at all times. Prices vary.

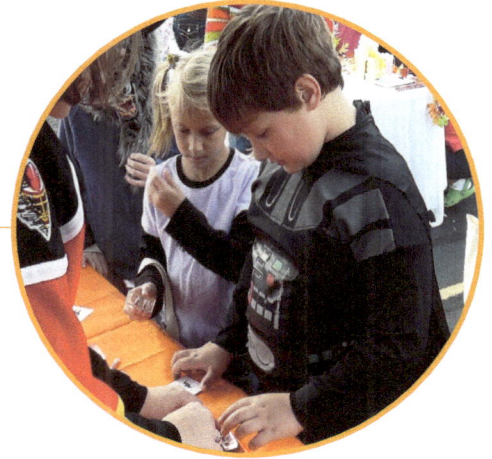

07

Scouts – As old as apple pie, the Girl Scouts, Boy Scouts, Brownies, Cadets, etc., have been around forever. I fondly remember my days as a Brownie. Scouting has always provided benefits to children, not only physically but emotionally. Your child will learn integrity, life skills, and will be engaged in social interaction with his/her peers.

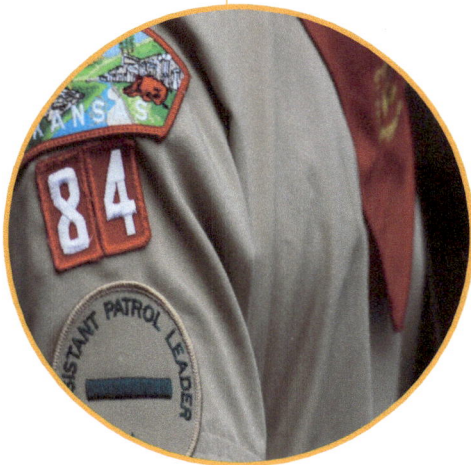

I hope these tips can get your sedentary offspring off the computer and onto getting physically fit. Remember, with your guidance, you can ensure your child a happy, healthy, active way of being!

DANCE
FREAKING ' TASTIC
FITNESS
THE BENEFITS OF DANCING CALORIES AWAY!

BY ANTHONY HEREDIA

Dancing is one of the highest calorie burns around, and in my opinion, one of the most beneficial. You have so many fun options!

Why dread exercise when you can have fun? Fitness is a critical necessity in our lives for countless reasons, but that doesn't mean it has to be a tedious chore. When fitness becomes "funness," it ceases to become a chore and is now a treat. We explore the monumental benefits of dance on your overall life and not just your waist. You see, the key is to enjoy your exercise to significantly increase your odds of keeping at it long enough to reach those encouraging goals. A better you is a marathon, not a sprint; so you need to find options that encourage you to maintain them over your lifetime. On average an individual will stick to a program or plan for eight weeks at best before giving up. I personally would attribute this to the individuals simply not enjoying what they are doing, which is fine. It's not about perfection. Try something that sounds fun; and if it loses its luster, then it's time to change it up to keep on track. Weight loss is simple usage of stored energy (those pesky pounds), and you accomplish this by exerting yourself above normal demand on the body. So why not exert with a beaming smile, lights above you, ambiance in the air, and music coursing as it stimulates your senses, releasing all those feel good hormones and burning pounds away?

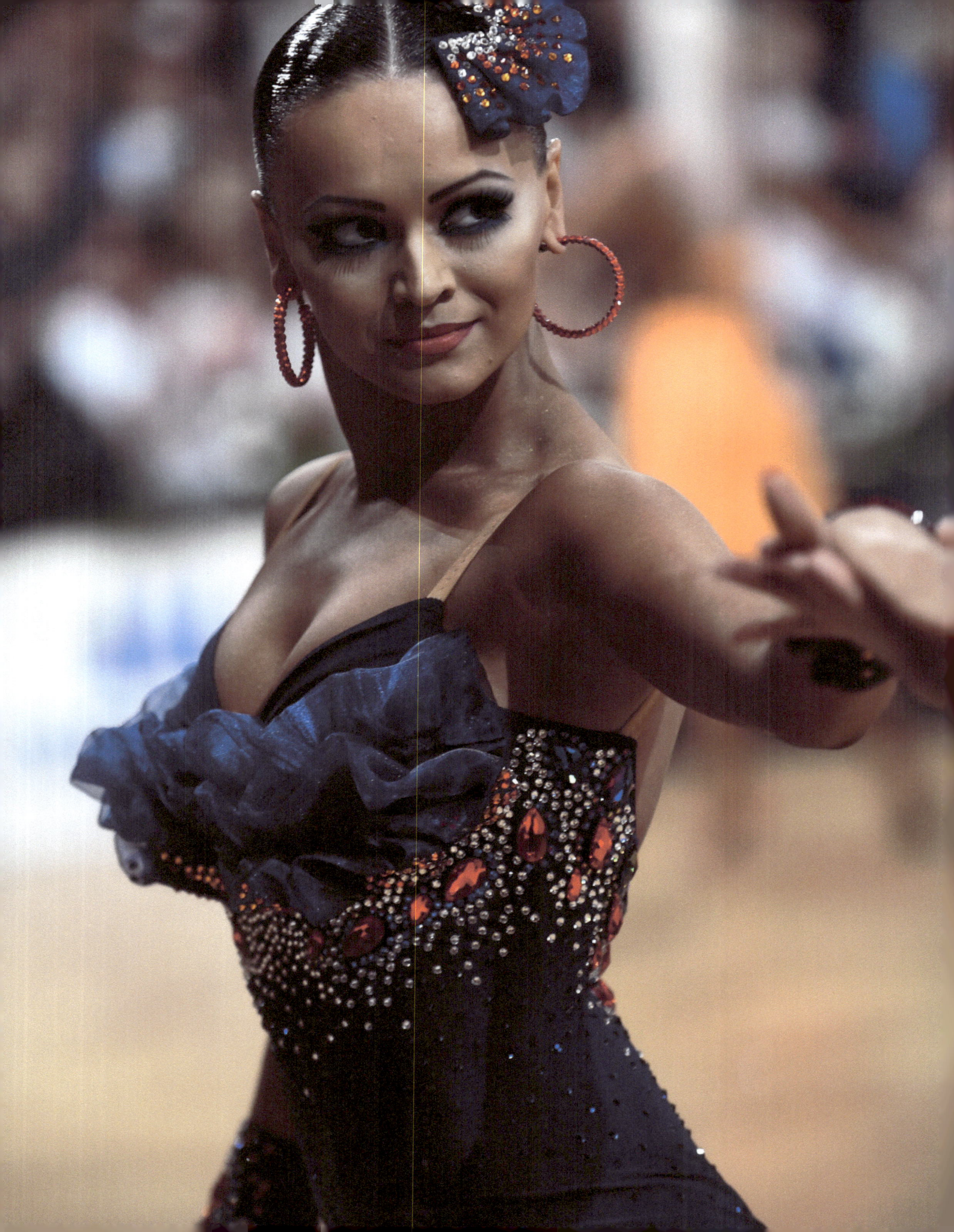

Studies have shown that one night of twirling on the dance floor can shave over 1000 calories, plus the calories burned as the muscles recover. A third of a pound in exchange for a night of fun . . . hmmm. . . . Let me think about that one. This is what I would love to open your eyes to, taking your workout, well . . . out! If you would like to know how many calories you burn during various other exercises, you can visit caloriecontrol.org. Dancing is one of the highest calorie burns around and, in my opinion, one of the most beneficial. You have so many fun options, like Zumba, Country, Belly Dancing, Salsa, Tap, Swing, even Pole Dancing. The bigger picture is that dancing helps to destroy stress, which is a plague upon our busy lives. Stress puts our bodies in self-defense mode and leads the body to store more body fat. Stress affects our mood, daily productivity, and our waist size by releasing high levels of cortisol into our system, which means more closet time for your little black dress, ladies, or that fitted suit for you gents. Remember that your body is not trying to give you a hard time. It is simply protecting itself, so let us work with it. Dancing reverses this whole ugly chain of events. Not a bad deal, wouldn't you say?

Let me put this all in perspective for you. One night of vigorous dancing (2-3 hours of semi-constant movement) can burn approximately 600-1000 calories, based on your weight and how much you're moving, of course. One pound of fat is 3500 calories, so that dazzling night of lights and feverish flavor just shaved off nearly a third of a pound with a huge smile on your face if you made an effort to move. Now, here is the bonus to all that twirling and laughing. I call it the "after burn." Let's reminisce if you will. I want you to go back to that one night where the drinks were flowing, the company was superb, every song was your song, and life just coursed through your every fiber. Remember how sore you felt the next day from all that dancing? Well, that's the "after burn." You see, your body isn't done working once you stop dancing. In fact, the work has just begun. Your body needs now to repair the muscles you just beat up from all your frivolity. You are now burning significantly more

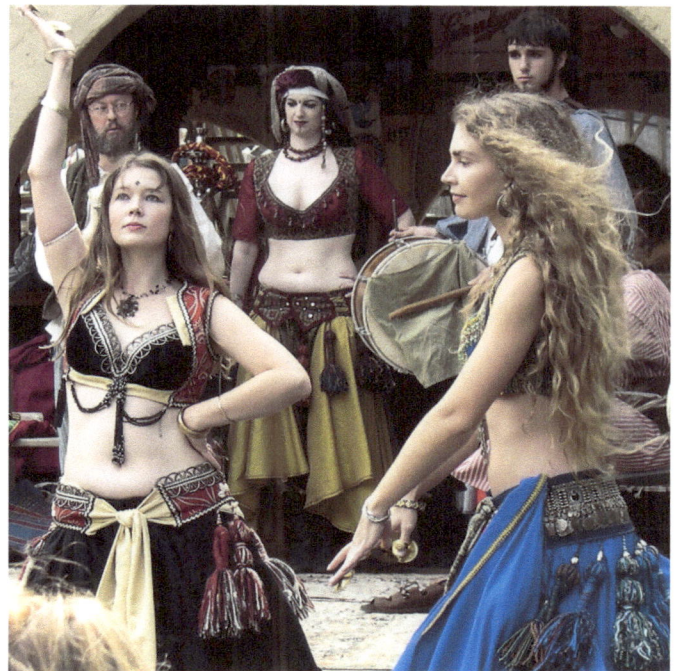

calories that night because your body is repairing the muscles while you sleep. You are burning higher fat while you sleep! Can it get any better than that? Well, actually it can, not to mention that from a good enough "workout," your metabolism is naturally heightened by up to 30% for the next three days as your body continues to do repairs from that one night.

Wow, do I really need to go on? To sum that all up, one night of fun equals nearly 900 calories, plus extra fat burned while you sleep, plus 30% metabolic boost for the next three days equals a grand total of anywhere between 1400-2000 calories burned from one night of fun. Please make a note not to forget about the crucial stress release you get from all this, which will really benefit your life all around by making you become more productive, sleep better, and enhance your moods and relationships overall. If you are not sold by now, then I quit. You see, the concept is to personalize exercise so that it becomes a way of life. If you find your niche, you might not need to "exercise" another day in your life. Wow, what a modern concept! I say it's time for us to take back our health by personalizing fitness to suit our passions, not what they tell us. I propose a toast to heavenly curves and a long healthy life with a smile on our faces! Cheers!

Yoga
Benefits

Photographed by Ash Gupta
with Diane Grinley for 838 Media Group
Clothing courtesy of Temple Flower Activewear
Modeled by Jasmina Hdagha
Written by Kaylene Peoples

Breathing is relaxing .

Yoga causes less stress and more calm. Certain
yogas incorporate meditation and relaxation,
which help you to focus better.

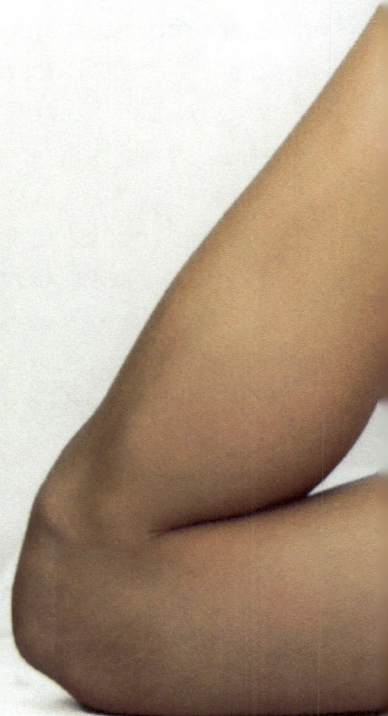

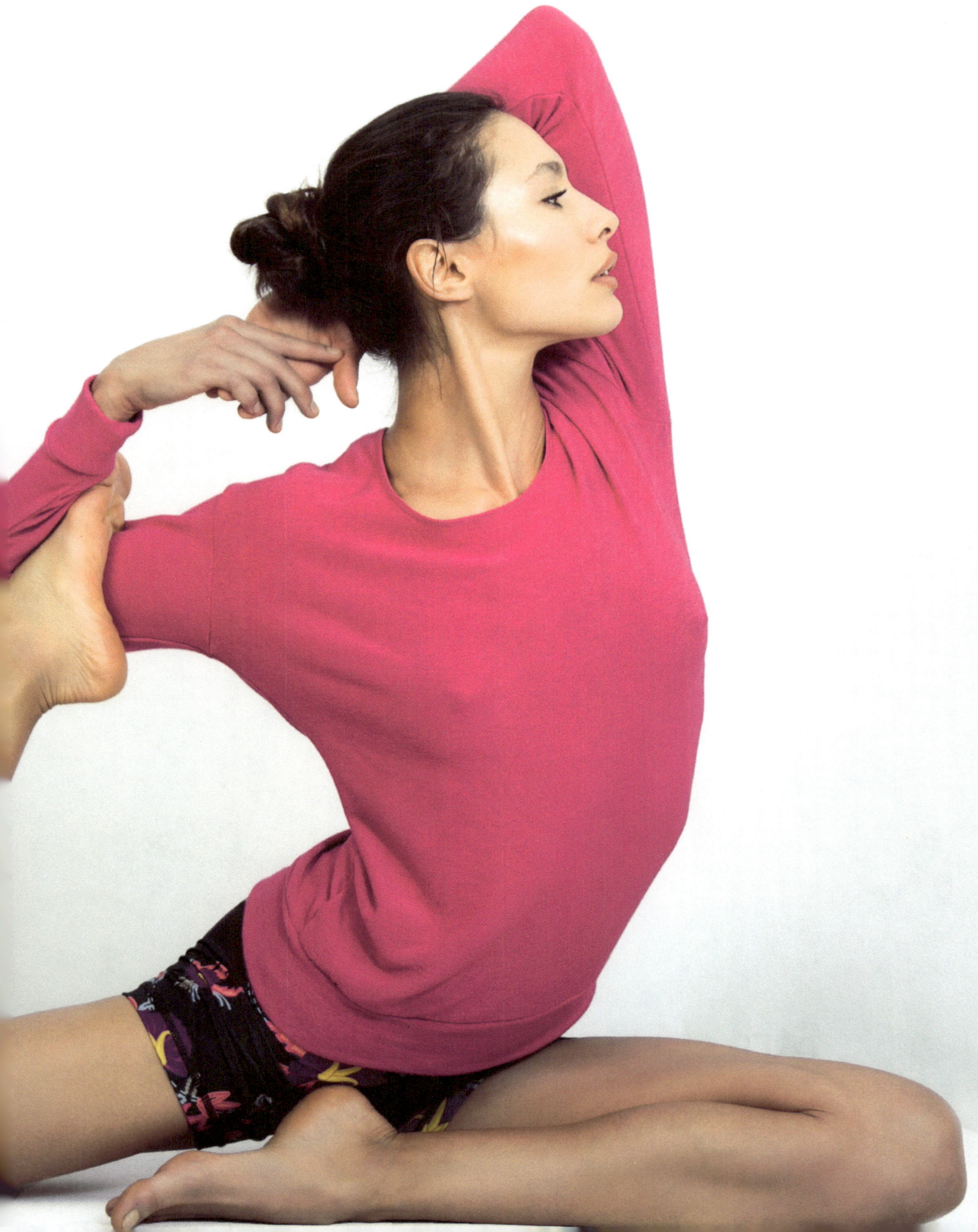

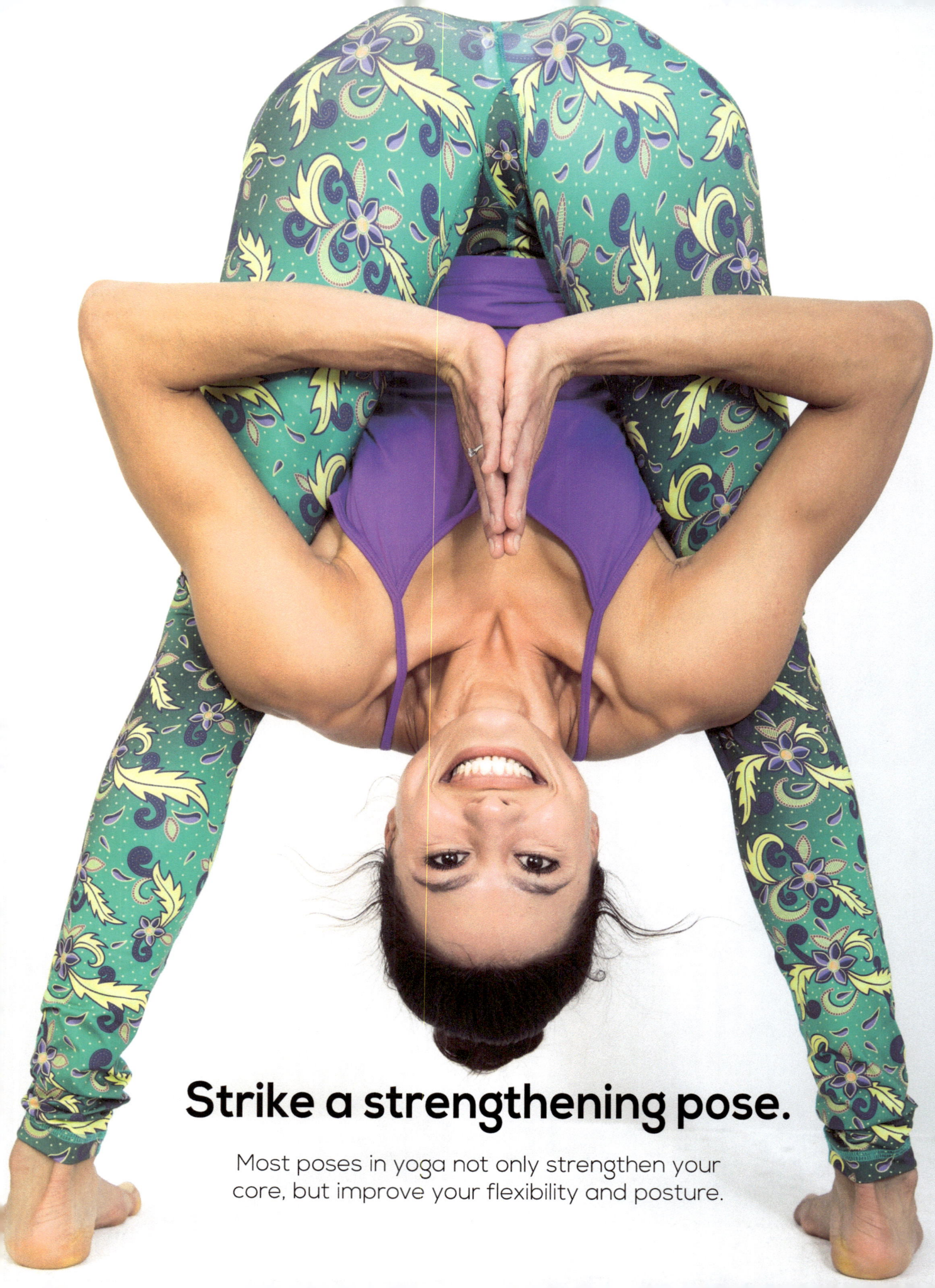

Strike a strengthening pose.

Most poses in yoga not only strengthen your core, but improve your flexibility and posture.

Maintains Heart Health

Yoga has been proven to lower blood pressure
and slow your heart rate, which is good for
those who suffer from high cholesterol.

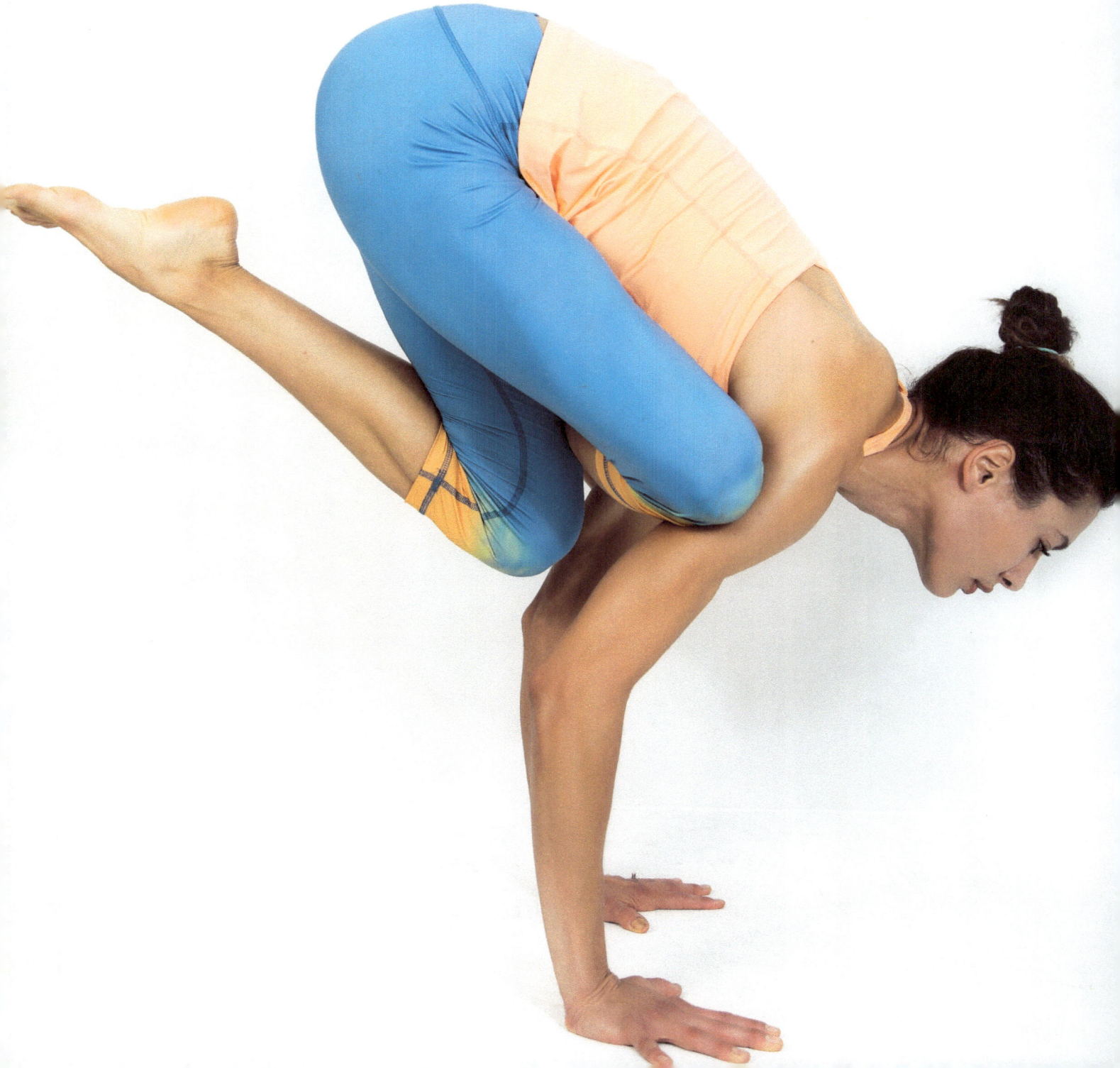

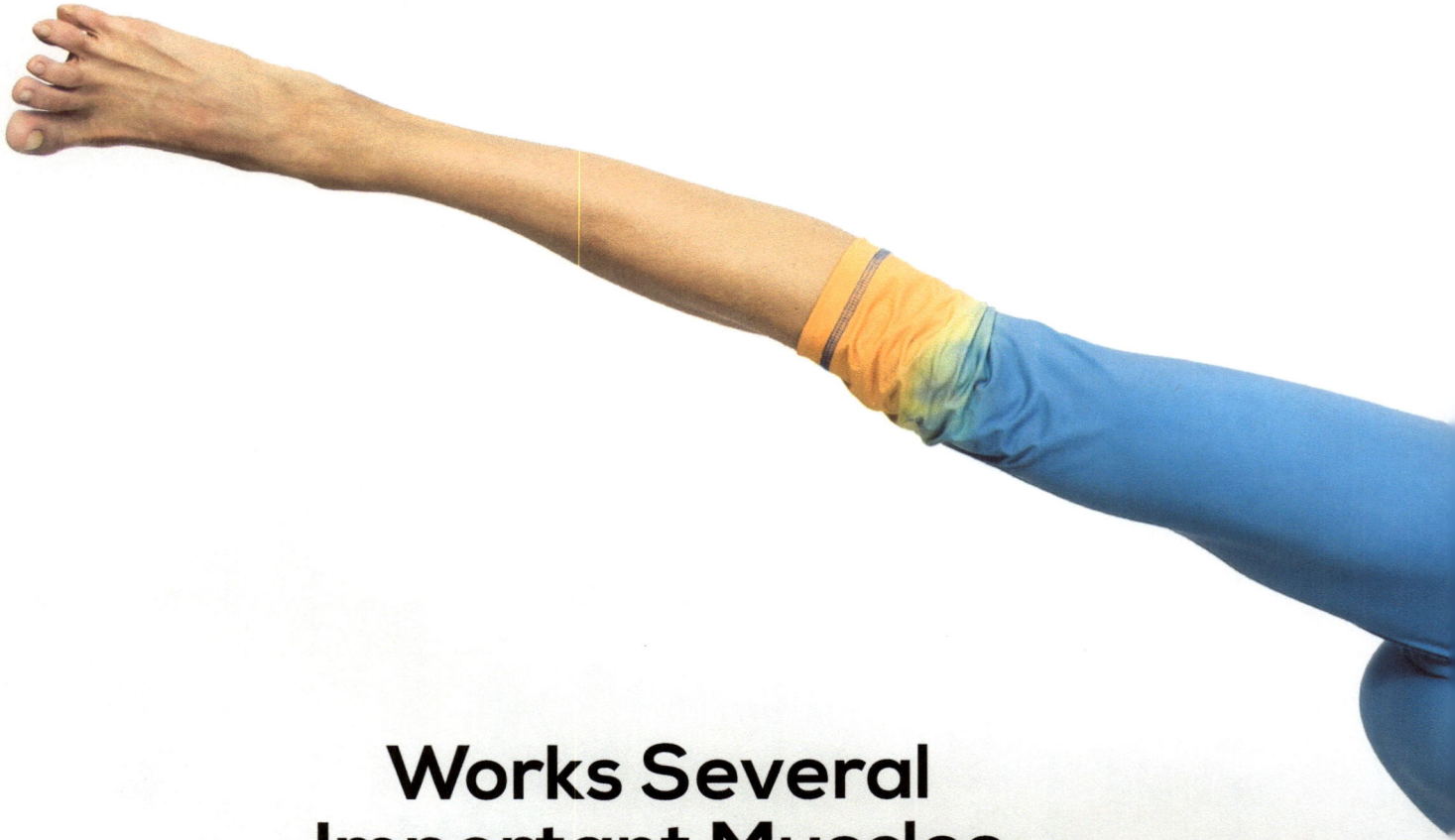

Works Several Important Muscles

Downward dog, upward dog, and the plank pose, build upper-body strength. The standing pose (after holding poses for several long breaths) build strength in your hamstrings, quadriceps, and abs. Poses that strengthen the lower back include upward dog and the chair pose.

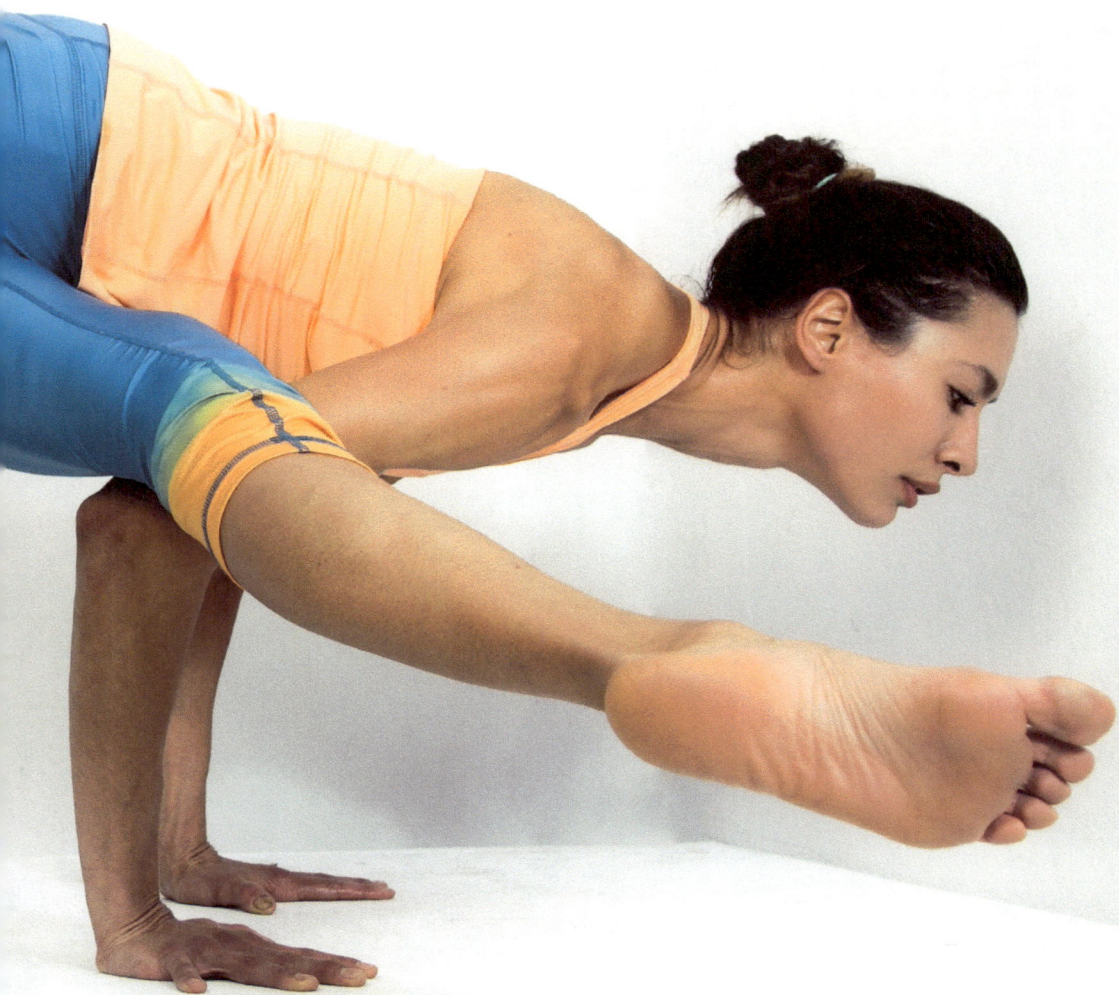

Improves posture.

Most standing and sitting poses develop core strength, since you need your core muscles to support and maintain each pose. With a stronger core, you will sit and stand "taller."

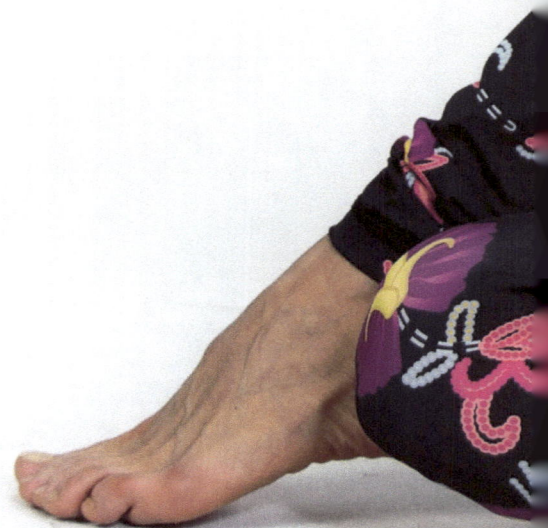

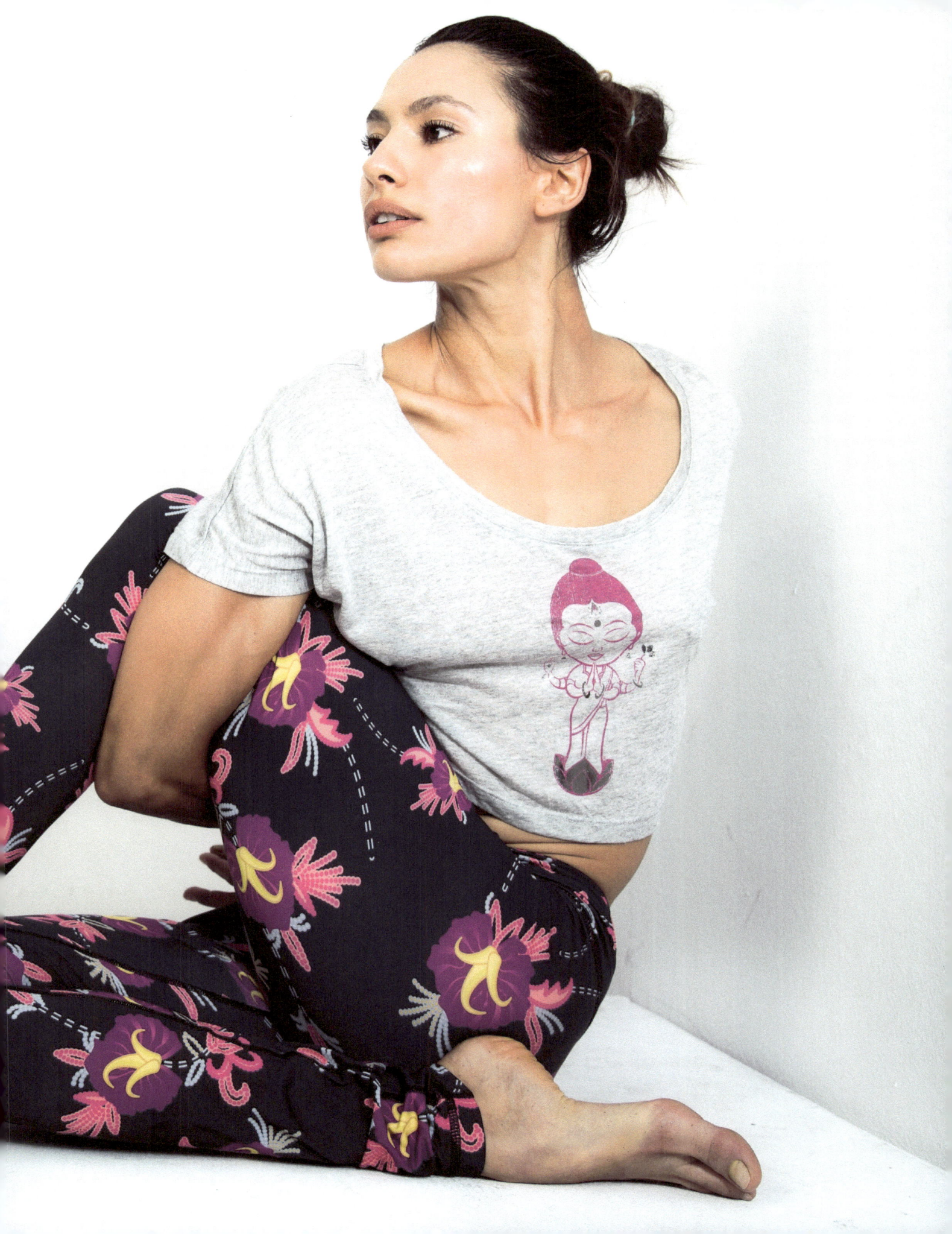

Something for Everyone

1. Ashtanga Yoga

You do a nonstop series of yoga poses. This type of yoga uses a special breathing technique to help focus the mind and control the flow of breath through the body.

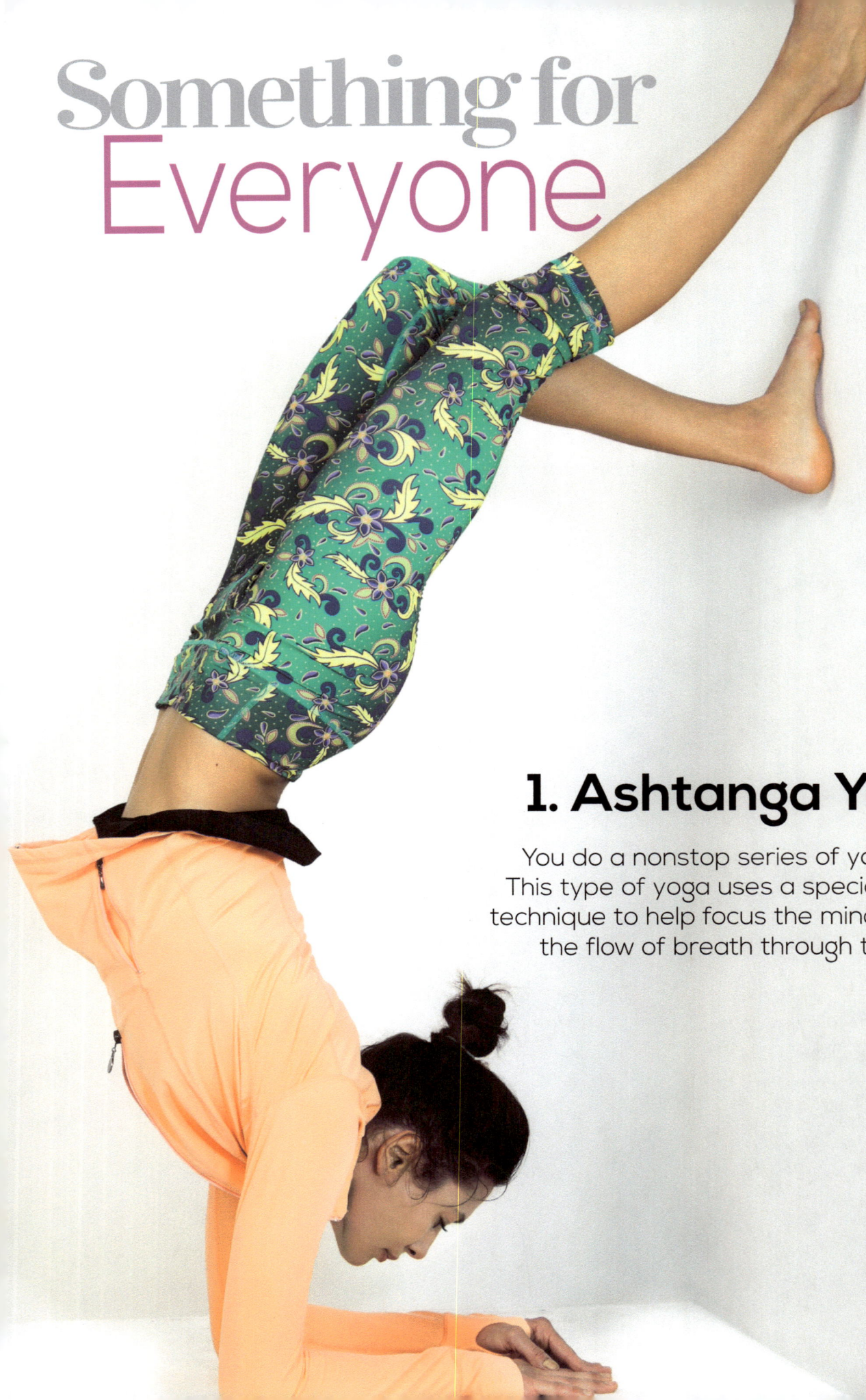

2. Bikram Yoga

You do a sequence of 26 yoga poses in a hot room, above 100 degrees.

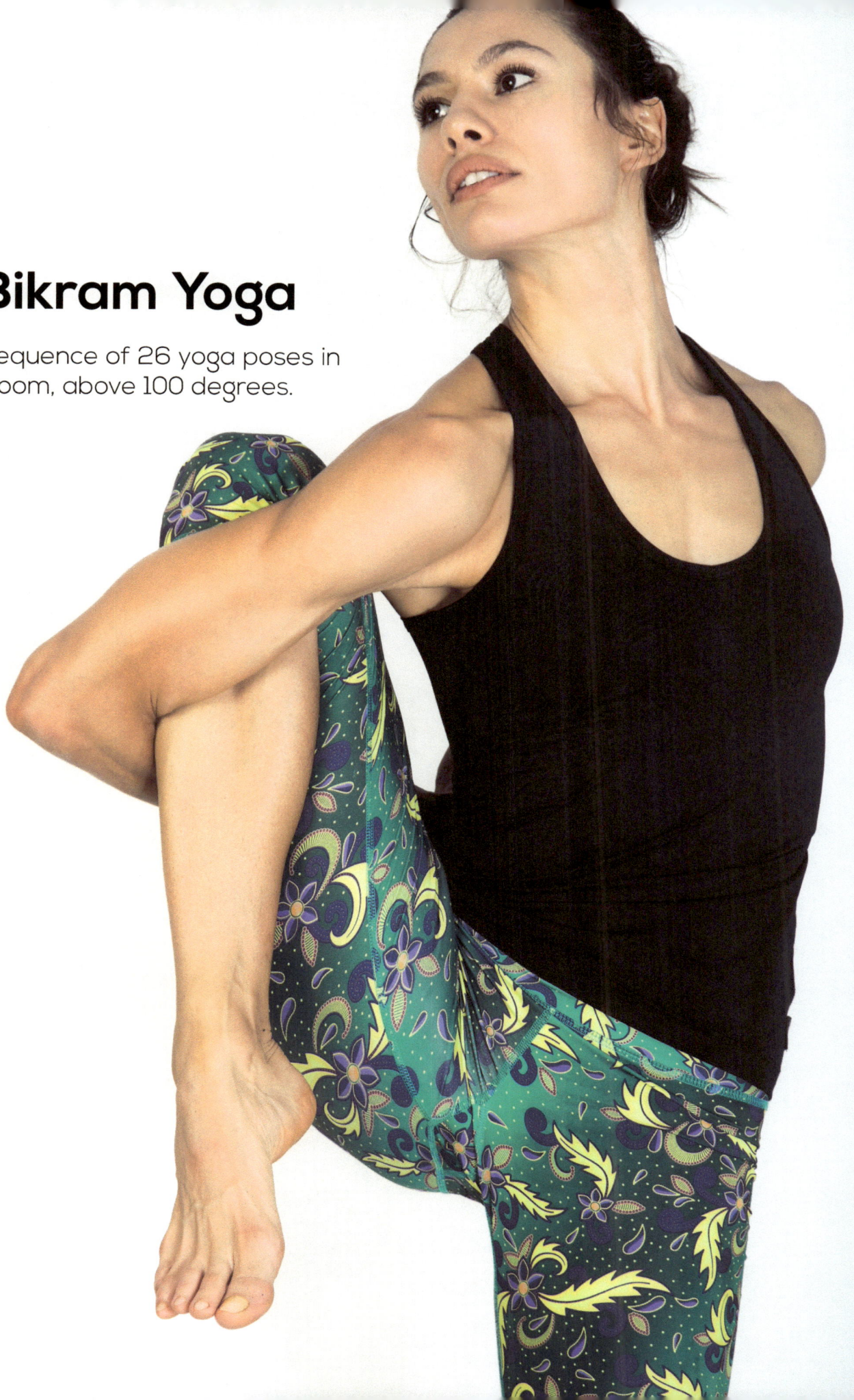

3. Hatha Yoga

"Hatha yoga" originally meant the physical practice of yoga: the poses, more than the breathing exercises, for instance. Today the term is often used when a few different yoga styles are combined to create a simple class that is ideal for beginners who are learning to do basic poses.

4. Inyengar Yoga

Iyengar yoga is detail-oriented and slow-paced, which is good for beginners.

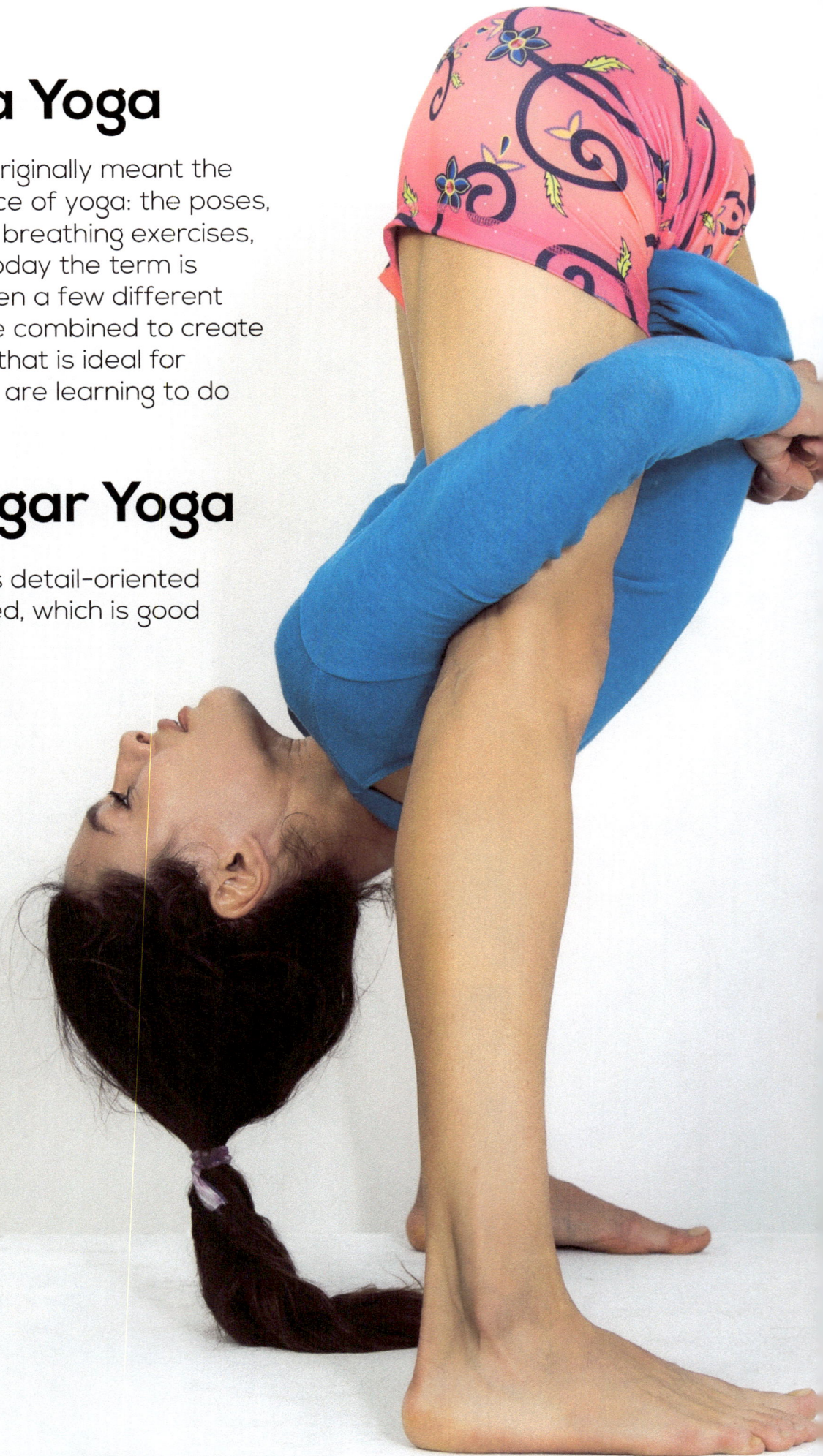

5. Kripalu Yoga

You do slow movements that barely cause a sweat, and progresses through three levels of deeper mind-body awareness.

6. Kundalini Yoga

You will experience the spiritual and philosophical approach of yoga. Classes include meditation, breathing techniques, chanting and yoga postures.

7. Power Yoga

This is the most physically intense and athletic forms of yoga. Based on the sequence of poses in Ashtanga yoga, power yoga builds upper-body strength as well as flexibility and balance. You flow from one pose to another.

8. Sivananda Yoga

This form of yoga has 13 poses. You lie down in between each pose. Most people can do this form of yoga regardless of their physical level.

9. Viniyoga

You focus on how your breath moves through your body and affects each pose. (It's not about precision on each pose.) With long, deep stretches this style of yoga is best suited for beginners and/or people who want to focus on flexibility, recovery from an injury, body awareness, and relaxation.

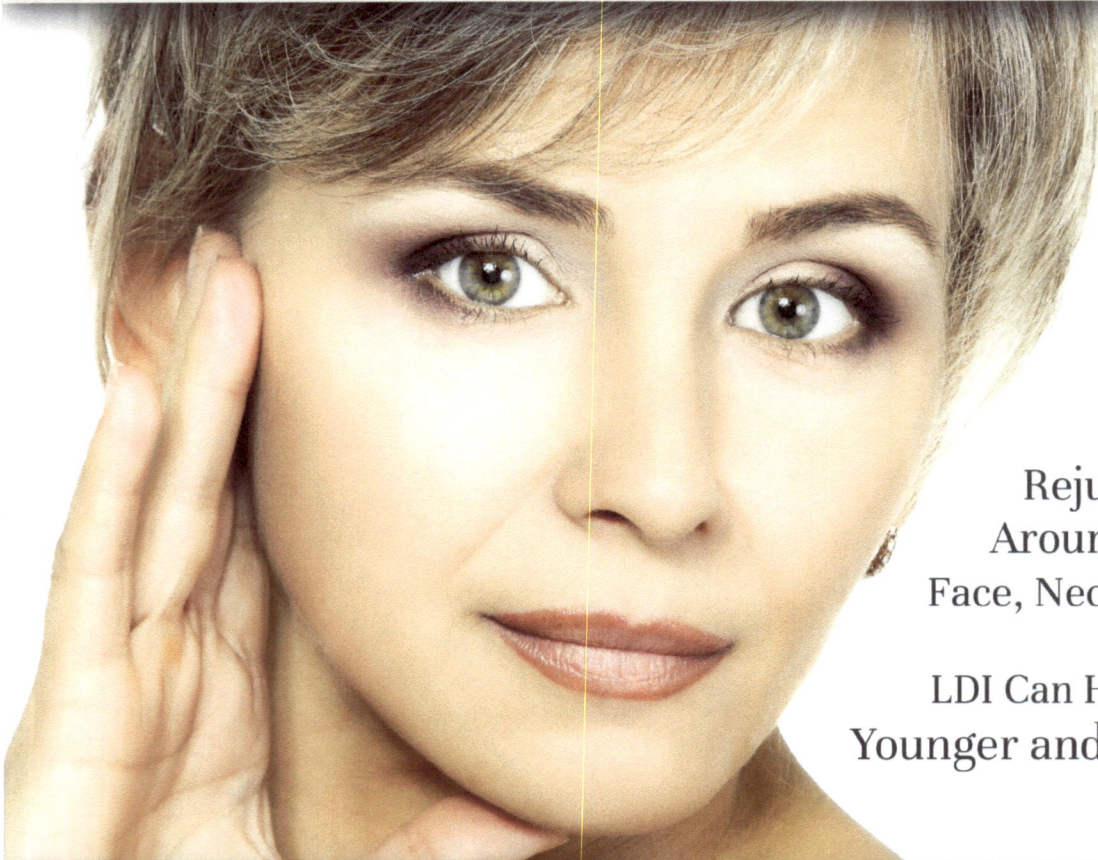

KEEPING
Your Dog Fit

HAVE YOU EVER SEEN AN OVERWEIGHT PET? THE FAT CAT, THE "ROLY-POLY" LAZY DOG AND ITS "ROLY-POLY" LAZY MASTER(S)— THE TWO USUALLY GO TOGETHER HAND IN HAND.

BY KAYLENE PEOPLES

Ever notice when you feed your dog just one extra scoop, his neck looks bigger? Well, maybe not just one scoop, but certainly extra generous portions? There is a reason the serving size on each dog food bag is there. Just speaking from experience, my dog Megan (a German Shepherd/Pit Bull mix) has been catching my husband and me unawares. First, she goes to him for a feeding very early in the morning. (I'm a night person, so I tend to wake up much later.) Then, right around 10:00 a.m. when I am cooking breakfast, there Megan is begging for cheese, or some turkey. I give her a small taste. I'm usually left a note informing me, "Megan has been walked and fed." That is my cue: don't feed her again. She's happy, and I can eat without her barking for her own scheduled feeding. But then there are those times when the routine goes awry. And since I have an older dog, I've seen some things over the years. Double feedings and fewer walks mean unhealthy weight gain.

I know a couple who was so extreme with exercise they strapped their German shepherd (Moses) onto a treadmill and worked him out for an hour almost daily. I don't recommend this. In fact, I believe this might have bordered on animal cruelty. But they have since moved away, and I no longer cringe at the thought. But their dog was fit! The husband was a chef and cooked a lot at home, fed his dog scraps constantly; and even though Moses got regular walks, those walks weren't enough to trim his burgeoning potbelly.

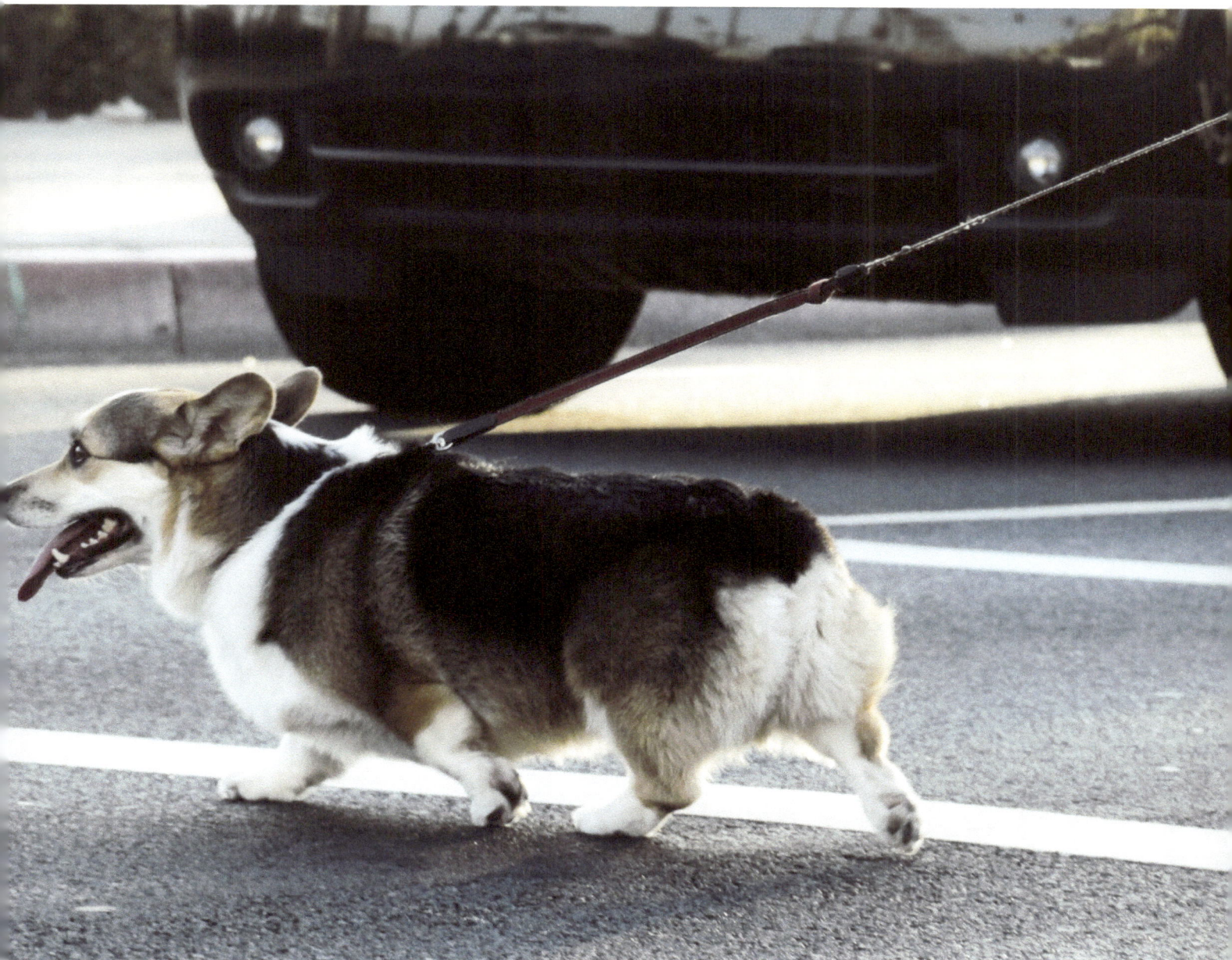

Shirley, the adorable poodle around the corner, gets her exercise in the family swimming pool. She splashes around with the kids and is a fit little pooch. Other dogs are taken on long hikes, to the beach, jogging excursions, and more. Living in Southern California, where the weather is sunny most of the time, creates the perfect setting for a slender dog. However, have you ever seen an overweight pet? The fat cat, the "roly-poly" lazy dog and its "roly-poly" lazy master(s)—the two usually go together hand in hand.

Don't feed your dog table scraps. If you want to give your dog a treat, a milk bone usually suffices.

You may wonder why your dog is overweight. It starts with diet. It's a good idea to follow the recommended portion sizes on your dog's wet or dry food. Don't feed him/her table scraps. If you want to give your dog a treat, a milk bone usually suffices, plus most packaged doggie treats have ingredients added for gum and teeth health. Is your dog getting enough exercise? Now, I'm not talking about lunges, treadmills, or sprinting on a track. I'm merely referring to a basic 15-minute dog walk. How many times a day does your dog get exercise? Most dogs when left to their own devices lie around the house and sleep, getting up only to go to relieve themselves, eat the postman, attack a cat, or intimidate motorcycle riders passing by. Two walks a day are ideal. If you're too lazy to walk your dog, hire a dog walker or the kid up the street to do it for you. Either way, just like us, dogs do better with exercise.

With regular exercise, aches and pains disappear, weight on the joints diminish, and your dog will keep that pep in his/her step. Not to mention the sun's vitamin D has been proven to be a much needed component for maintaining good health. Don't be like me. Megan has tricked me into double feedings, which went on for weeks. I noticed she was putting on a few extra pounds and realized I'd been out-smarted. I cut back her portions and doubled her daily walks, and her weight fell off fast.

Keeping your dog fit is a lot easier than keeping yourself fit. Dogs have no preconceived notions about food, rarely are they allergic to gluten, and their meals are routine. With a little bit of care, your four-legged companion will live a long and healthy life, and be by your side while you do your own set of lunges and crunches!

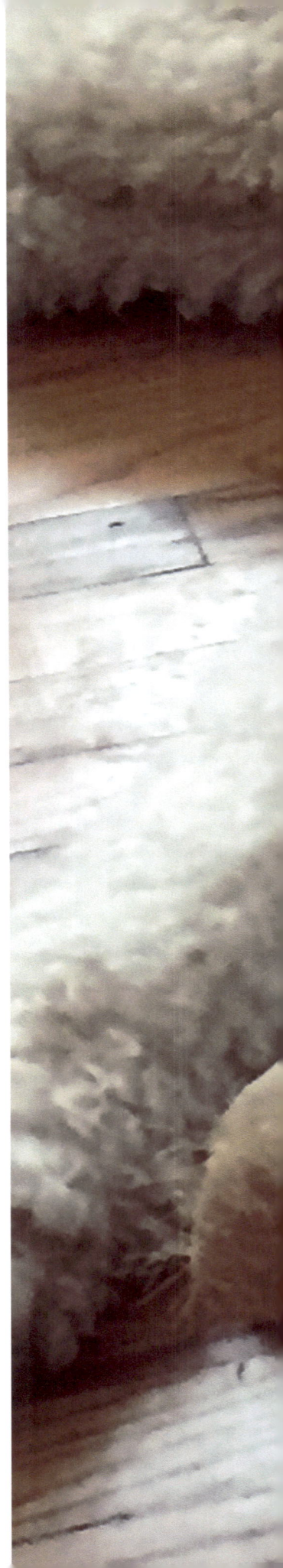

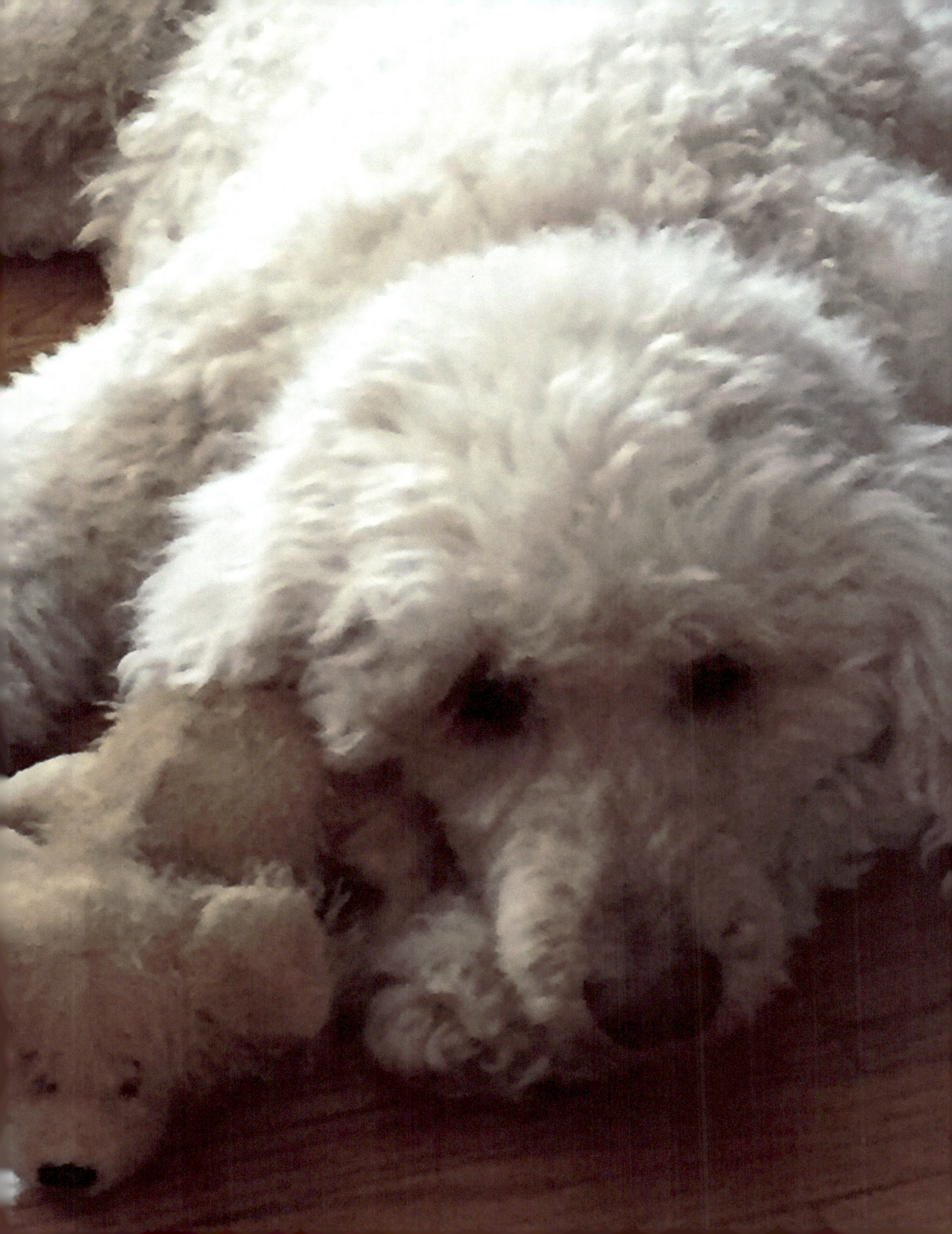

Swimsuit
Facts

Photographed by Ash Gupta
with Siddhesh Rane
for 838 Media Group
Model: Isabella Leon
Written by Kaylene Peoples

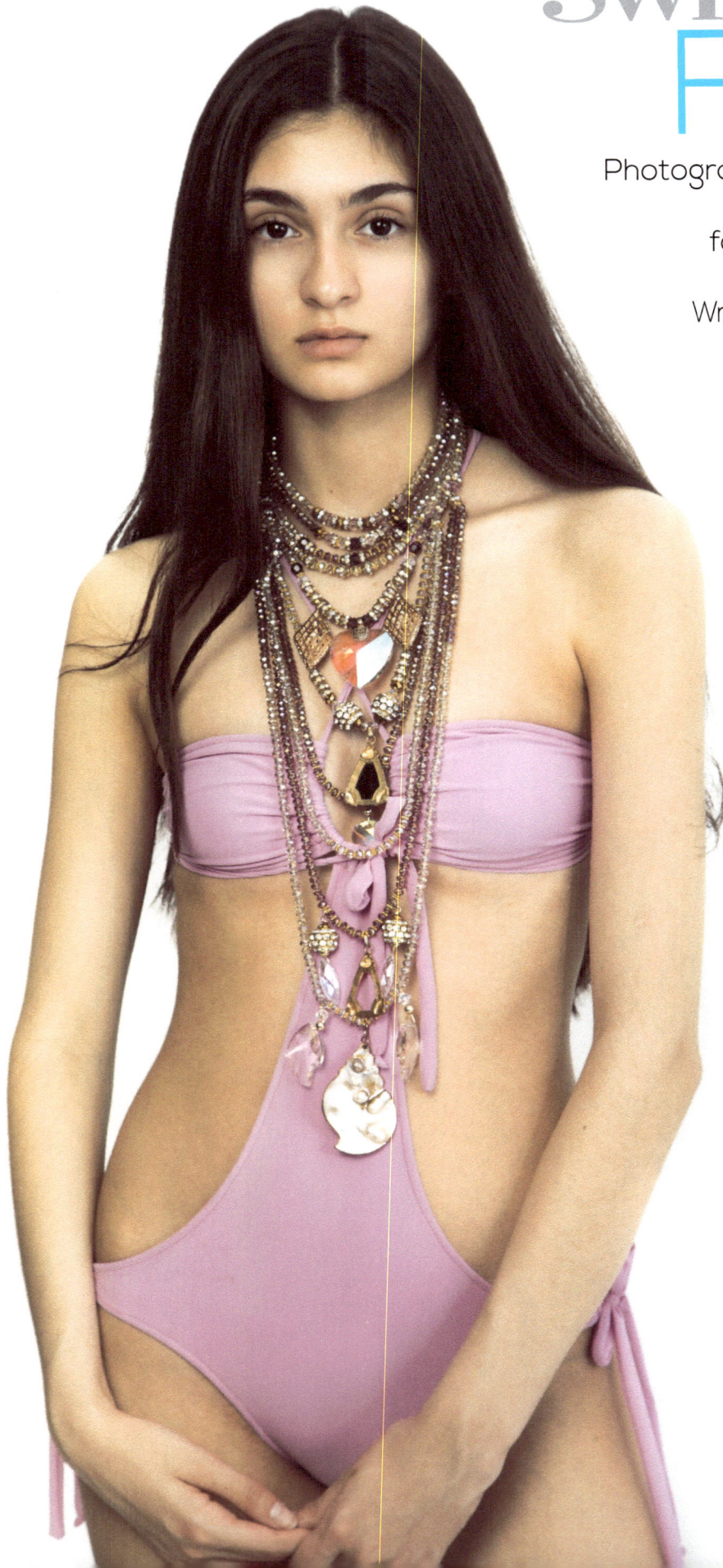

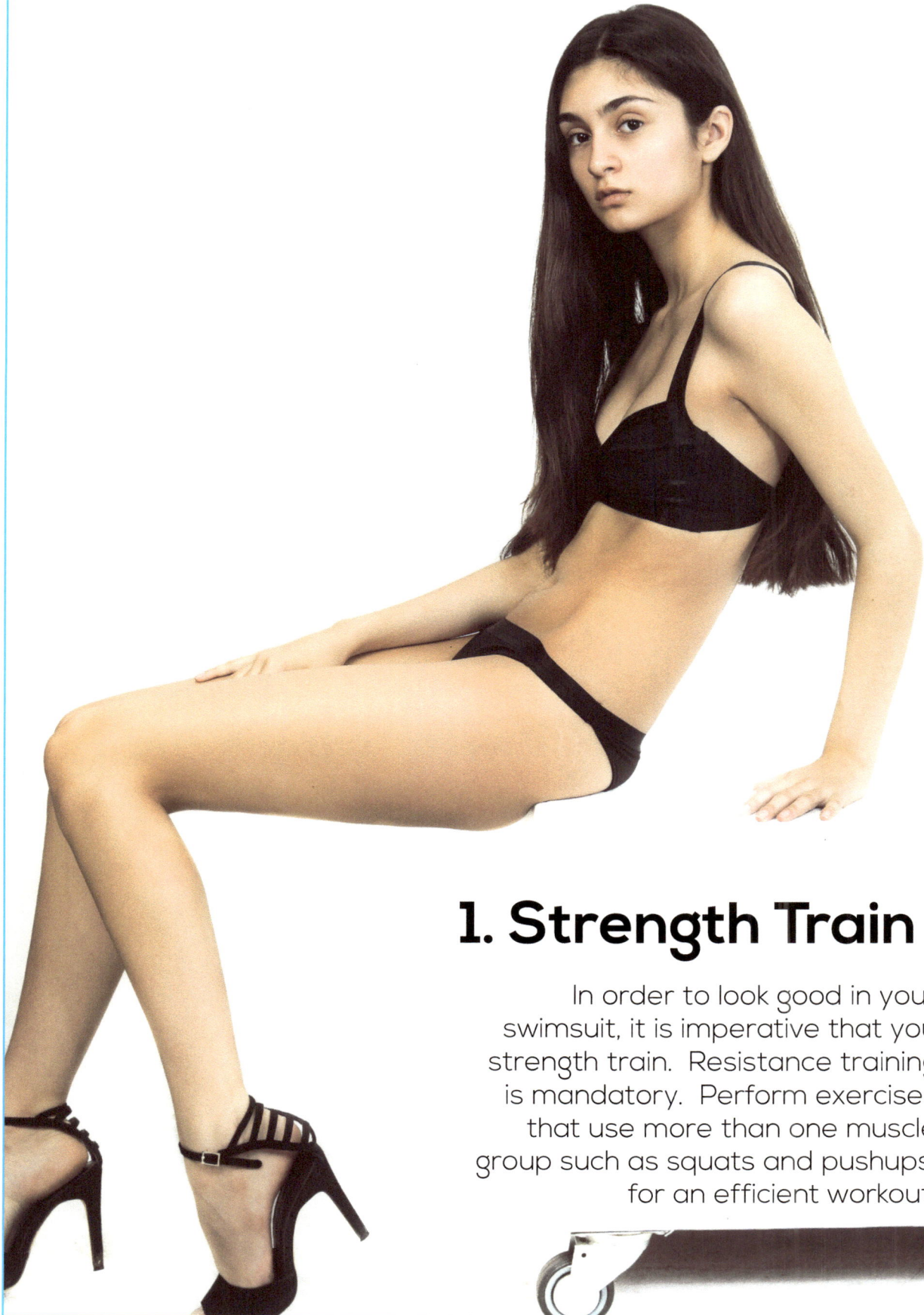

1. Strength Train

In order to look good in your swimsuit, it is imperative that you strength train. Resistance training is mandatory. Perform exercises that use more than one muscle group such as squats and pushups, for an efficient workout.

2. Morning Workouts

Work out in the morning to speed up your metabolism for the entire day.

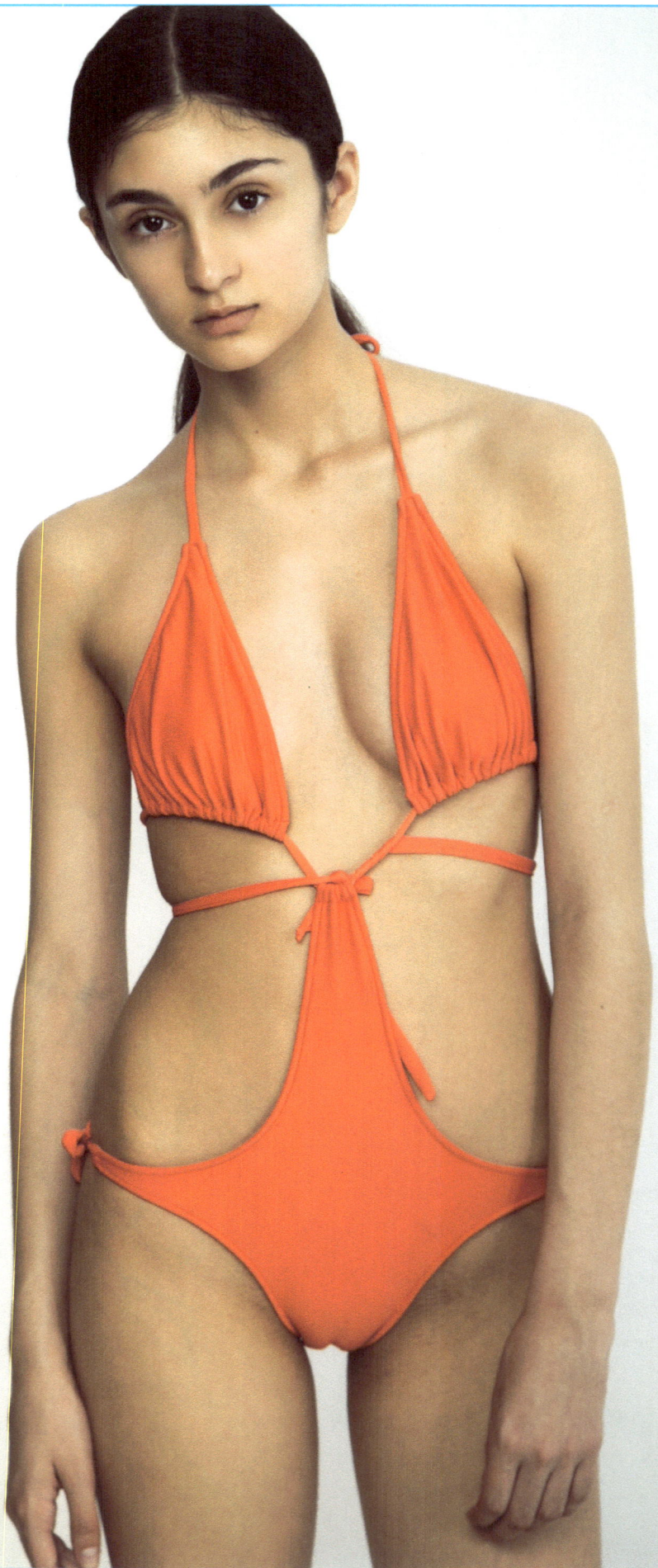

3. Firm That Derrière

Prevent saggy glutes from ruining your bikini bottom look. Try doing squats, lunges, and deadlifts.

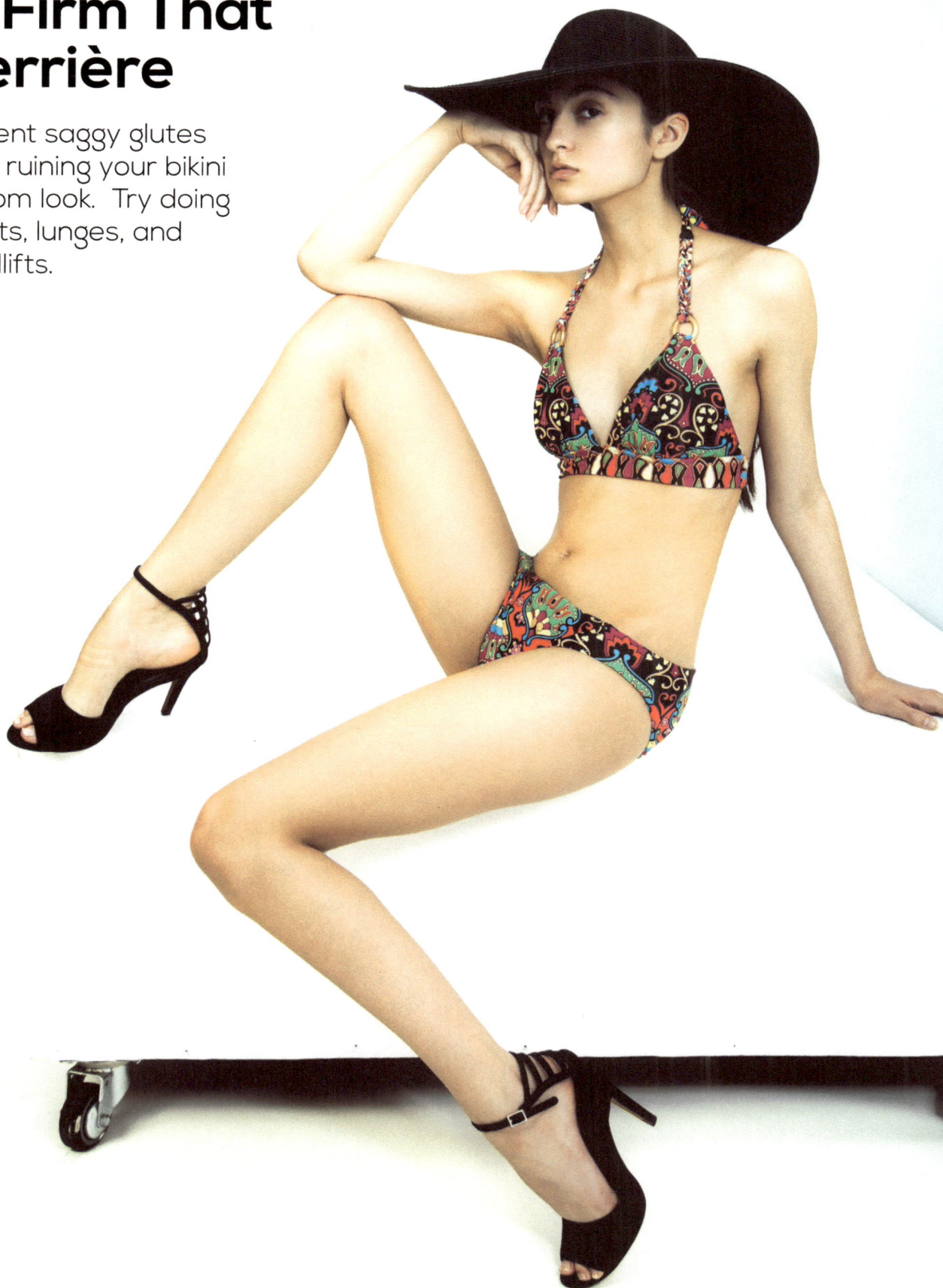

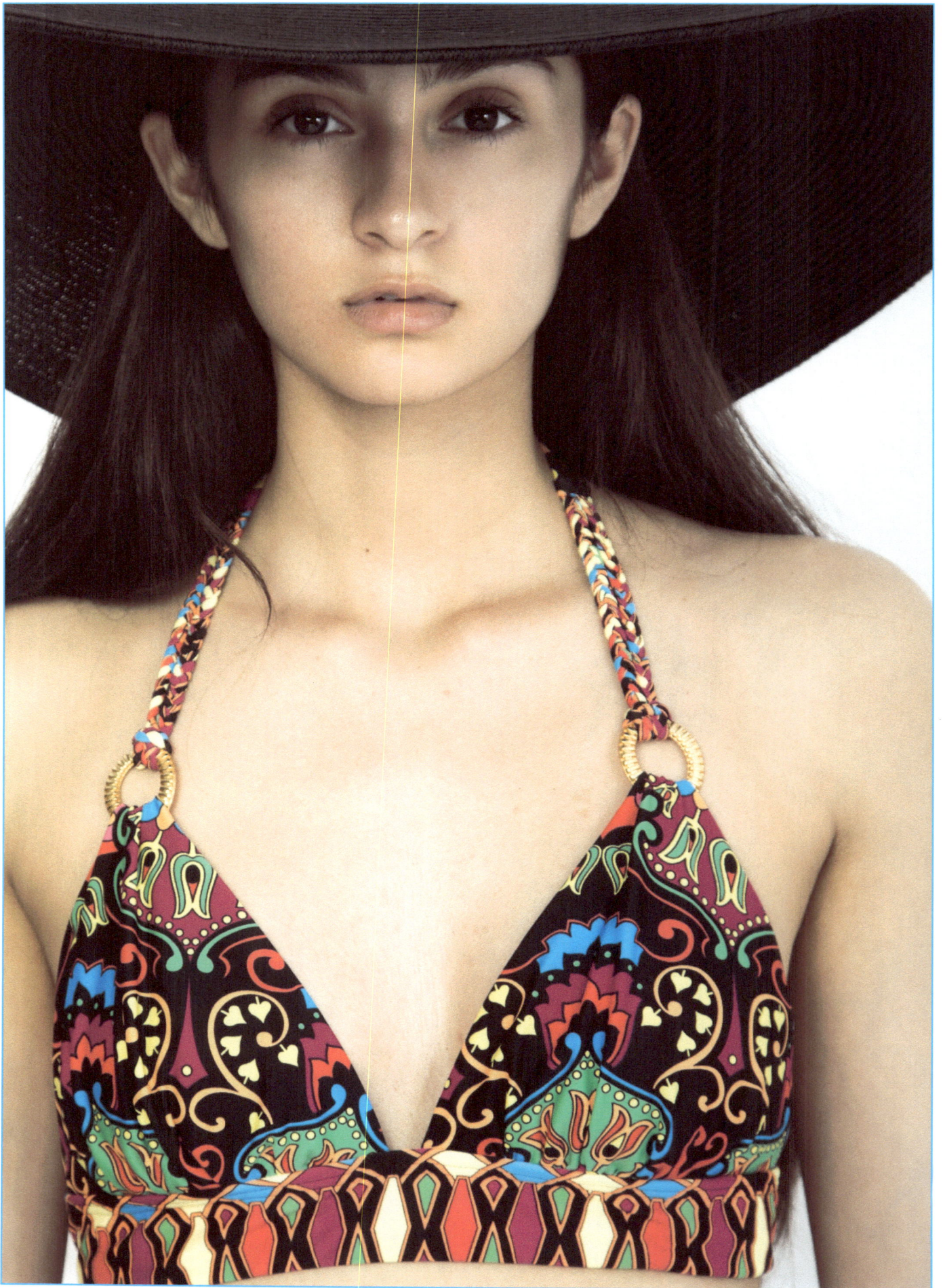

4. Eat Natural Diuretics

Increasing your intake of diuretics helps your body de-bloat. What are the foods that work? Cucumbers, green tea, lemon, asparagus, and anything with a higher concentration of magnesium, potassium, vitamin C, and/or caffeine.

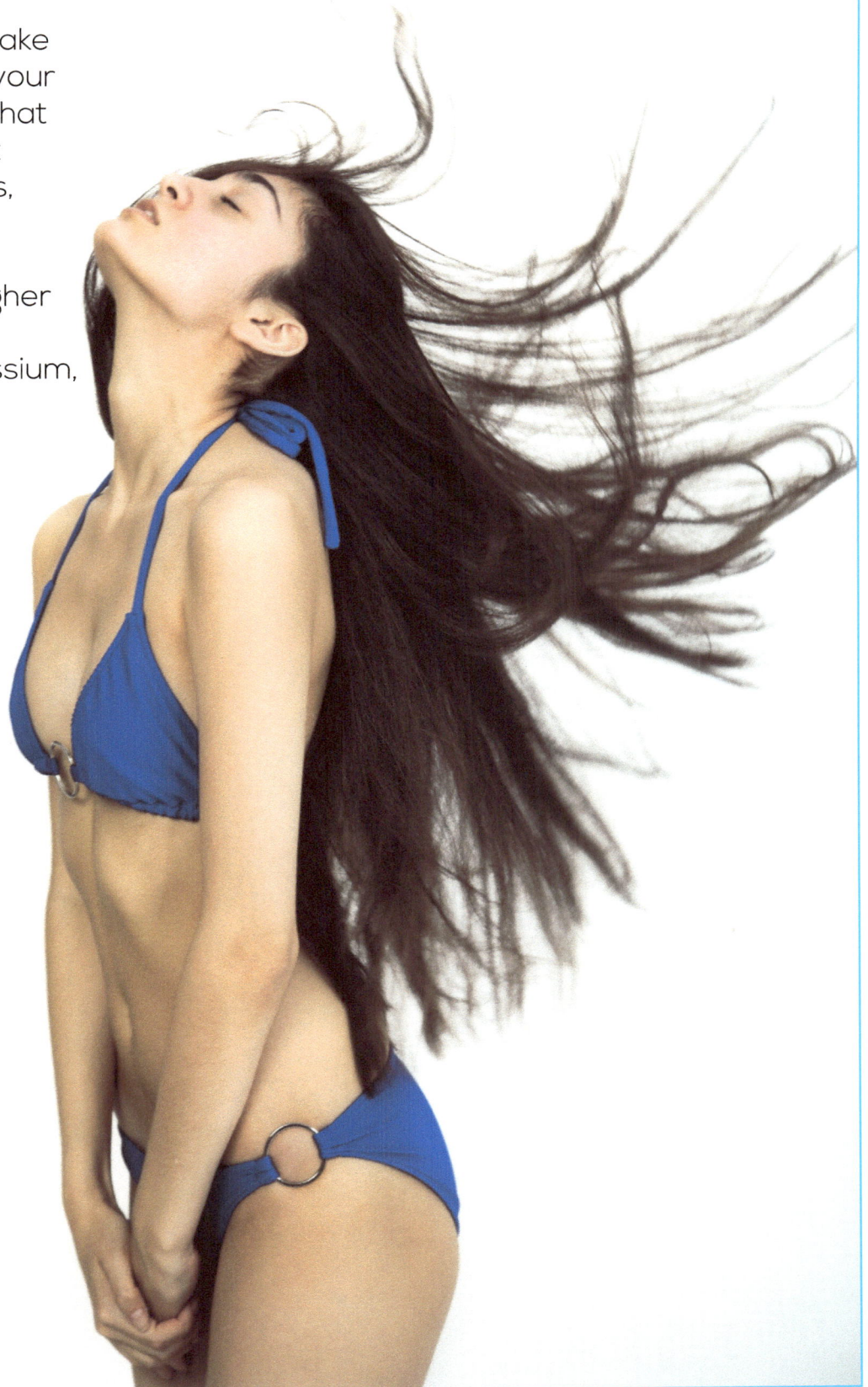

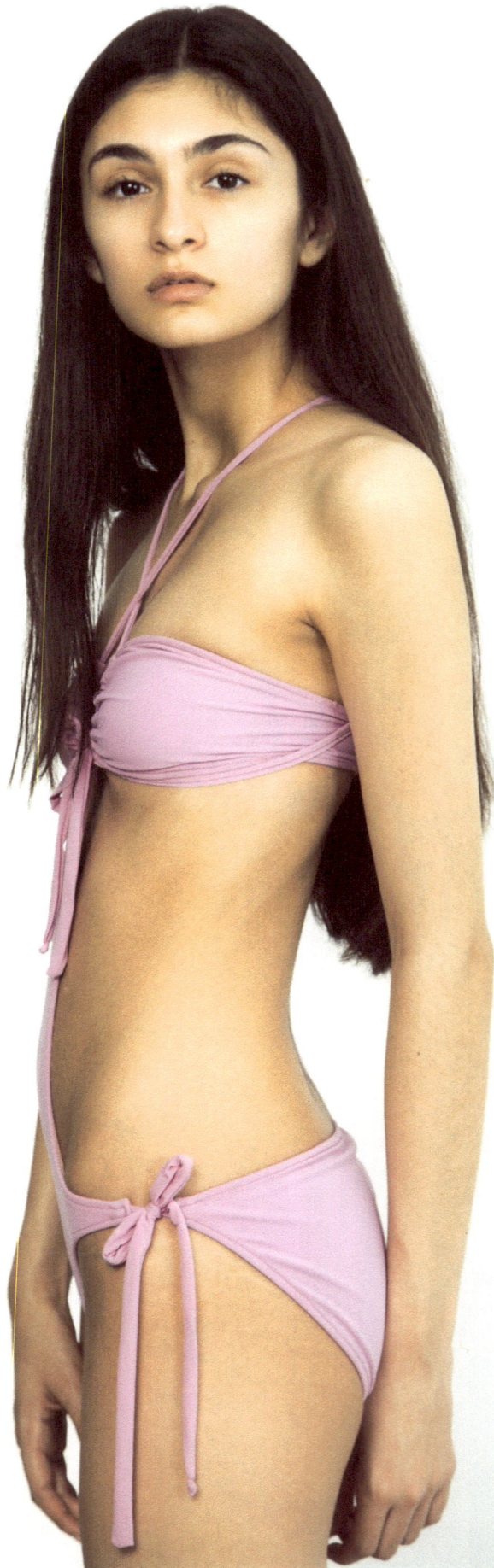

5. Drink Water

Don't fall into the trap of becoming dehydrated, which can derail the effectiveness of your workouts. Drinking water is the easiest way to rid yourself of excess body water weight by flushing the water out.

6. Reduce Processed, Starchy Carbohyrdates

Foods that contain processed, starchy carbs have way too much sodium and preservatives, which cause you to bloat. Great replacements are fresh fruit and vegetables..

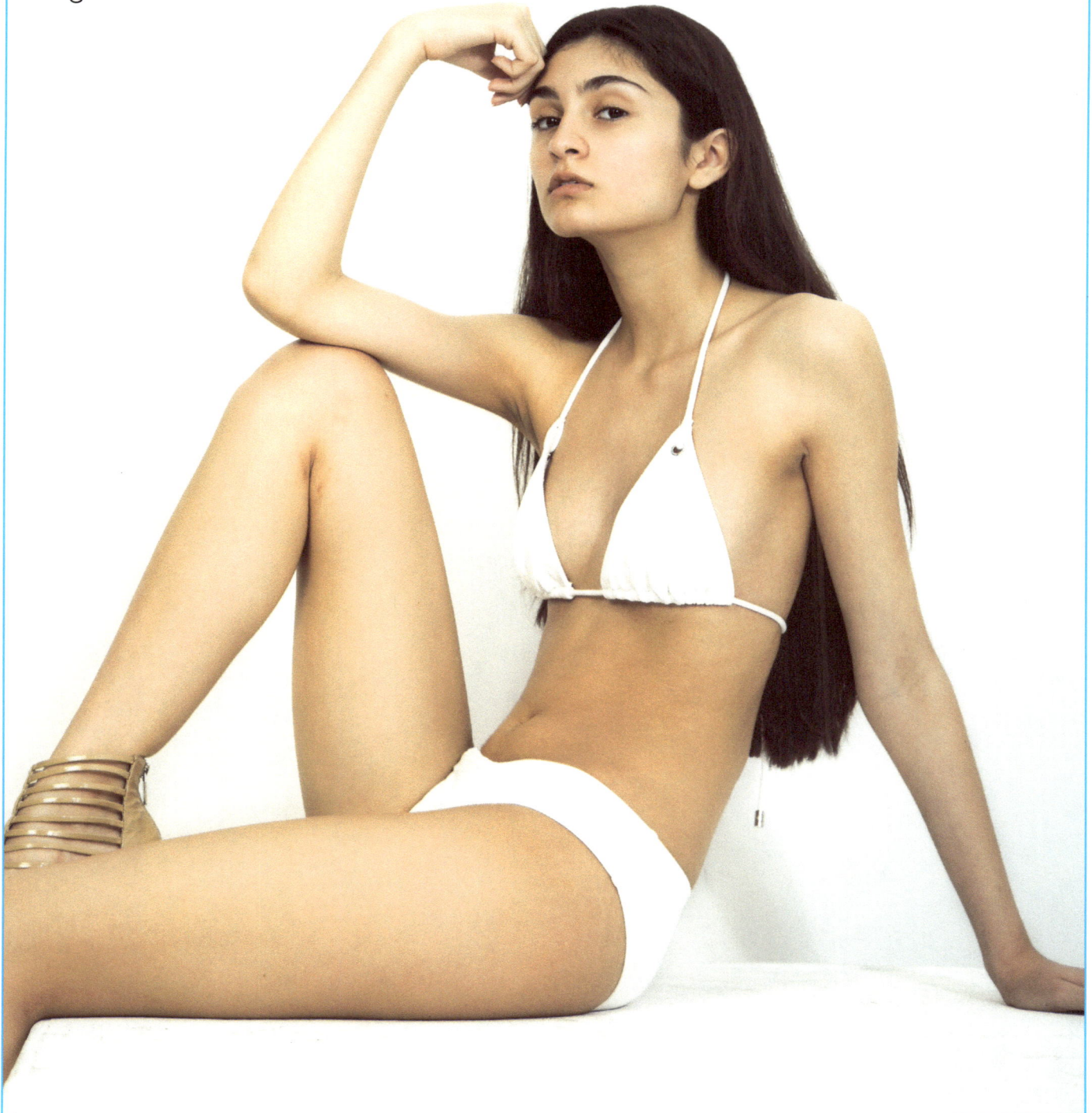

7. Reduce Your Sugar Consumption

Read food labels and beware of hidden sugar in salad dressings, sauces, bread, and juices. Avoiding eating out at restaurants is a good idea until you have at least reached your goal of your ideal swimsuit body.

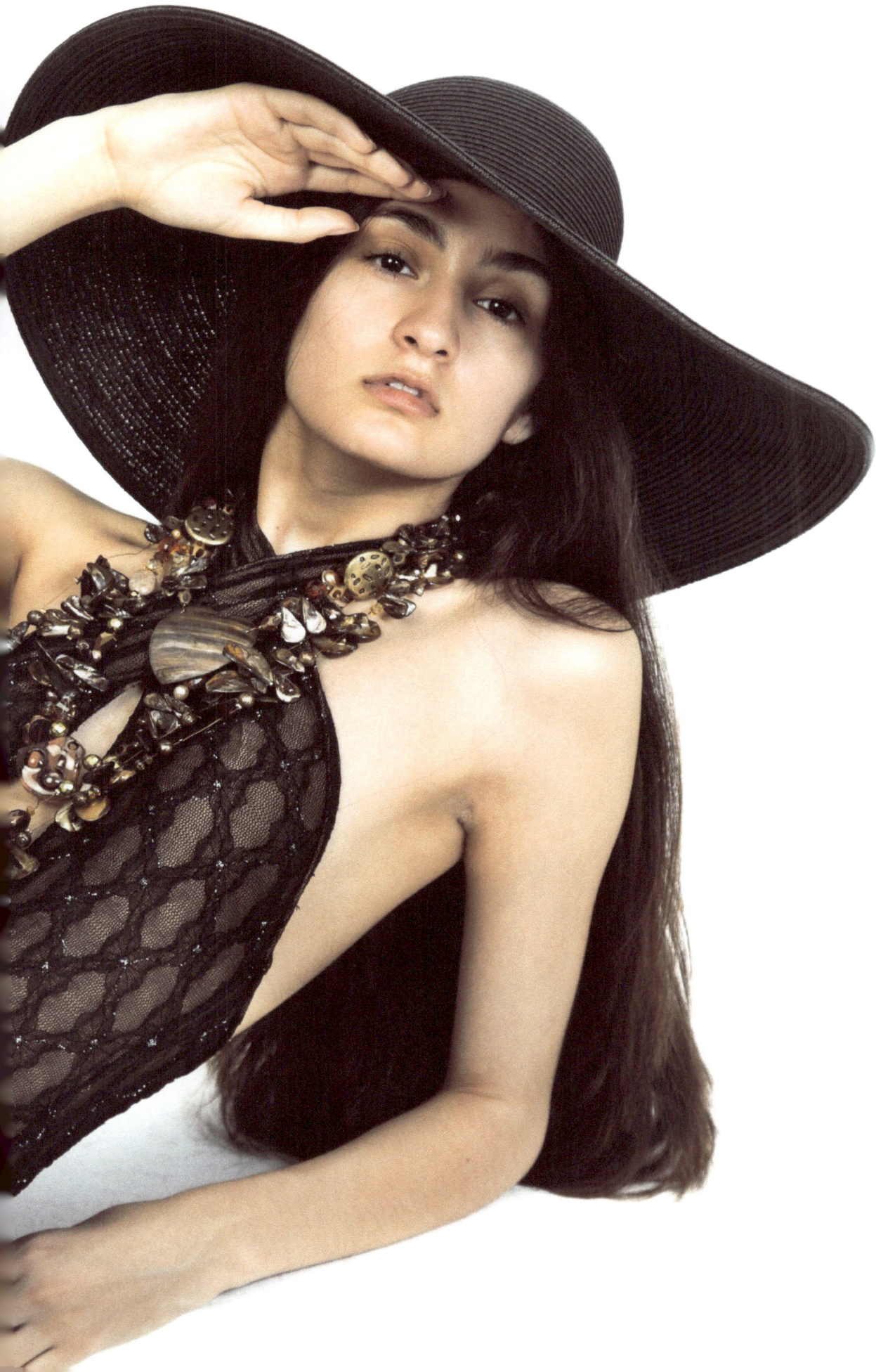

8. Less Alcohol, Please

There is very little nutritional value in drinking alcohol, not to mention loaded with calories. Red wine has been credited with minor positive effects, but white wine is loaded with sugar; and hard liquor is just filled with empty calories. If you want to be svelte in your bikini, it's best to just avoid all forms of alcohol entirely.

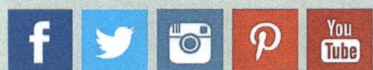

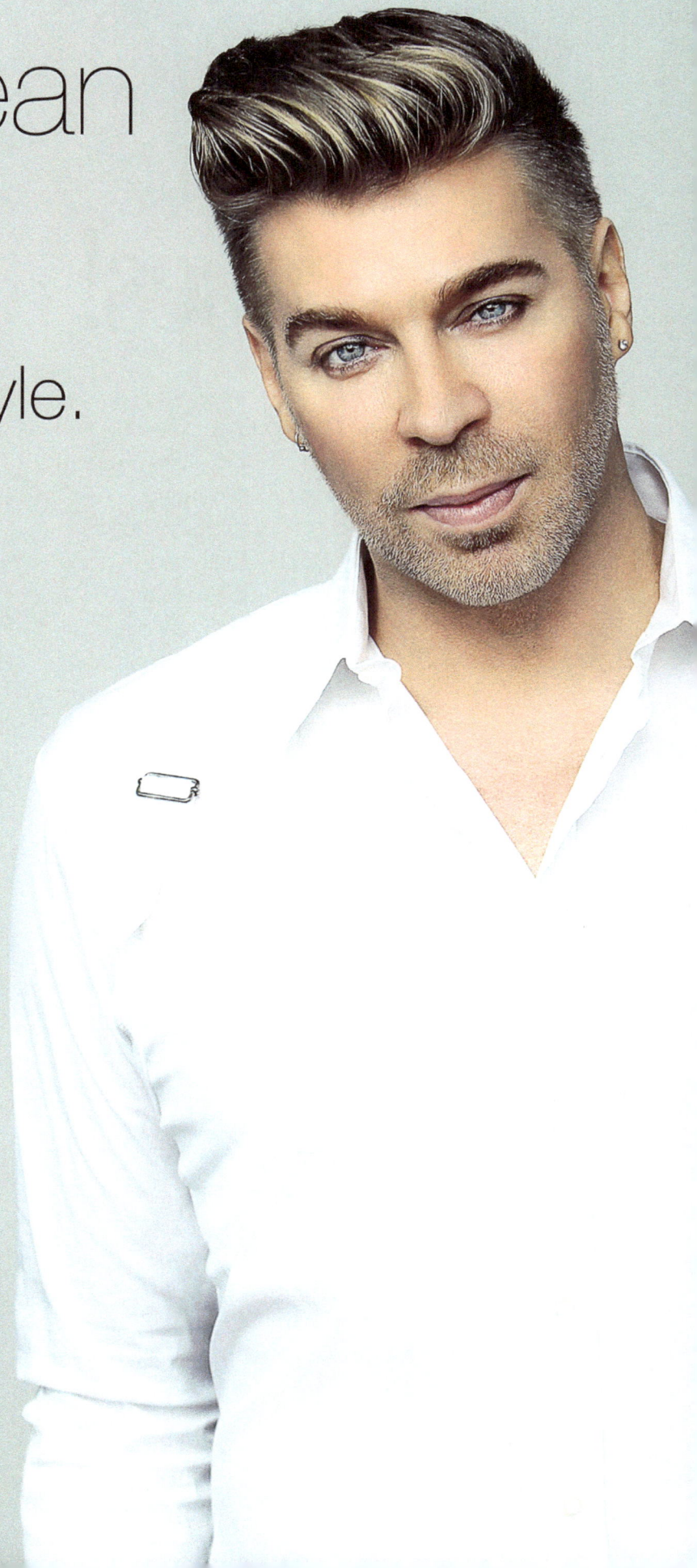

Home Made into Gym Routine:
No Excuses!

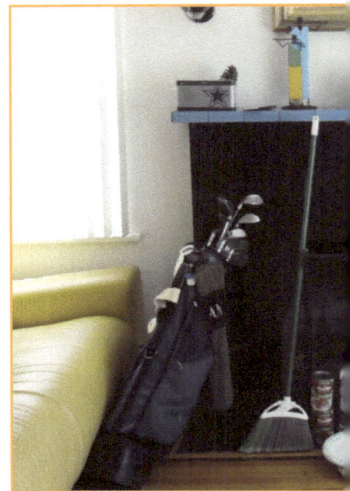

BY ANTHONY HEREDIA
Photographer: Devino Tricoche
Model: Mikala Muhammad

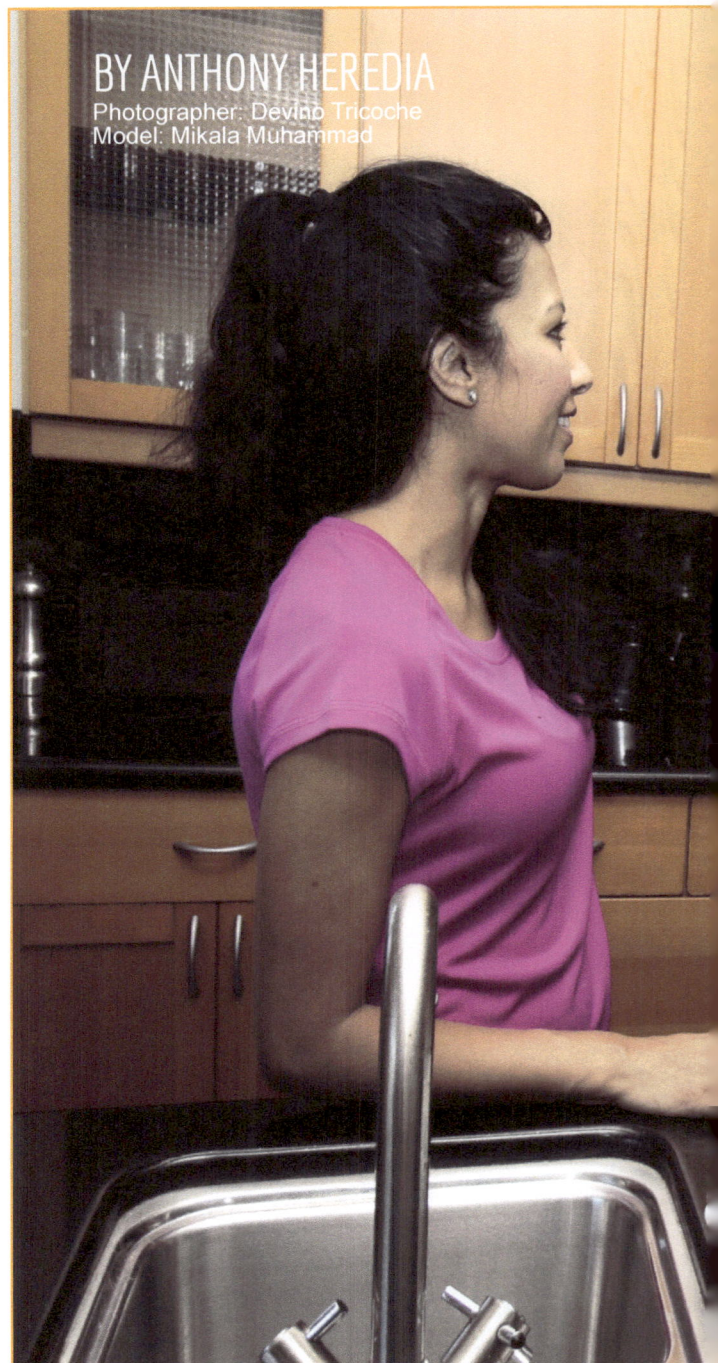

Who needs a gym to get in shape when you have a house full of amazing equipment right at your fingertips? You can replicate just about any piece of large gym equipment with everyday items you use in not so everyday ways, until now, that is. The key to getting a slim, sexy body is consistency and using as many muscles as possible for max results. No one is going to deny you have a crazy busy life, but if you wait for your life not to be hectic to take your fitness into your own hands, you can honestly admit that it will never happen. It is not about avoiding the chase but working around it, or better yet, through it. The number one gripe about working out is not having time to head to the gym, so make a gym out of your home, and ditch the excuses for not having time to get fit.

On the next few pages is a great beginner's full body workout for those days you just cannot make it to the gym or to your normal routine. This routine should only take you about 30 minutes at a good pace, doing just the resistance portion, or up to an hour should you add the recommended bouts of cardio between the resistance training. If you don't have time, stick to powering through the resistance routine alone; but if you can squeeze a bit more time out, add in the cardio for max fat burn. As you get stronger and better at this, simply try to complete the cardio and resistance training with the minimum rest time for a hardcore short kick in the fitness butt. Rather than miss a workout day, just run through this routine to give yourself the gift of consistency. You will thank me in the summer.

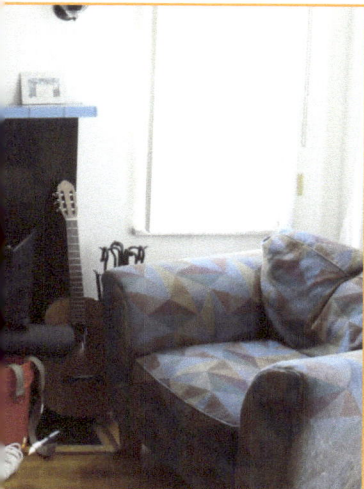

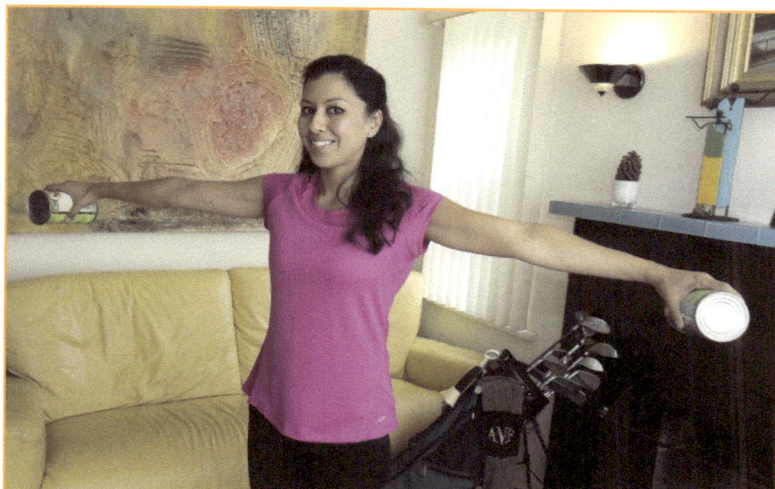

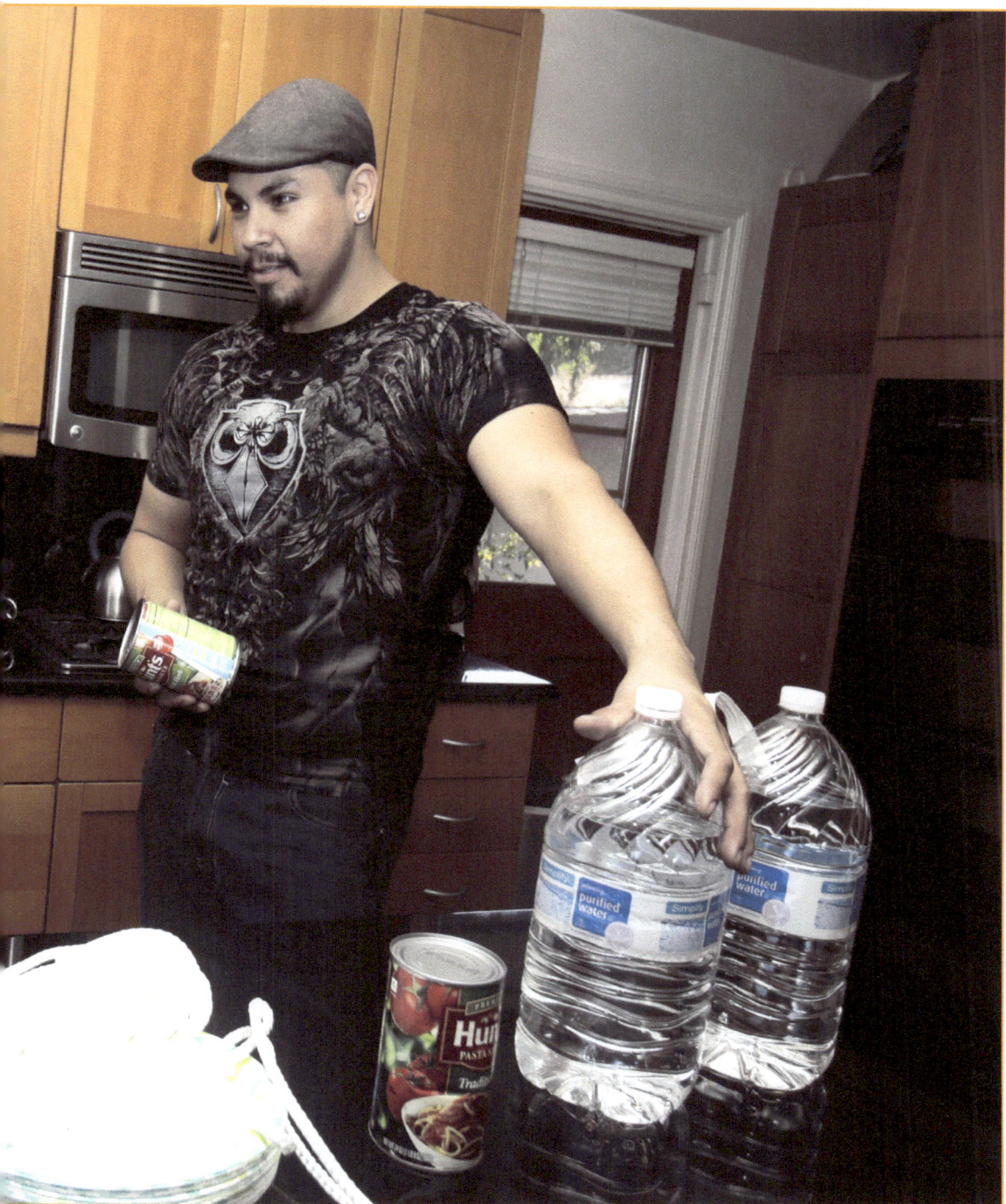

HOW IT WORKS

The idea of this routine is to get full body attention in a short period of time, using home objects and your body weight as tools. Start in the order provided. This works you from head to toe once completely; and then complete the full circuit again a second time to be done. Adjust the items you use and positions/angles you place your body in to be safe but still challenging. If you can complete 12-15 repetitions with ease, then you are not challenging yourself enough for max results. Aim for a range of 6-12 reps. To increase the size of a muscle, you use more weight and complete fewer reps (6-8 reps); or for strength and long, lean muscle with less bulk, you would use just enough weight to last 12-15 reps. Remember not to be afraid of using more weight. You don't magically bulk up overnight like the Hulk. Size takes so much time and effort, but you burn so many more calories challenging yourself more.

Make sure, please, to breathe and not hold your breath during this; your muscles need oxygen for maximum power. Take a 30-90 second break between each exercise. Try working your way toward as short a break as possible, but listen to your body. Pushing through to the next exercise before you are ready can lead to you passing out from just not having enough oxygen to feed the needy muscles. Lastly, as an optional component to kick this up a few notches, you add a 60-second speedy, running in place between each of these for ultimate fat burn. Kick your knees up to waist level and aim for speed. So you would finish a resistance set, take a break, 60-second speed run in place, and then another rest before you move on to the next resistance set. You can use this for the sporadic days you don't have time for your typical routines or as a standalone workout short with no cardio or full burn with it. As a standalone routine, begin by doing this every other day. Make sure to do your favorite form of cardio (hiking, running, treadmill, swimming, etc.) on the days you don't do this for at least 30-60mins.

WHAT YOU WILL NEED

Broom/mop/sturdy long stick

Two water/milk/juice gallon jugs

Yoga mat

Ottoman or bucket with a pillow for comfort

Large soup/veggies/sauce cans

Motivating music

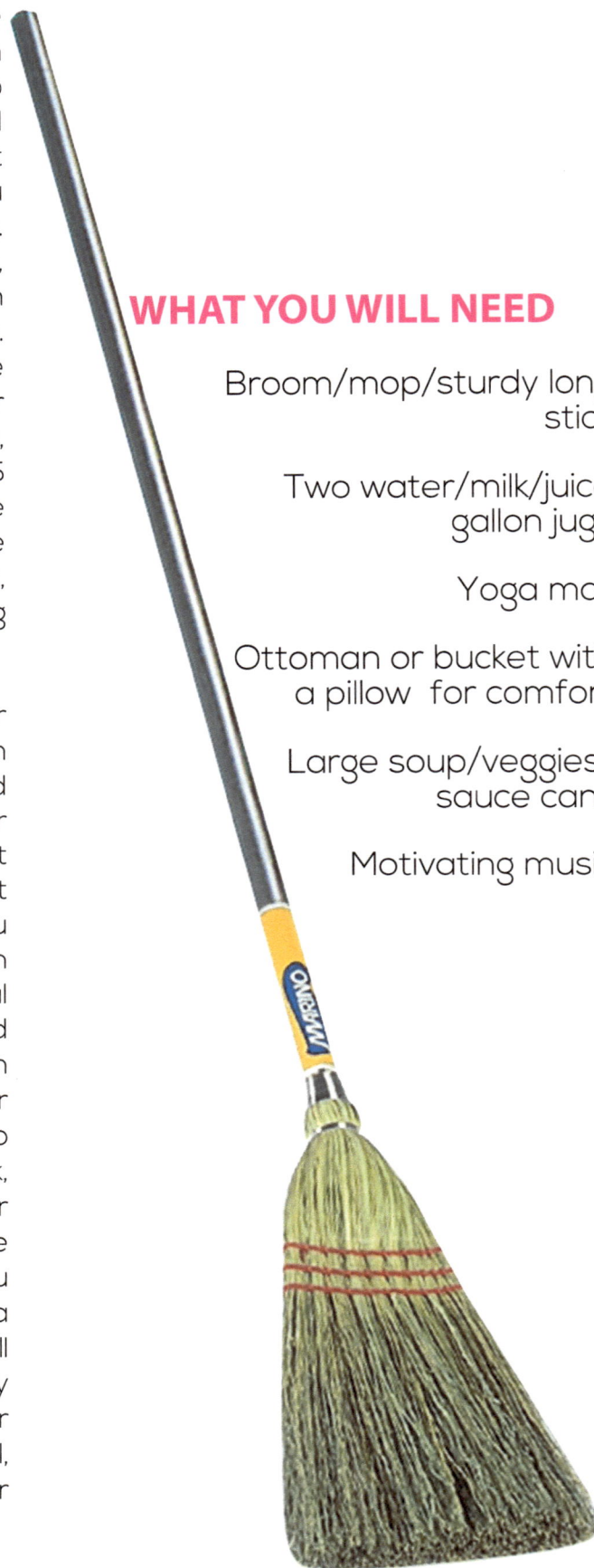

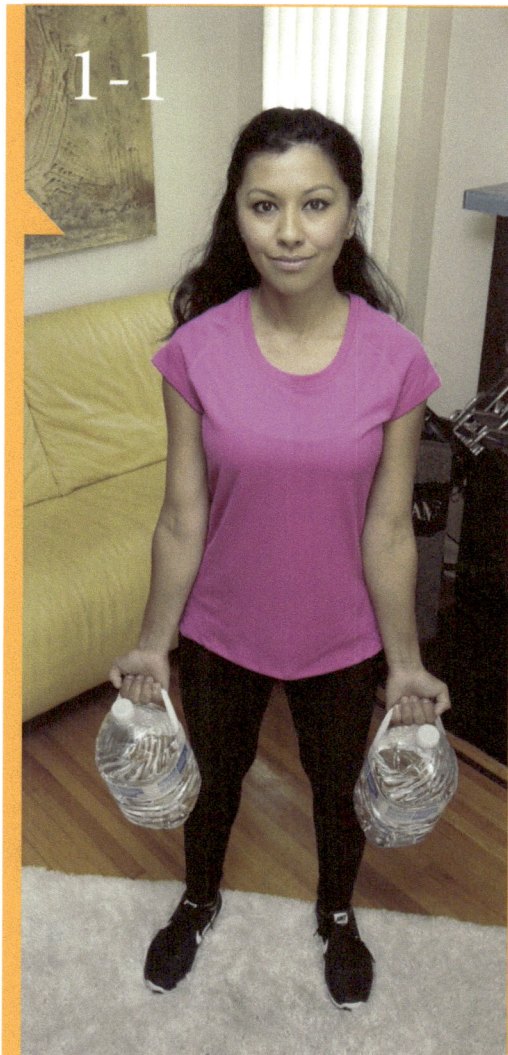

1) Water Gallon Curls

A one-gallon container of liquid (water, milk, juice, etc.) weighs about 8 lbs, or you can fill an empty gallon container with dirt or sand, which will take the weight to about 13 lbs. Start with the jugs hanging beside you, palms facing outward and forward. Keep your elbows pointing toward the ground and curl the jugs upward slowly, making sure not to swing them up or bend forward for assistance. The only part that should be moving is your elbow to your hands. Bring fists up to near shoulder position, and then slowly bring them back down. If you don't feel the muscles you are focusing on doing most of the work (biceps), then you need to adjust until you do, or risk wasting your time, or worse, getting hurt.

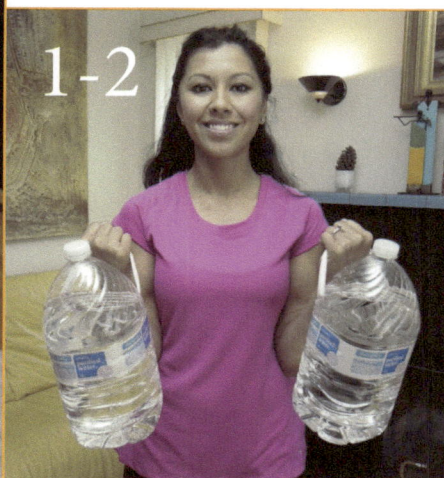

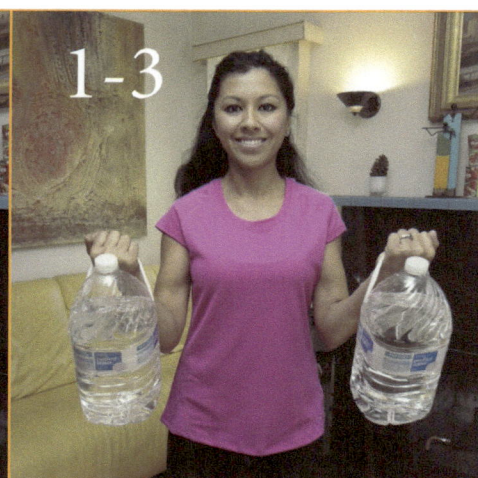

2) Water Gallon Shoulder Press

Open up your arms and have your knuckles pointing toward the ceiling, making sure to have straight wrists so as not to hurt them. Keep your neck muscles down so as not to shrug toward your neck when you press. When ready, press the jugs up slowly, making sure they go up evenly and with your chest open and arms in a straight line. You don't want to pull your elbows inward, or you stop using the correct muscles. Press to above your head and begin to descend in the same open-chested manner.

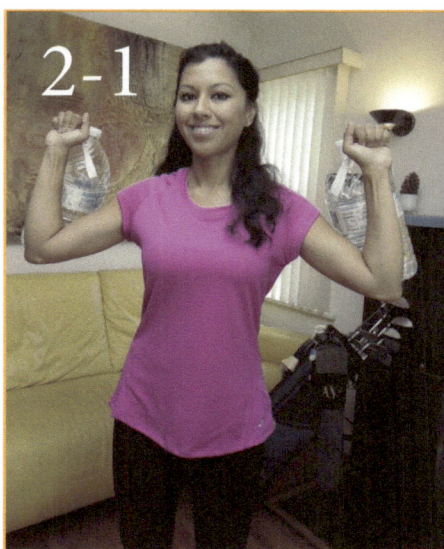

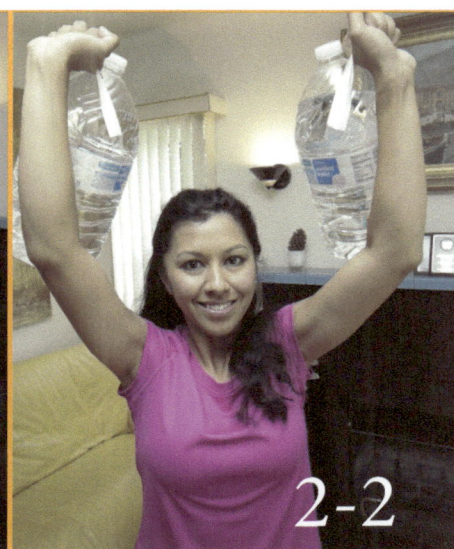

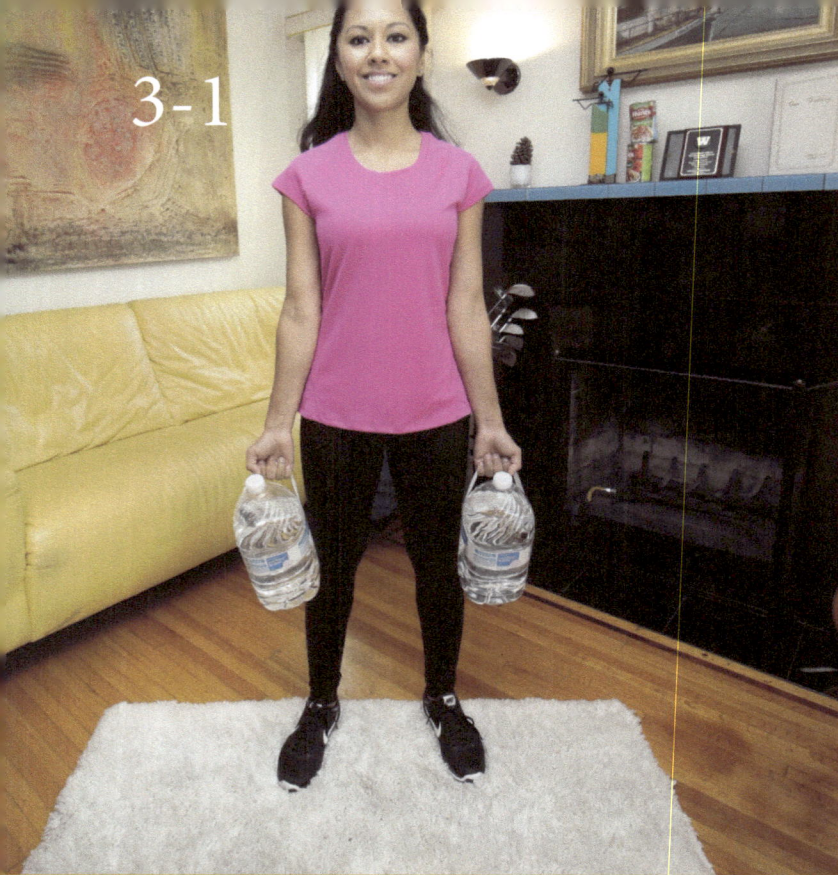

3-1

3) Water Gallon Deltoid Raises

Your shoulders should mostly be stabilizing, and the teardrop ball of your shoulder, known as the deltoid, is what you should be feeling here. As this muscle is not very strong, if the weight is too heavy, you will begin to shrug your neck muscles up to help, which will cause problems down the road; so drop the weight down to large cans of food to make sure you use the tight muscles and not compromise your form. Start with arms straight down at your sides and simply raise them straight out until fully horizontal and shoulders non-active, neck muscles relaxed. Bring back the same just to your sides with neck muscles never activating.

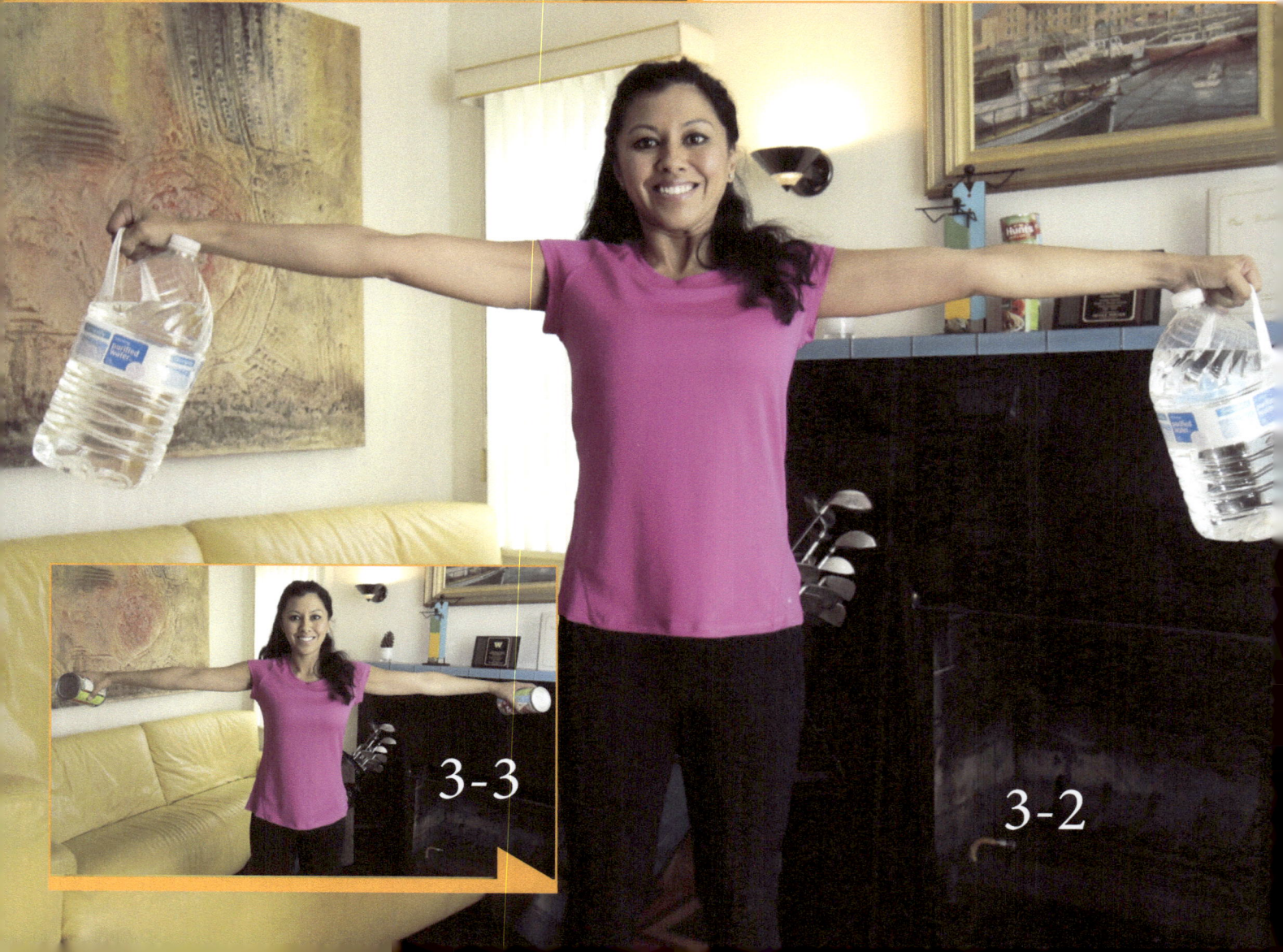

3-2

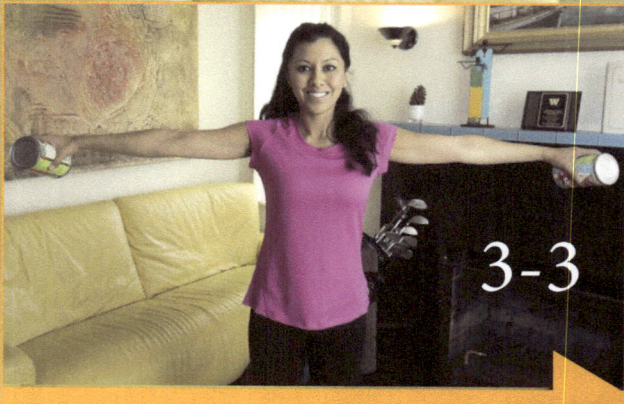

3-3

4) Chair Tricep Dips

Bring two chairs of same height together with enough room between them that you can dip your body comfortably. Grip the front of the chairs so knuckles face forward, elbows point backward, and arms are straight to start. To start with less intensity, bend your knees as if getting ready to sit and keep them close to you as you dip; to increase intensity, simply extend your legs farther and farther out until they are straight. Again, ensure that your neck is not strained; your shoulders and arms are what should be keeping you up. When ready, dip straight down between your hands, allowing your elbows to flare back and muscles under your arm get to shine and tighten up. Dip down as far as your upper arms, reaching horizontally; and then back up you go to start position.

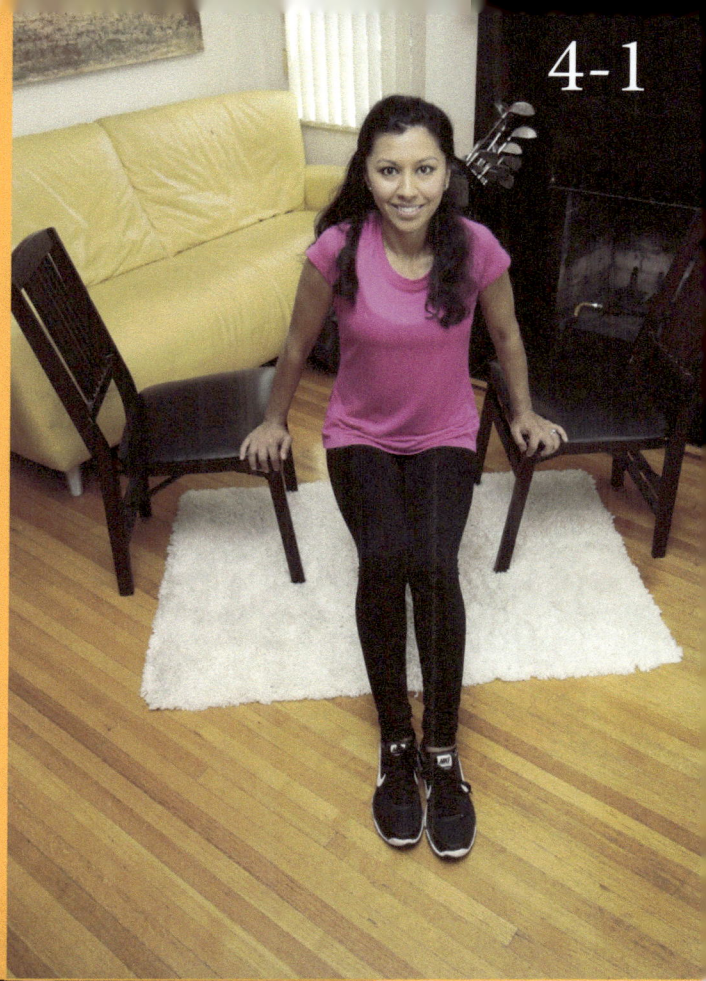

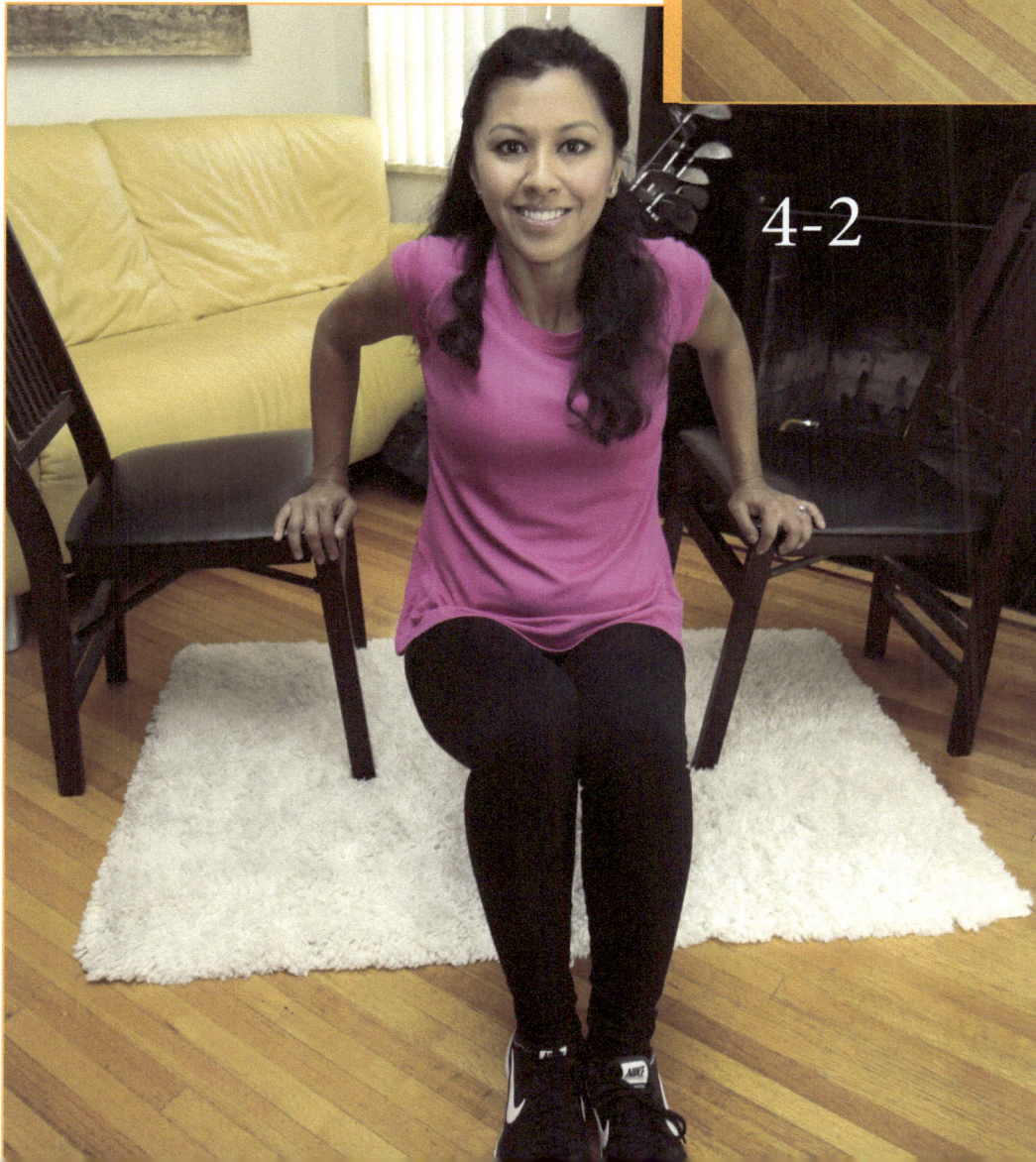

4-1

4-2

5) Broom Upper Back Rows

Start with your broom about chest height on the opposite side of the doorway, and pull back on it for tension. As you get enough tension to support your weight, begin to slowly inch your feet forward as you lean back until your body is at a nearly full lean and supported by the broom. Arms should be straight. Bring your hands all the way over to touch the doorway for added support and to keep the bar from slipping. Once you're comfortably at a lean, pull yourself in toward the middle of the broom, making sure you pinch your shoulder blades back as if someone had his/her thumb on your spine and you were trying to pinch it. Once fully pulled in, slowly go back, ensuring you are mostly using your back and shoulders to do this and not all arms, or else you will be getting the wrong kind of results, not to mention those arms should be tired by now.

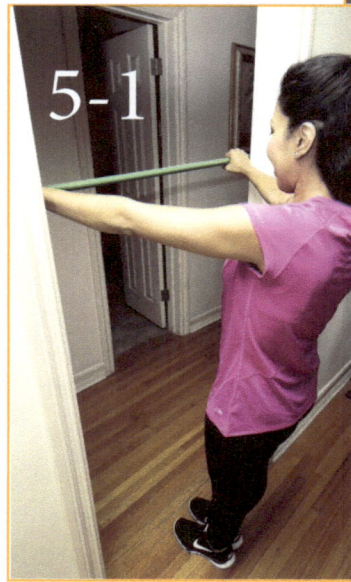

5-1

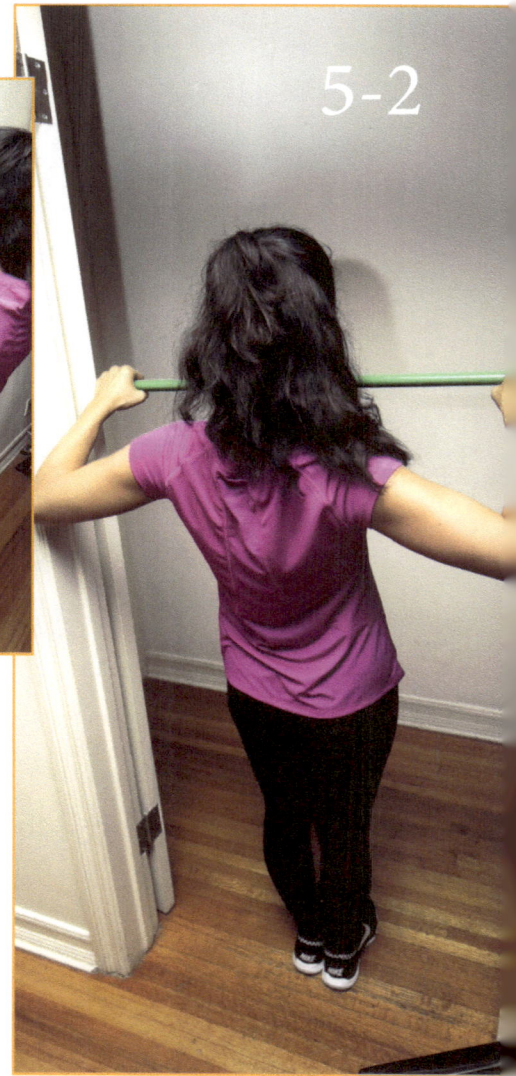

5-2

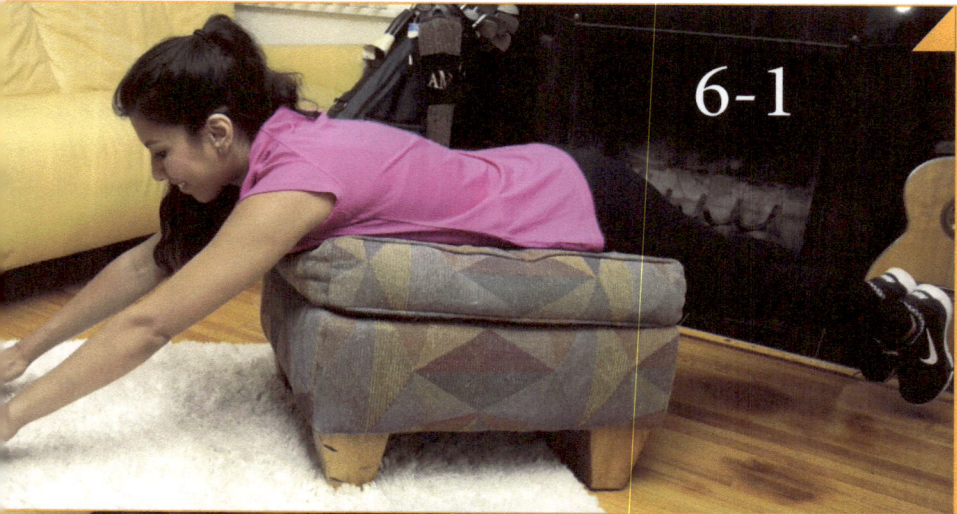

6-1

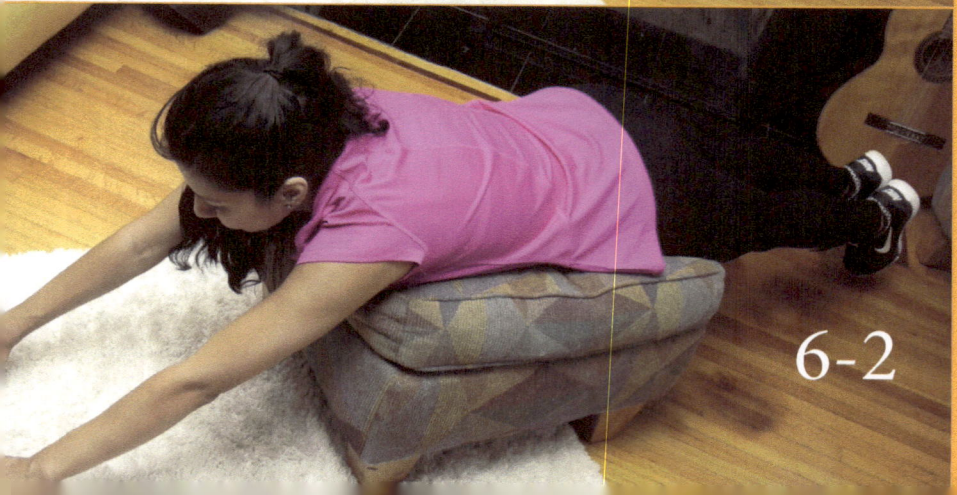

6-2

6) Ottoman Superman (Low Back)

Find yourself an ottoman, a large open chair, or even a bucket with a pillow on it. Lie downward with arms extended forward and legs back. Center yourself comfortably for balance, and ensure you are high up enough that your body can curve down like a "C." Once ready, aim arms up and tighten low back to pull legs up so you now become an upward "C," or looking as if you are Superman/-woman, and bring them back down slowly. Don't drop your weight, but carry it back down, using those muscles.

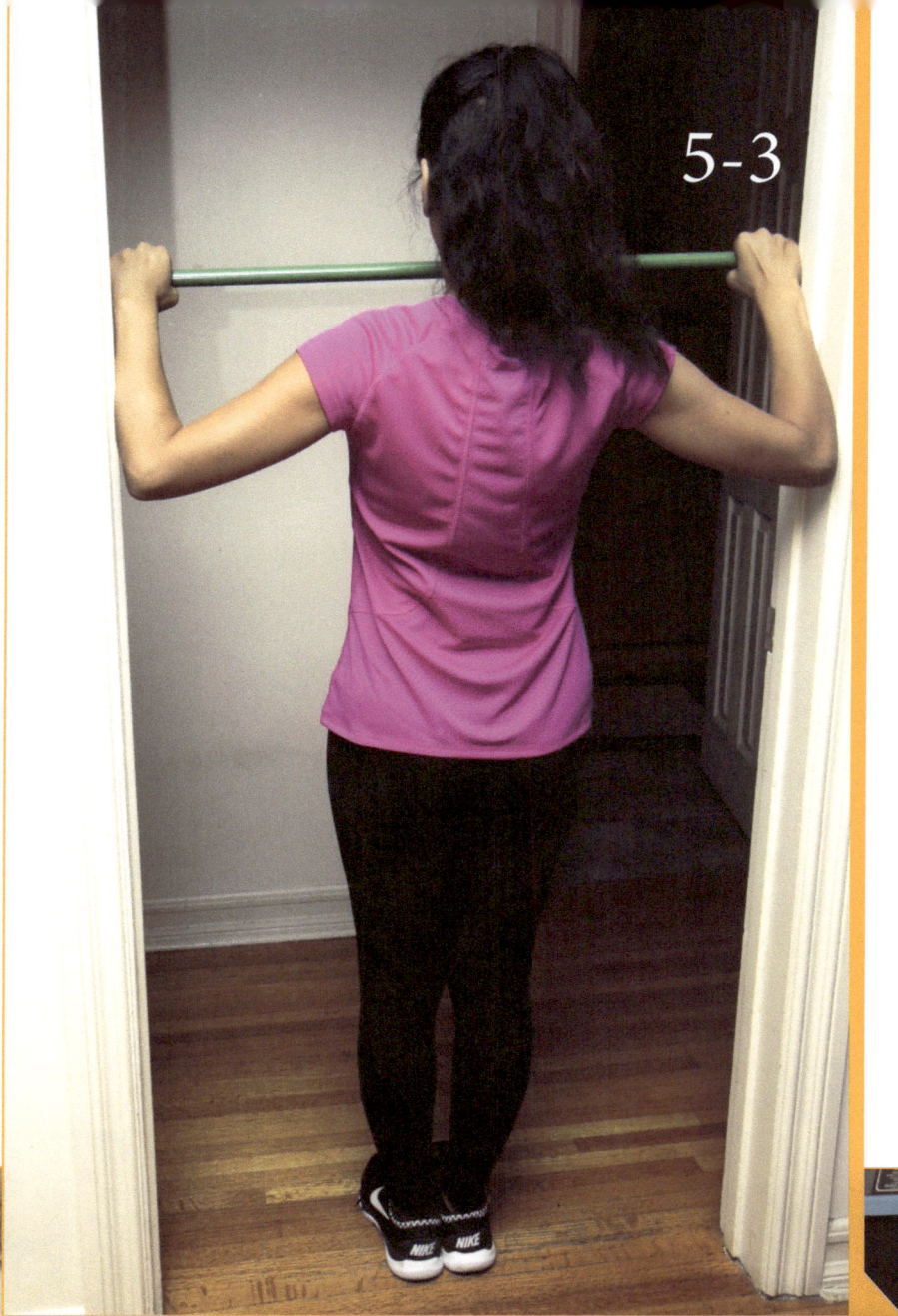

5-3

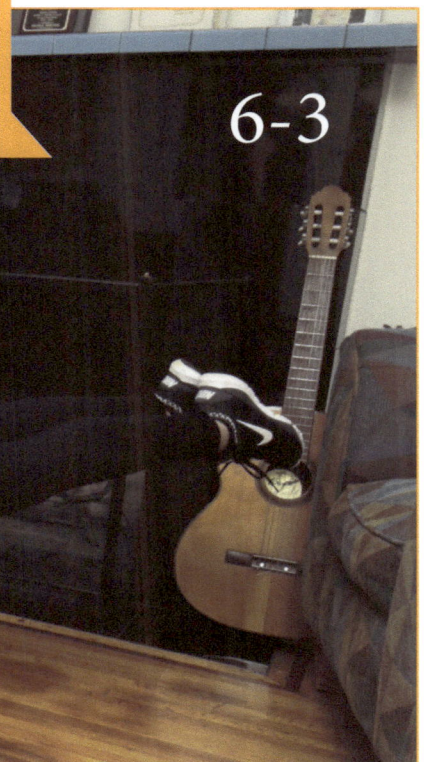

6-3

7) Ottoman Crunches

Lie with mostly your back on the ottoman, gripping the bottom of it for balance and leaving your hips and legs hanging off to have room to bend them. Once ready, tighten your core and bring your legs straight up with your abs as far as you can so you become a "V"; slowly bring them back down with your core still tight. Do not drop your legs.

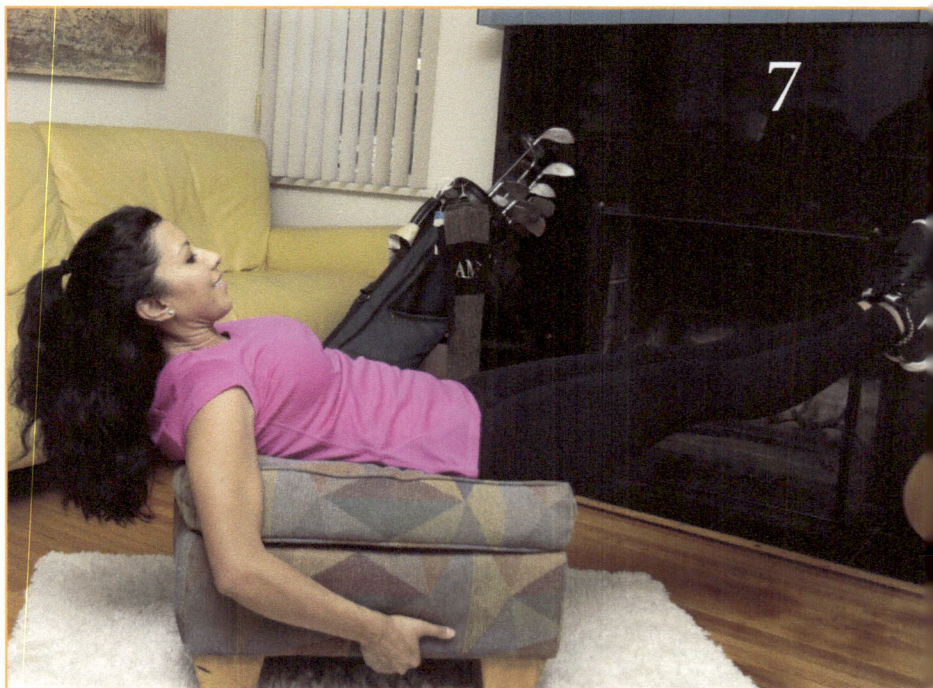

8) Ottoman Oblique Crunches

Lie sideways on ottoman with hips and legs out with room to bend again. The arm closer to the floor should be on the ground for balance, and the other arm should be supporting the back of your neck, not pulling your neck, but just supporting it. Once ready, pivot onto your side and bend/crunch your entire core together, making a V-shape on your side, bending your knees into your core and pulling your elbow toward your hips. Once at max V shape, slowly extend back out, carrying the weight.

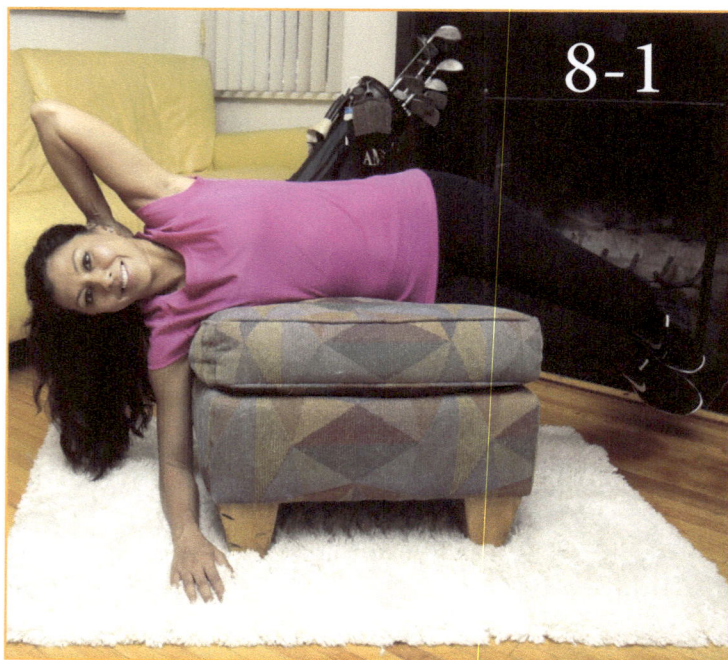

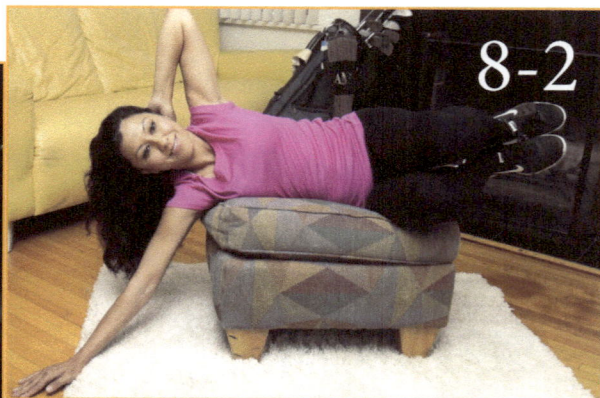

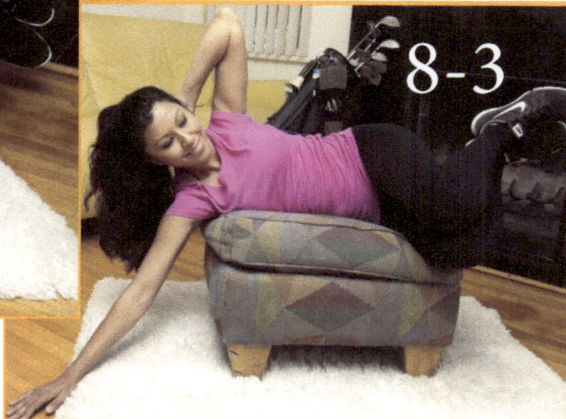

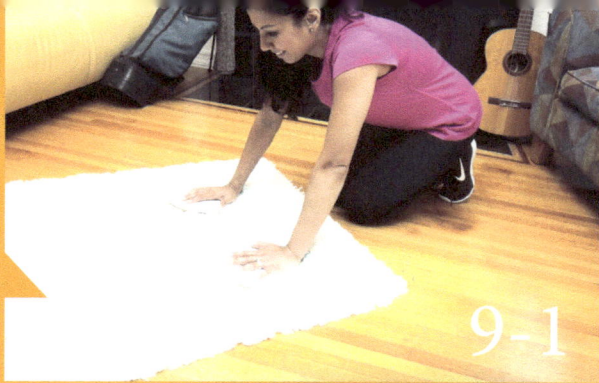
9-1

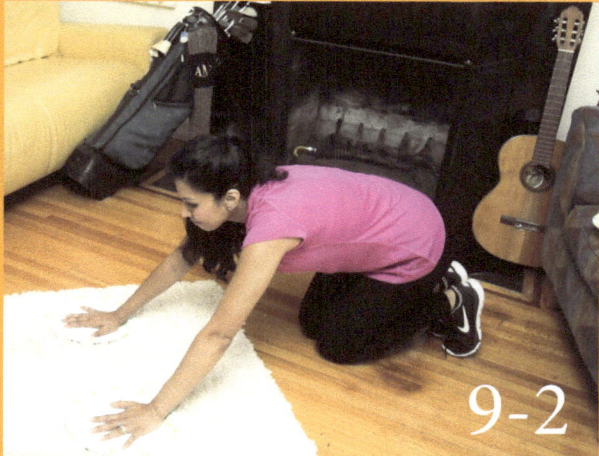
9-2

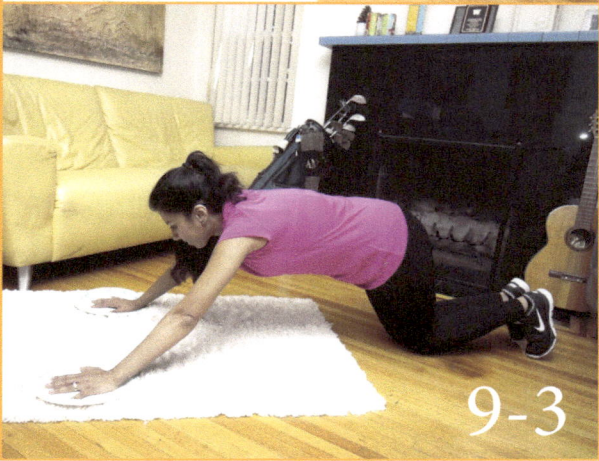
9-3

9)Paper Plate Sliders

This works best on carpet, so grab two paper plates and make your way to a carpet. Get yourself on your knees with paper plates under each hand and arms extended out. When ready, begin to slide forward, allowing your core to tighten in order to extend yourself out and use your core to pull you back to start position. If you are feeling ambitious, you can do this same form, but slide to the far right or to the far left to work out those side ab muscles for extra definition.

10) Tuck and Extend Glute Press

Stay on the carpet, facing down on your hands and knees. Widen your hands a bit for stability, and tuck one knee into your chest as shown.

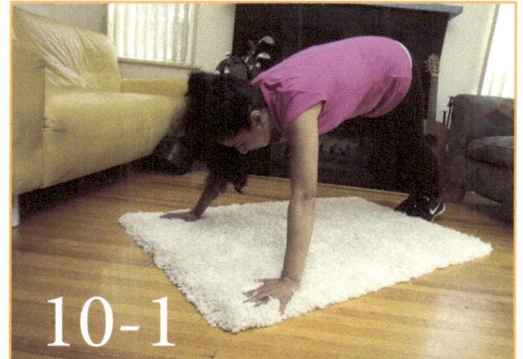
10-1

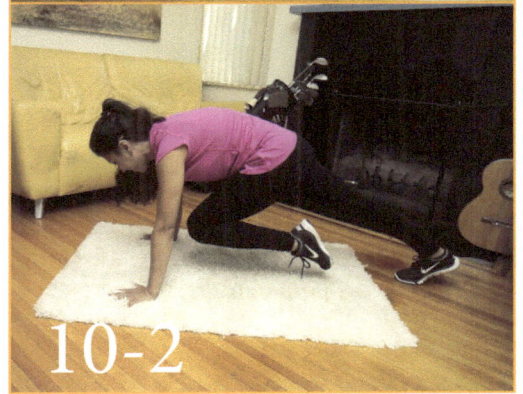
10-2

Take your tucked knee and extend out to point while using your glutes to pull it as far back into the ceiling as possible. Bring the knee back into tuck, and keep going back and forth until finished.

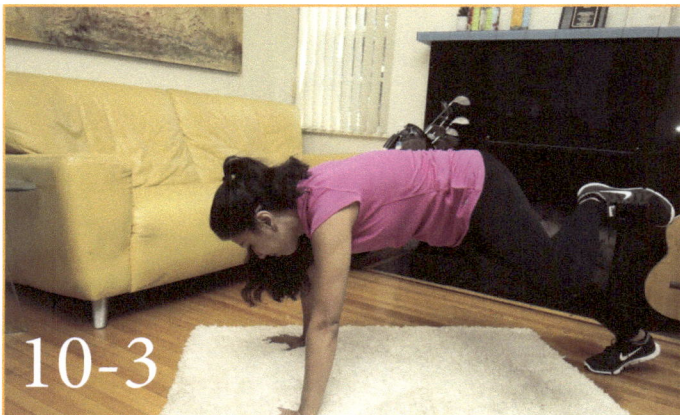
10-3

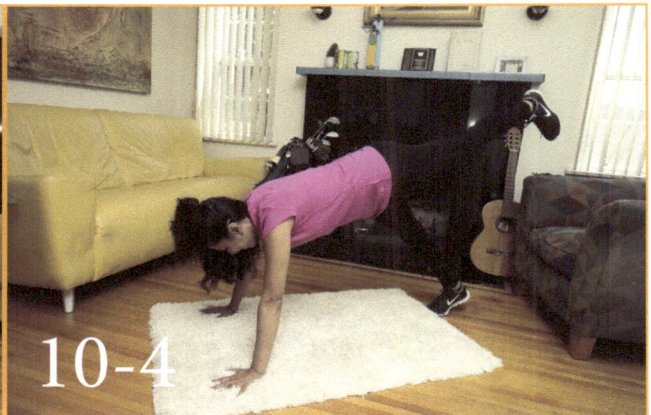
10-4

11) Wall Glute Bridges

Find yourself a nice blank wall, and lie with your back on the floor and legs flat against the wall. Widen your hand next to your side to create a wide base for balance to start. Now, as you are in an L shape against the wall, raise your hips up toward the sky by tightening your glutes to bring your body into a flat plank position away from the floor, and bring back down using glutes. To increase intensity and results, first slide hands closer to body for less stability, and then for even more of a challenge, try holding a weight (such as a water jug) on your hips while lifting your hips upward.

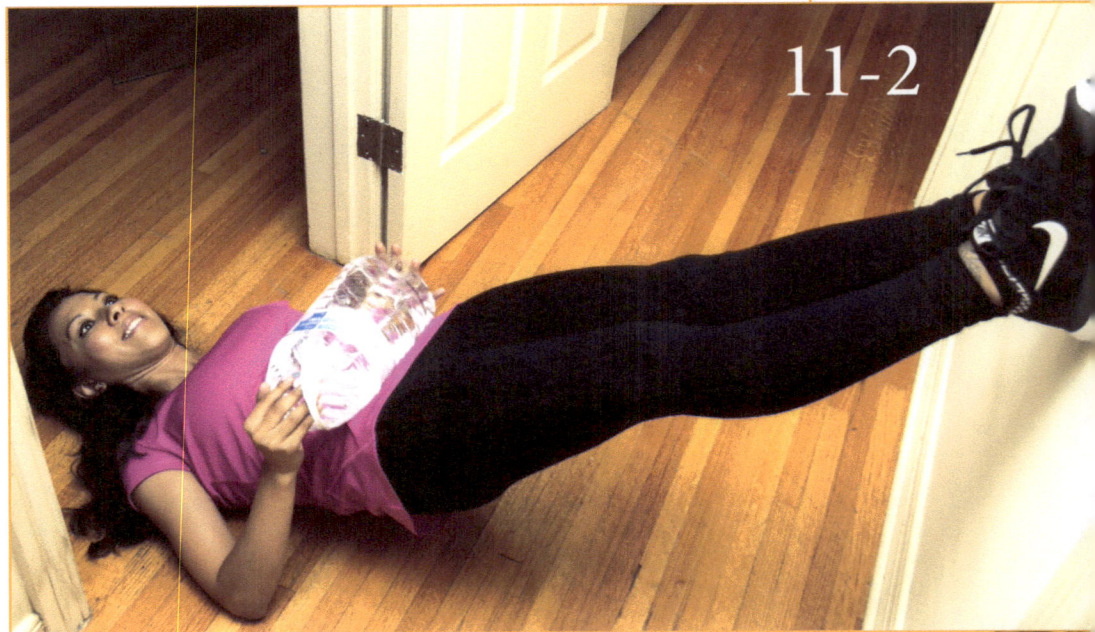

11-2

12) Stair Step Calf Raises

All you need is a stair for this one. Even a stepping stool or sturdy box will do as long as it's tall enough for you to dip down and up with your heels. Stand on the edge of the step ledge with your toes pointed up and heels hanging down and off (as shown) while you hold onto anything for stability. When ready, simply lift up onto your toes as high as you can and let the muscles set you back down to start position.

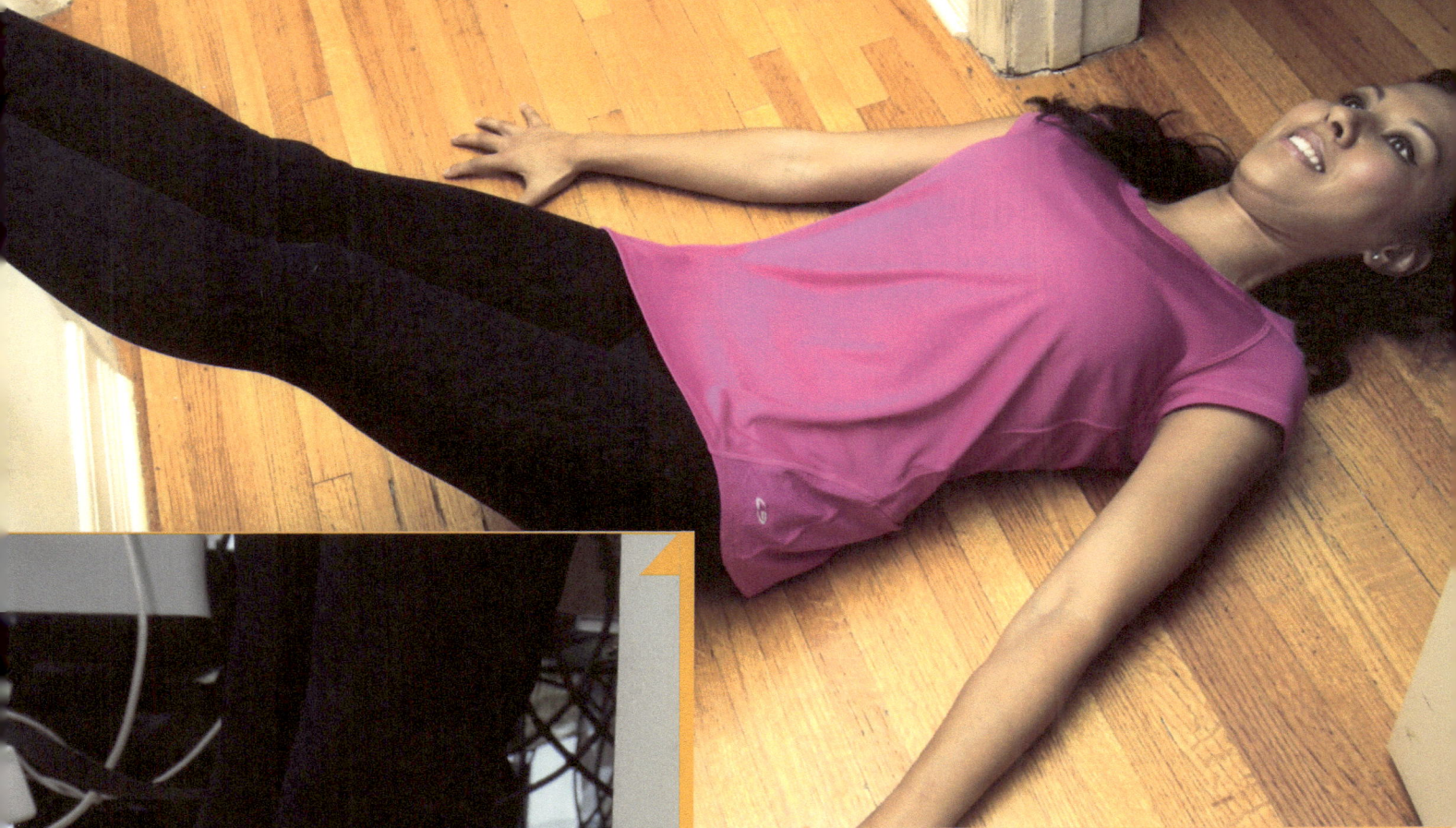

11-1

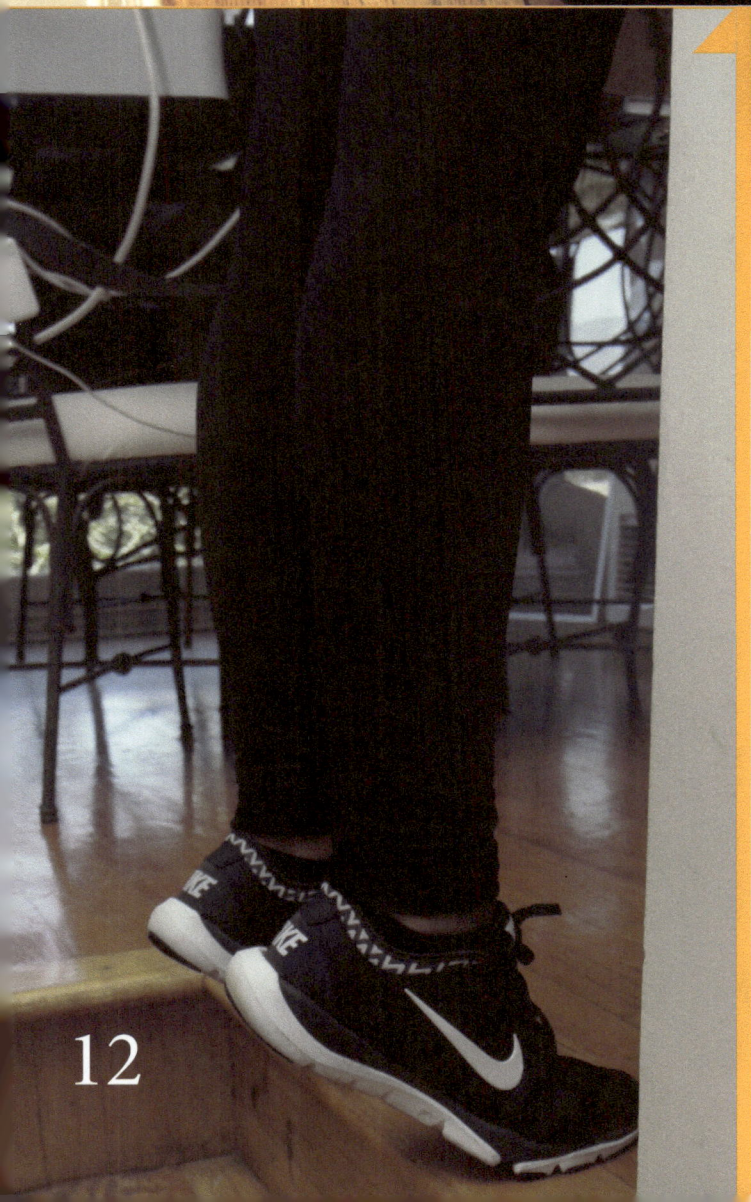

12

Health 101
Basics to Weightloss

BY ANTHONY HEREDIA

HOW DO I LOSE WEIGHT, HOW MUCH SHOULD I EAT, WHEN SHOULD I EAT IT, AND WHAT ABOUT WORKING OUT?" THESE ARE ALL VERY GOOD QUESTIONS. PLEASE READ.

There are many reasons why we gain weight and why we can't lose it, so please don't let me oversimplify anything. There is no single magic bullet or one size fits all approach, but there are universal changes you can make that will result in that trim, lean look you covet.

The trick to weight loss is simply to burn more energy than you take in (both food and stored fat being examples of energy). There is a catch to eating less, though. Cutting calories does not mean starvation, which can actually make things much worse for you. You should not eat less than your body's minimal need, called your BMR (basal metabolic rate). This is basically how many calories you would burn if you were to be at rest for a 24-hour period. If you are not active at all, eating close to your BMR calories is a good start until you are more active. Please remember that if you are taking medication or have any serious problems going on, you should first consult your doctor before drastically modifying your calories. This is general advice for a relatively healthy adult, so with that said, let me teach you how to find out your BMR.

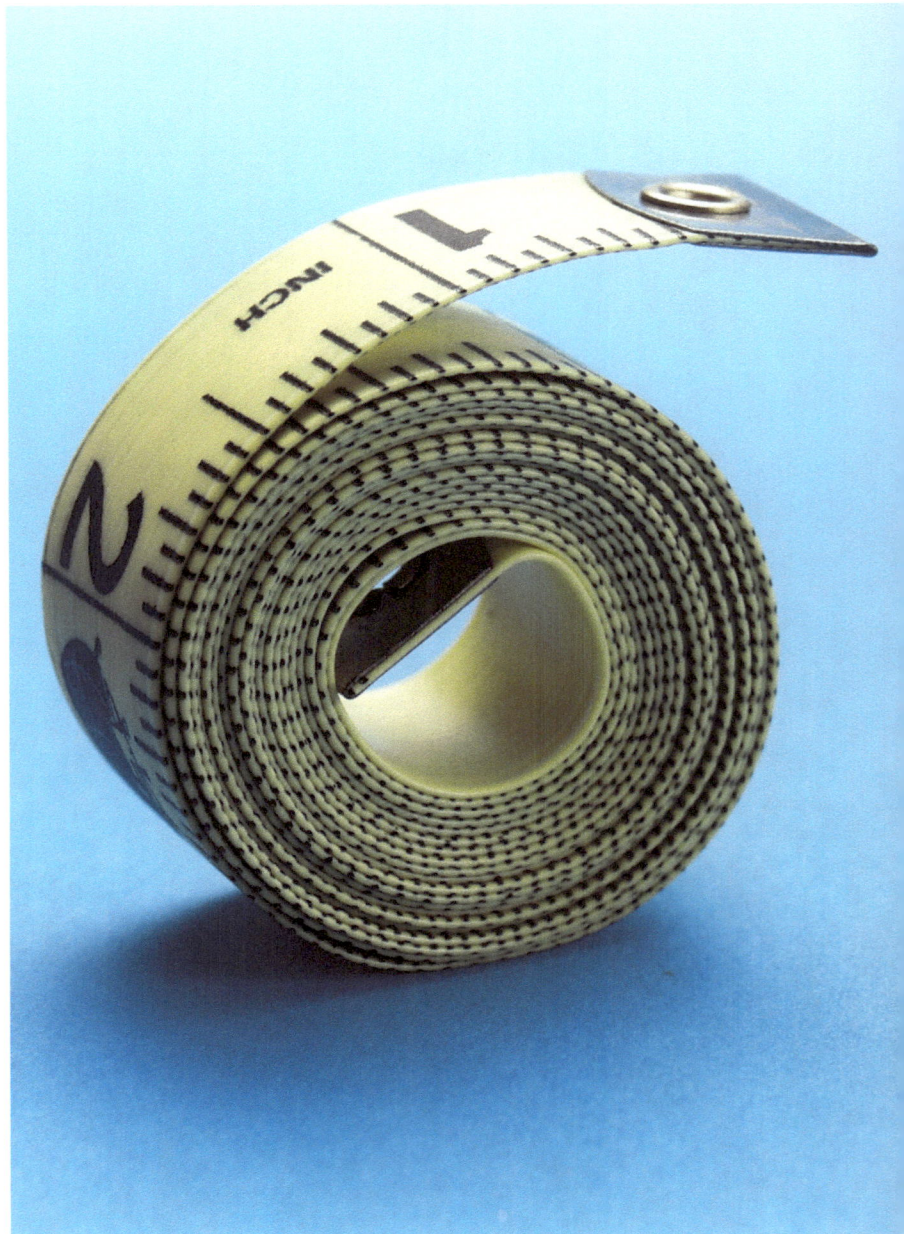

To find your BMR, simply multiply your body weight times 10, and that will give you a great estimate (for example, 150 lbs x 10 = 1500 calories). If you are fairly active (1-3 workouts a week), add 2-300 calories on top of your BMR to keep everything working properly. If you are very active (4-5 workouts a week), add 4-500 calories so that your body can take the beating. Please note that when you're very high in activity, your body needs a lot more. If you give it less than what it needs, it will simply rebel by slowing you down to conserve energy. Working out extremely hard and not eating more is the same as not working out at all and starving. It's a form of starvation that results in your body breaking itself down, so work with it and not against it. I would recommend getting some professional help to modify some things so that you get the best out of your workouts, if things get hard. If you just want something to calculate your calories for you, go to www.caloriecontrol.org/calcalcs.html, and the work is done for you.

Now that you have your calories, remember to spread them evenly throughout the day over at least 5 to 6 meals to switch to fat burning mode. I must urge you not to cut meals, looking for more weight loss. It will make your goals more difficult, triggering your body's self defense. To get faster results eat better quality foods, work out harder or more often, but don't eat fewer meals. Training hard under fueled leads to metabolic rebellion; less fat is burned. A car without enough gas will just stop, but your body will fatigue you sooner, make you sleepier more often, and drain your good moods. A big reason metabolism slows down from under eating while training hard lies in the recovery. You cause damage while you work out, tissues break down that need to be rebuilt; but if your body doesn't have what it needs to rebuild because you didn't take it nutritionally, it will just break down other healthy tissues to fix the broken ones. In other words, you lose hard-earned muscle from your legs (which burn a lot of fat) to fix the muscle on your arms. Muscles are huge fat burning engines that keep you beautiful, and you want to make sure to hold onto every drop if you can.

Now that you have your calories, remember to spread them evenly throughout the day over at least 5 to 6 meals to switch to fat burning mode.

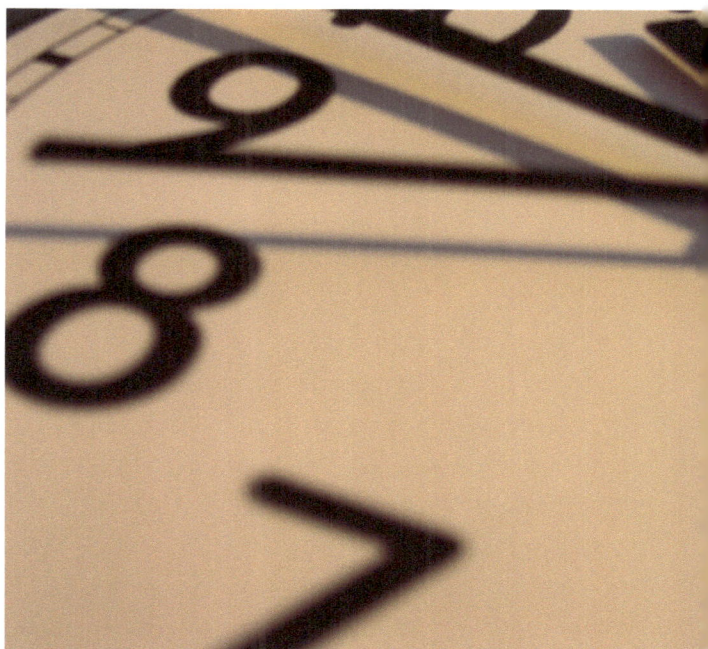

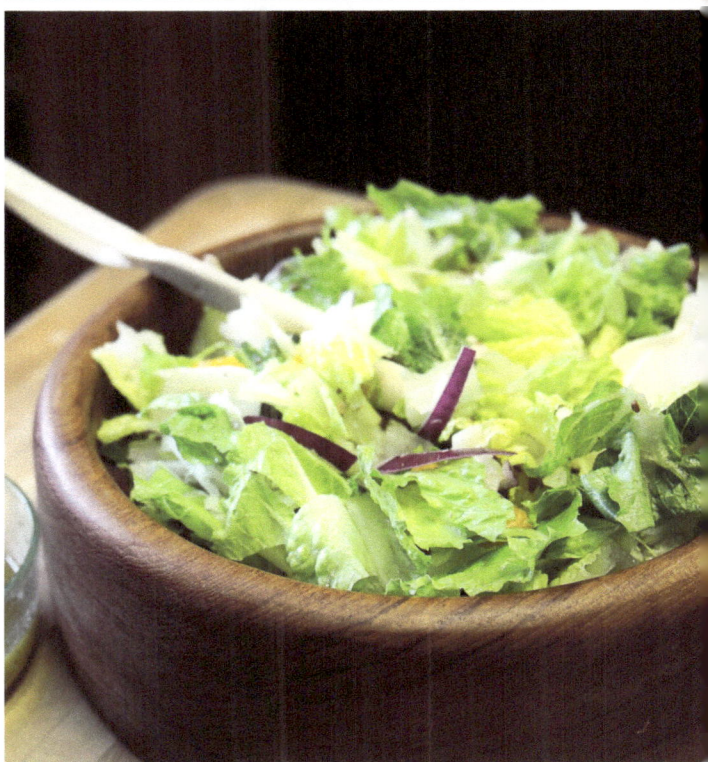

Now that we've got you scared into eating, let us address activity a bit more and how hard you should push. This is where many go wrong and have no clue what they are doing wrong. The human body responds best when it is pushed. It's marvelous! You see, your body is great at doing as little as possible (go figure). Its primary purpose is to be as efficient as possible at consistent balance (homeostasis).

Why use 300 calories for that run if we can get it down to 100 calories? If you run a mile January 1st and that same exact mile under the same conditions consistently by midyear, you are burning a fraction of the calories because your body got great at using less energy to do the same. That's what your body was designed to do, so the best approach to activity is consistent challenge by pushing one notch past comfort. As soon as you get good at it or it becomes easy, kick it up a notch. Problem is that in general we have a tendency not to push ourselves hard enough. You know that's true, so don't even start with me. We push as much as we can, and when we get to that comfort border, we stop and take a break until we get back down to the lower end of the comfort gauge. The best and quickest results are past that sweaty border you hate to cross. No challenge yields low results. The best way to overcome this is to take a class at your gym, any class that you want, but stay for the whole class no matter how tired or out of place you feel. You need accountability, and someone (like a workout buddy) to push you past your normal sensors that want to quit too early. This isn't about being perfect; it's about progress. The point is to get an idea of what that border is and learning to push past it, even if it takes getting yelled at for an hour to do it. This is almost always the best way to start. If that isn't enough, take a boot camp course or get a credentialed and experienced trainer.

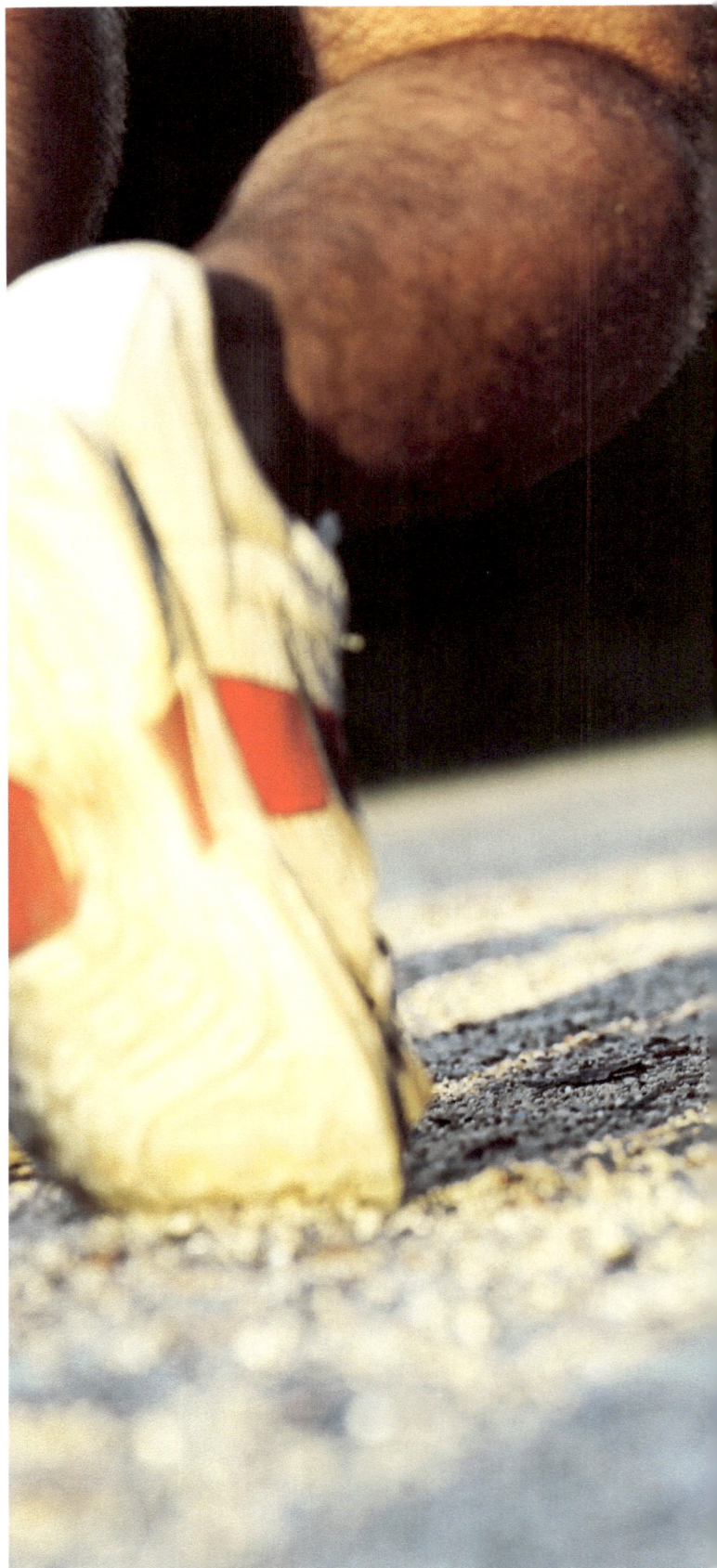

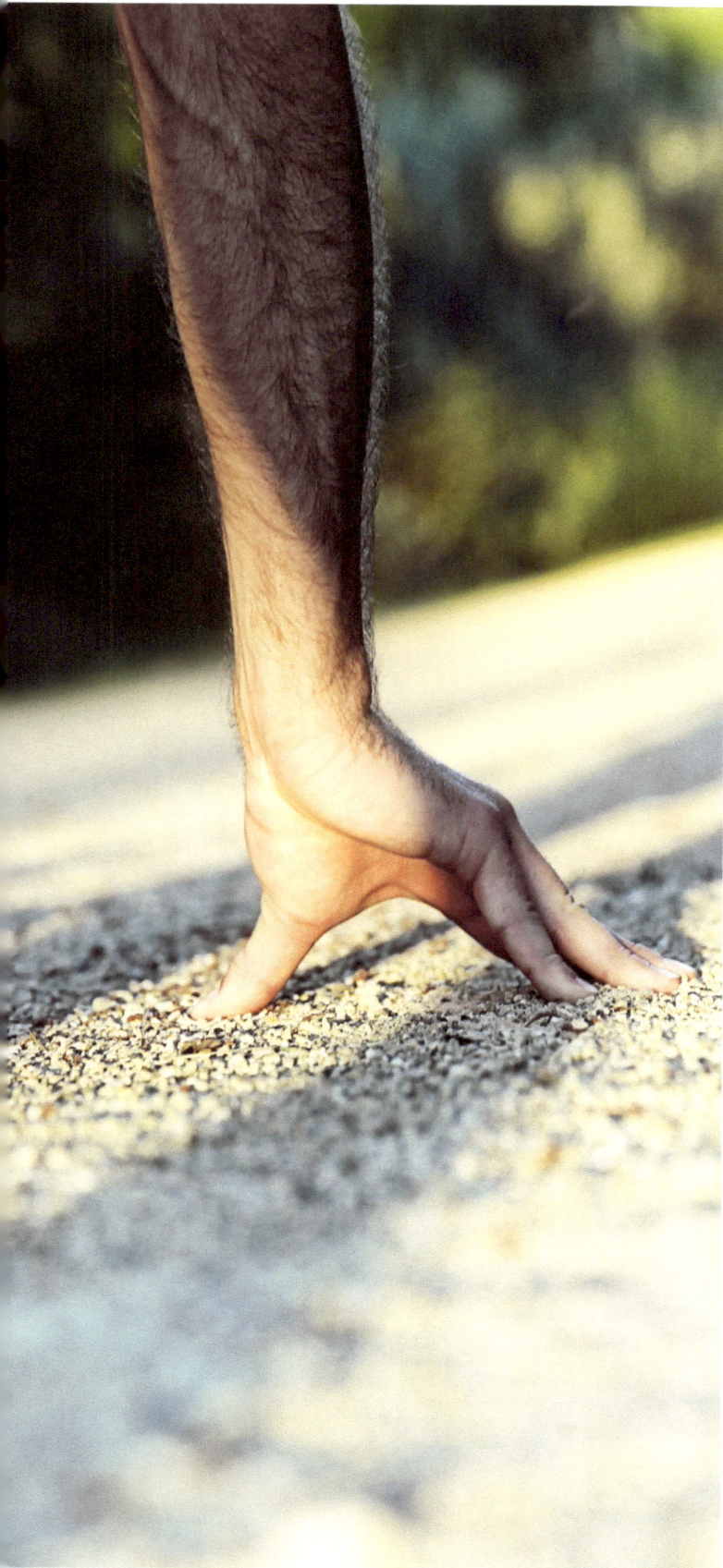

No challenge yields low results. The best way to overcome this is to take a class at your gym, any class that you want, but stay for the whole class.

Now let's get more specific on intensity. In general if you are in good health (please consult your physician before beginning a hard regimen), you should be getting your heart rate up between 70-80% of your heart rate for cardio workouts and try to keep it there for as long as you can for now. To find that out simply subtract your age from 220 and that will give you your 100%. Multiply that by 0.7 and 0.8 to give you that range (i.e., 220 – 35 yrs = 185 max heart rate, then 185 x 0.7 and 0.8 = a target heart range of 130-148 for a kick-butt fat-shredding workout). Buy yourself a heart monitor if you don't want to be held to a machine, or you can always use the one built into the machines if that is where you plan to be. Weight training in itself is a whole other article that we will approach later, but for now, find a great class, boot camp, or trainer who will do the trick. The best fitness for you is one that is challenging, keeps you coming back, pushes you past your comfort, and keeps your heart pumping well into your goals.

These are the basics to kick starting weight loss. Eat more and not less with balanced calories spread over the day. Find fun in your fitness or you'll get discouraged. Challenge yourself by pushing for that target heart rate for the best results; that will be enough to give you a great kick start to shredding the fat off your body. Fuel your body and challenge your physical limits, and I promise it will reward you with a physique to die for.

The End.